Managing Failed Anti-Reflux Therapy

Mark K. Ferguson and M. Brian Fennerty (Eds)

Managing Failed Anti-Reflux Therapy

With 76 Illustrations, 14 in Full Color

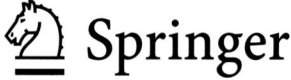 Springer

Mark K. Ferguson, MD
Professor of Surgery, Head, Thoracic Surgery
Service, Department of Surgery, University of
Chicago, Chicago, IL, USA

M. Brian Fennerty, MD
Professor of Medicine, Division of
Gastroenterology, Department of Medicine,
Oregon Health & Science University, Portland,
OR, USA

A catalogue record for this book is available from the British Library

Library of Congress Control Number: 2005926816

ISBN 10: 1-85233-909-8   Printed on acid-free paper
ISBN 13: 978-1-85233-909-8

Printed in Singapore   (BS/KYO)

9 8 7 6 5 4 3 2 1

SpringerScience+BusinessMedia
springeronline.com

Preface

Although GERD was initially described in the early 19th century, it is essentially a consequence of our modern day largesse. Dietary factors and associated obesity have combined with as yet other unknown factors (e.g. a decrease in the prevalence of *H. pylori*?) to make GERD one of the most common diseases affecting western society. It is estimated that up to 20 million adults in the United States suffer from GERD, and treatment of these individuals consumes approximately $10 billion annually, the majority of it for prescription drugs used to manage the disease and its symptoms. Fortunately, despite challenges presented by co-factors resulting in GERD (diet, obesity, etc.), therapy of GERD is largely successful. However, even a low failure rate for a therapy used in the management of GERD still results in large numbers of affected patients because of the high prevalence of this disease. Use of a conservative estimate of a failure rate of 5% translates to 1 million ineffectively treated and unhappy patients. How to manage these patients is the subject of this book.

Why is publication of this book important now? Several factors prompted us to work on this project. Mature results for proton pump inhibitor use are available, making this an appropriate time to review outcomes of PPI therapy of GERD. Similarly, mature results are now available for minimally invasive surgical therapy for GERD. In fact, results are sufficiently promising in the mid-term that some authors are recommending surgery over PPI use even for patients with only moderate GERD disease. In addition to defining the success of these therapies, the long-term results also illustrate important failure rates and help define characteristics of patients who are less likely to benefit from conventional treatment options.

Use of alternative therapies is now becoming quite common, particularly endoscopic treatments such as bulking agents, radiofrequency therapy, and plication procedures. The exact role of these modalities in the management of the typical patient with GERD will be defined in the next few years. A greater challenge is whether and how to use these techniques for patients who have already failed conventional therapy for GERD.

Given the complexity of causes underlying failures of GERD therapy, the approach to managing these patients should be multidisciplinary. For patients who have persistent GERD symptoms despite aggressive therapy, too often a single therapeutic approach is used to an extreme without consideration of alternative modalities, or even whether the symptoms are actually related to reflux. This may be because of the training, philosophical orientation, or lack of knowledge of the treating physician. To overcome some of these shortcomings, we felt the time was propitious to produce a book describing management of medical and surgical failures from both medical and surgical perspectives.

The objectives of this book are to review current medical and surgical management of GERD, define what constitutes failure of such therapy, and describe approaches to management of such patients. We have enlisted a group of authors whose reputations in their specialties are universally recognized. Given the widespread incidence of GERD throughout western society, chapters are written for an international audience. Our goal was to outline a comprehensive approach to managing failed GERD therapy. However, ongoing advances in the pharmaceutical, endoscopic, and surgical instrumentation industries will always make such an effort incomplete. Our hope is that the reader is left with a framework for approaching these complex patients, and that any new information that arises can be fitted into this framework.

Mark K. Ferguson, MD
M. Brian Fennerty, MD

Acknowledgments

The editors would like to thank Eva Senior, our Senior Editorial Assistant, and Melissa Morton, our Editor, at Springer for their invaluable contributions to this text.

Contents

Contributors

John A. Bonino, MD
Department of Internal Medicine, University of Kansas School of Medicine, Kansas City, KS, USA

Jose M. Clavero, MD
Division of General Thoracic Surgery, Mayo Clinic College of Medicine, Rochester, MN, USA

Jean-Marie Collard, MD, PhD, FACS, MHon AFC
Upper Gastrointestinal Surgery Unit, St. Luc Academic Hospital, Louvain Medical School, Brussels, Belgium

Federico Cuenca-Abente, MD
Department of Surgery, University of Washington Medical Center, Seattle, WA, USA

Myriam J. Curet, MD
Department of Surgery, Stanford University, Stanford, CA, USA

Steven R. DeMeester, MD
Department of Surgery, Keck School of Medicine, University of Southern California, Los Angeles, CA, USA

Claude Deschamps, MD
Division of General Thoracic Surgery, Mayo Clinic College of Medicine, Rochester, MN, USA

Kenneth R. DeVault, MD, FACG
Department of Gastroenterology and Hepatology, Mayo Clinic College of Medicine, Jacksonville, FL, USA

André Duranceau, MD
Department of Surgery, Université de Montréal, Division of Thoracic Surgery, Centre Hospitalier de l'Université de Montréal, Montréal, Canada

M. Brian Fennerty, MD
Professor of Medicine, Division of Gastroenterology, Department of Medicine, Oregon Health & Science University, Portland, OR, USA

Mark K. Ferguson, MD
Professor of Surgery, Head, Thoracic Surgery Service, Department of Surgery, University of Chicago, Chicago, IL, USA

Éric Fréchette, MD, FRCS
Department of Surgery, Université de Montréal, Division of Thoracic Surgery, Centre Hospitalier de l'Université de Montréal, Montréal, Canada

Gianmattia del Genio, MD
Upper Gastrointestinal Surgery Unit, St Luc Academic Hospital, Louvain Medical School, Brussels, Belgium

John G. Hunter, MD
Department of Surgery, Oregon Health and Science University, Portland, OR, USA

David A. Johnson, MD, FACP FACG
Department of Gastroenterology, Eastern VA School of Medicine, Digestive and Liver Diseases, Norfolk, VA, USA

Peter J. Kahrilas, MD
Division of Gastroenterology, Department of
Medicine, Northwestern University, Feinberg School
of Medicine, Chicago, IL, USA

Jennefer A. Kieran, MD
Department of Surgery, Stanford University,
Stanford, CA, USA

Brant K. Oelschlager, MD
Department of Surgery, University of Washington
Medical Center, Seattle, WA, USA

John E. Pandolfino, MD
Division of Gastroenterology, Department of
Medicine, Northwestern University, Feinberg School
of Medicine, Chicago, IL, USA

Carlos A. Pellegrini, MD
Department of Surgery, University of Washington
Medical Center, Seattle, WA, USA

David W. Rattner, MD
Division of General and Gastrointestinal Surgery,
Massachusetts General Hospital and Department of
Surgery, Harvard Medical School, Boston, MA, USA

Prateek Sharma, MD
Division of Gastroenterology and Hepatology,
University of Kansas School of Medicine,
Department of Veterans Affairs Medical Center,
Kansas City, MO, USA

Carrie A. Sims, MD
Department of Surgery, Massachusetts General
Hospital, Boston, MA, USA

Philippe Topart, MD
Service de Chirurgie Viscérale, Centre Hospitalier
Universitaire, Brest, France

1

The Epidemiology and Pathophysiology of Gastroesophageal Reflux Disease

Peter J. Kahrilas and John E. Pandolfino

Gastroesophageal reflux disease (GERD) is present in individuals with a symptomatic condition or histopathological alteration resultant from episodes of gastroesophageal reflux. Reflux esophagitis is present in a subset of GERD patients with lesions in the esophageal mucosa. However, reflux often causes symptoms in the absence of esophagitis.

Although GERD is widely reported to be one of the most prevalent clinical conditions afflicting the gastrointestinal tract, incidence and prevalence figures must be tempered with the realization that there is no "gold standard" definition of GERD. Thus, epidemiological estimates regarding GERD make assumptions; the most obvious being that heartburn is a symptom of GERD and that when heartburn achieves a certain threshold of frequency or severity, it defines GERD. A cross-sectional study surveying hospital employees in the United States in the 1970s found that 7% of individuals experienced heartburn daily, 14% weekly, and 15% monthly.[1] Ten years later, a Gallup survey of 1000 randomly selected persons found a 19% prevalence of weekly GERD symptoms.[2] Ten years later yet, a survey in Olmstead County found a 20% prevalence of at least weekly heartburn.[3] With respect to age, the Olmstead County data showed no correlation[3] whereas a recent report by El-Serag et al.[4] showed a slight correlation with advancing age ranging from a 24% weekly heartburn prevalence among 18–24 year olds to a 33% prevalence in those >55 years of age.

With respect to esophagitis, even though endoscopic changes in the esophageal mucosa represent objective diagnostic criteria, it is less clear what proportion of heartburn sufferers are so affected. Early reports using ambulatory esophageal pH monitoring to define GERD found that 48–79% of patients with pathologic acid exposure had esophagitis.[5,6] More recent reports, perhaps less subject to selection bias, have suggested that the prevalence of esophagitis among the GERD population is lower, ranging from 19 to 45%.[7] Very recently, a population-based study found endoscopic esophagitis in 22% of 226 individuals with heartburn at least once weekly.[4] Similar to esophagitis, the prevalence of Barrett's metaplasia is difficult to determine in the absence of a characteristic symptom profile or population studies. Illustrative of this, an autopsy study suggested that fewer than one in six patients with Barrett's metaplasia was recognized clinically prior to death.[8]

GERD is equally prevalent among males and females, but there is a male preponderance of esophagitis (2:1 to 3:1) and of Barrett's metaplasia (10:1).[7] Pregnancy is associated with the highest incidence of GERD with 48–79% of pregnant women complaining of heartburn.[9] All forms of GERD affect Caucasians more frequently than other races. However, this trend may be changing in the United States suggesting it is at least partially influenced by geography.[4] In fact, there is substantial geographic variation in prevalence with very low rates in

Africa and Asia and high rates in North America and Europe.[10]

The role of Helicobacter pylori in GERD deserves special attention given the striking inverse time trends in the prevalence of GERD and H. pylori related peptic ulcer disease.[11] Epidemiological data reveal that GERD patients with esophagitis are less likely to have H. pylori infection.[12] H. pylori infection is also associated with a decreased prevalence of Barrett's metaplasia and esophageal adenocarcinoma.[13–15] Thus, epidemiological data clearly suggest a relationship between H. pylori and GERD. However, the details of that relationship are strongly dependent on the associated pattern of gastritis. If the dominant H. pylori strains within a population primarily result in corpus-dominant gastritis as in Japan,[14] the prevalence of GERD in that population will be lower than it would be in the absence of H. pylori infection. These epidemiological data have led some to believe that H. pylori should not be eradicated in patients with GERD. However, H. pylori is a risk factor for the development of peptic ulcer and gastric cancer causing many practitioners to be uncomfortable with that recommendation.

GERD Pathophysiology

The fundamental abnormality in GERD is exposure of esophageal epithelium to gastric secretions resulting in either histopathological injury or in the elicitation of symptoms. However, some degree of gastroesophageal reflux and esophageal epithelial acid exposure is considered normal or "physiological." GERD results when esophageal epithelial exposure to gastric juice exceeds what the epithelium can tolerate.

Under normal conditions, reflux of gastric juice into the distal esophagus is prevented as a function of the esophagogastric junction (EGJ). The EGJ is an anatomically complex zone whose functional integrity as an anti-reflux barrier has been attributed to a multitude of mechanisms. Quite possibly each of these potential mechanisms is operant under specific conditions and the global function of the EGJ as an anti-reflux barrier is dependent on the sum of the parts. The greater the dysfunction of the individual mechanisms of competence, the worse the overall anti-reflux integrity of the EGJ. By extension, the greater the degree of EGJ incompetence, the worse the severity of GERD.

Functional Constituents of the EGJ

Conceptualized as an impediment to reflux, the EGJ is generally viewed as a high-pressure zone at the distal end of the esophagus that isolates the esophagus from the stomach. The anatomy of the EGJ is complex. The tubular esophagus traverses the diaphragmatic hiatus and joins the stomach in a nearly tangential fashion. Thus, there are several potential contributors to EGJ competence, each with unique considerations: the intrinsic lower esophageal sphincter (LES), the influence of the diaphragmatic hiatus, and the muscular architecture of the gastric cardia that constitutes the distal aspect of the EGJ high-pressure zone.

The LES is a 3- to 4-cm segment of tonically contracted smooth muscle at the EGJ. Resting LES tone varies among normal individuals from 10 to 30 mm Hg relative to intragastric pressure, and continuous pressure monitoring reveals considerable temporal variation. Large fluctuations of LES pressure occur with the migrating motor complex; during phase III, LES pressure may exceed 80 mm Hg. Lesser fluctuations occur throughout the day with pressure decreasing in the postcibal state and increasing during sleep.[16] The genesis of LES tone is a property of both the smooth muscle itself and of its extrinsic innervation.[17] At any given moment, LES pressure is affected by myogenic factors, intraabdominal pressure, gastric distention, peptides, hormones, various foods, and many medications (Table 1.1).

To maintain the delicate balance between forward and backward flow, the LES has a complex neurological control mechanism involving both the central nervous system and peripheral enteric nervous system. Lower esophageal sphincter pressure is modulated by vagal afferents as well as both vagal and sympathetic efferents.[18] Efferent function is mediated through myenteric plexus neurons that can effect either LES contraction or relaxation. Synapses between the efferent vagal fibers and

Table 1.1. Factors that influence the LES pressure and tLESR frequency.

	Increase LES Pressure	Decrease LES Pressure	Increase tLESRs	Decrease tLESRs
Foods	Protein	Fat Chocolate Ethanol Peppermint	Fat	
Hormones	Gastrin Motilin Substance P	Secretin Cholecystokinin Glucagon Gastric inhibitory polypeptide Vasoactive intestinal polypeptide Progesterone	Cholecystokinin	
Neural agents	α-Adrenergic agonists β-Adrenergic antagonists Cholinergic agonists	α-Adrenergic antagonists β-Adrenergic agonists Cholinergic antagonists Serotonin	L-Arginine	Baclofen L-NAME Serotonin
Medications	Metoclopramide Domperidone Prostaglandin F$_{2\alpha}$ Cisapride	Nitrates Calcium channel blockers Theophylline Morphine Meperidine Diazepam Barbiturates	Sumatriptan	Atropine Morphine Loxiglumide

the myenteric plexus are cholinergic. The post-ganglionic transmitter effecting contraction is acetylcholine whereas nitric oxide is the dominant inhibitory transmitter with vasoactive intestinal polypeptide serving some type of modifying role.[19,20]

Physiological studies clearly demonstrate that the EGJ high-pressure zone extends distal to the squamocolumnar junction (SCJ) thereby implying that the contributory structures reside in the proximal stomach as opposed to the distal esophagus.[21] Elegant anatomical studies attribute this distal portion of the EGJ high-pressure zone to the opposing sling and clasp fibers of the middle muscle layer of gastric cardia.[22] In this region, the lateral wall of the esophagus meets the medial aspect of the dome of the stomach at an acute angle, defined as the angle of His. Viewed intraluminally, this region extends within the gastric lumen, appearing as a fold that has been conceptually referred to as a flap valve because increased intragastric pressure would force the fold against the medial wall of the stomach, sealing off the entry to the esophagus[23,24] (Figure 1.1). Of note, this distal aspect

of the EGJ is particularly vulnerable to disruption as a consequence of anatomical changes at the hiatus because its entire mechanism of action is predicated on maintaining its native geometry.

Surrounding the LES at the level of the SCJ is the crural diaphragm, most commonly the right diaphragmatic crus. Two flattened muscle bundles arising from the upper lumbar vertebra incline forward to arch around the esophagus, first diverging like a scissors and then merging anterior with about a centimeter of muscle separating the anterior rim of the hiatus from the central tendon of the diaphragm[21,25] (Figure 1.2). The hiatus is a teardrop-shaped canal and is about 2 cm along its major axis. Recent physiological investigations have advanced the "two sphincter hypothesis" for maintenance of EGJ competence, suggesting that both the intrinsic smooth muscle LES and the extrinsic crural diaphragm serve a sphincteric function. Independent control of the crural diaphragm can be demonstrated during esophageal distension, vomiting, and belching when electrical activity in the crural diaphragm is selectively inhibited despite continued respiration.[26,27] This reflex inhibition of crural activity is eliminated with vagotomy. However, crural diaphragmatic contraction is augmented during abdominal compression, straining, or coughing.[28] Additional evidence of the sphincteric function of the hiatus comes from manometric recordings in patients after distal esophagectomy.[29] These patients still exhibited an EGJ pressure of about 6 mm Hg within the hiatal canal despite having sustained surgical removal of the smooth muscle LES.

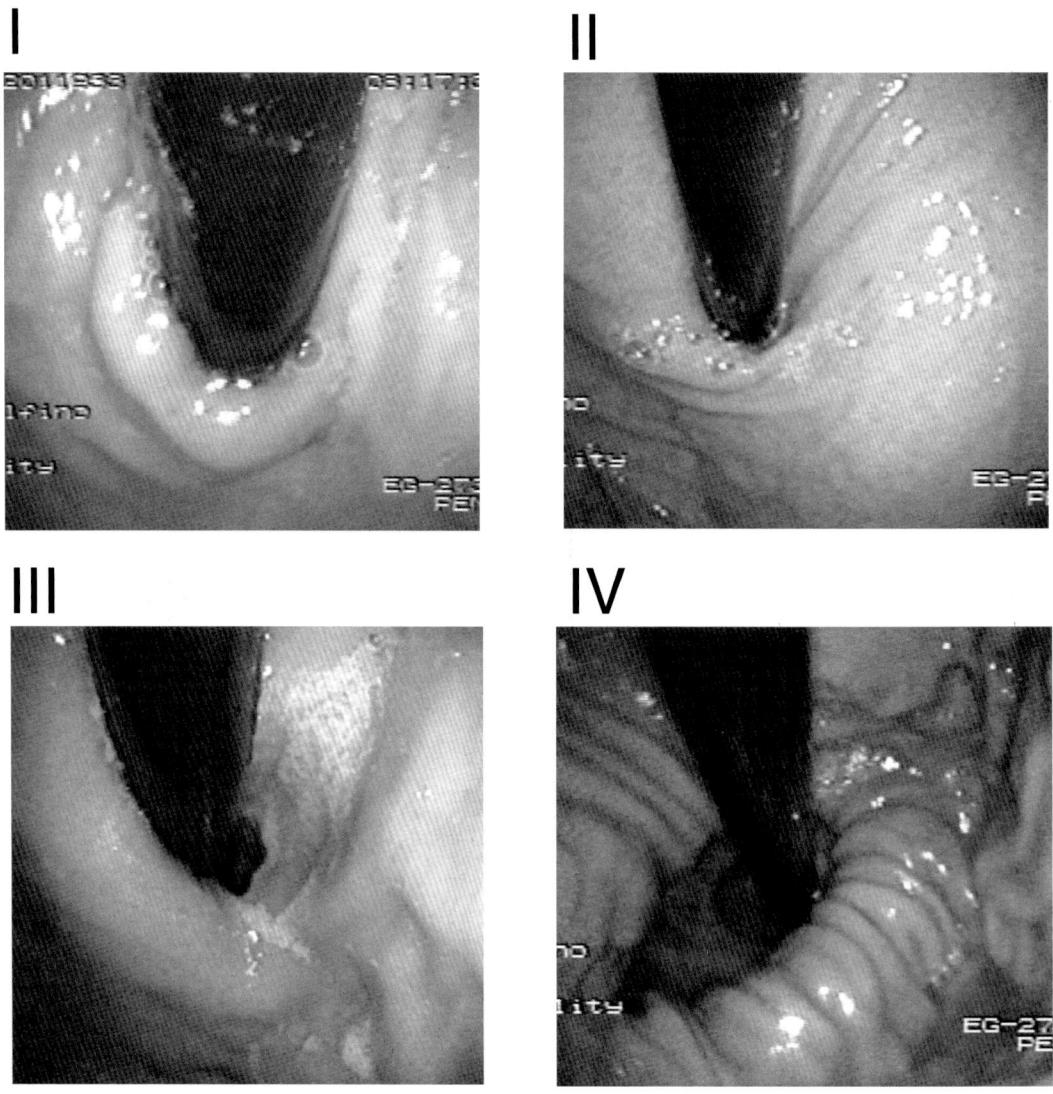

Figure 1.1. Three-dimensional representation of progressive anatomical disruption of the gastroesophageal flap valve as viewed with a retroflexed endoscope. Grade I, Normal ridge of tissue closely approximated to the shaft of the retroflexed scope. Grade II, The ridge is slightly less well defined and opens with respiration. Grade III, The ridge is barely present and the hiatus is patulous. Grade IV, There is no muscular ridge and the hiatus is wide open at all times (Reprinted from Hill et al.,[24] Copyright 1996, with permission from the American Society for Gastrointestinal Endoscopy.)

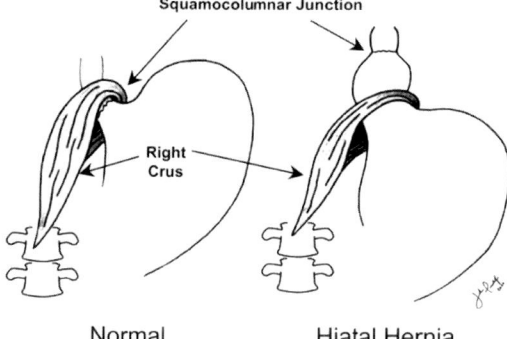

Squamocolumnar Junction

Right
Crus

Normal   Hiatal Hernia

Figure 1.2. Anatomy of the diaphragmatic hiatus. The right crus makes up the muscular component of the crural diaphragm. Arising from the anterior longitudinal ligament overlying the lumbar vertebrae. A single muscle band splits into an anterior and posterior muscular band, which cross each other to form the walls of the hiatal canal and then fuse anteriorly. With hiatus hernia the muscle becomes thin and atrophic limiting its ability to function as a sphincter. (Reprinted with permission from Pandolfino and Kahrilas.[81])

Mechanisms of EGJ Incompetence in GERD

Physiologically, the EGJ must perform seemingly contradictory functions. During swallowing it must facilitate the esophagogastric flow of swallowed material while at the same time preventing reflux of gastric content into esophagus that is otherwise favored by a positive abdomen-to-thoracic pressure gradient. During rest the EGJ must, again, contain caustic gastric juice but also be able to transiently relax and permit gas venting. These functions are accomplished by the delicate interplay of anatomical elements and physiological responses of the EGJ.

The dominant mechanism protecting against reflux varies with physiological circumstance. For example, the intraabdominal segment of the LES may be important in preventing reflux associated with swallowing, the crural diaphragm may be of cardinal importance during episodes of increased intraabdominal pressure, and basal LES pressure may be of primary importance during restful recumbency. As any of these protective mechanisms are compromised, the deleterious effect is additive resulting in an increasing number of reflux events and conse-

quently increasingly abnormal esophageal acid exposure.

Investigations have focused on three dominant mechanisms of EGJ incompetence: 1) transient LES relaxations (tLESRs), without anatomic abnormality, 2) LES hypotension, again without anatomic abnormality, or 3) anatomic distortion of the EGJ inclusive of (but not limited to) hiatus hernia. Which reflux mechanism dominates seems to depend on several factors including the anatomy of the EGJ. Whereas tLESRs typically account for up to 90% of reflux events in normal subjects or GERD patients without hiatus hernia, patients with hiatus hernia have a more heterogeneous mechanistic profile with reflux episodes frequently occurring in the context of low LES pressure, straining, and swallow-associated LES relaxation.[30] These observations support the hypothesis that the functional integrity of the EGJ is dependent on both the intrinsic LES and extrinsic sphincteric function of the diaphragmatic hiatus. In essence, gastroesophageal reflux requires a "two hit phenomenon" to the EGJ. Patients with a normal EGJ require inhibition of both the intrinsic LES and extrinsic crural diaphragm for reflux to occur: physiologically this occurs only in the setting of a tLESR. In contrast, patients with hiatal hernia may exhibit preexisting compromise of the hiatal sphincter. In that setting reflux can occur with only relaxation of the intrinsic LES, as may occur during periods of LES hypotension or even deglutitive relaxation.

Transient LES Relaxations

Compelling evidence exists that tLESRs are the most frequent mechanism for reflux during periods of normal LES pressure (>10 mm Hg). Transient LES relaxations occur independently of swallowing, are not accompanied by peristalsis, are accompanied by diaphragmatic inhibition, and persist for longer periods than do swallow-induced LES relaxations (>10 seconds).[31,32] Of note, prolonged manometric recordings have not consistently demonstrated an increased frequency of tLESRs in GERD patients compared with normal controls.[33] However, the frequency of acid reflux (as opposed to gas reflux) during tLESRs has been consistently reported to be greater in GERD patients.[34]

Recognizing the importance of tLESRs in promoting reflux, investigators have attempted to define this reflex using physiological and pharmacological manipulations. The dominant stimulus for tLESRs is distension of the proximal stomach, not surprising given that tLESR is the physiological mechanism for belching.[35] Transient LES relaxation can be experimentally elicited by either gaseous distension of the stomach or distension of the proximal stomach with a barostat bag. Furthermore, the degree to which tLESR frequency is augmented by gastric distension is directly related to the size of hiatus hernia, suggesting that the associated anatomical alteration affects the function of the afferent mechanoreceptors responsible for eliciting this reflex.[36] The most likely candidate for the afferent receptor is the intraganglionic lamellar ending, or IGLE.[37] Intraganglionic lamellar endings are found at the receptor end of vagal afferents innervating the gastric cardia and can be shown physiologically to fire in direct proportion to applied tension.[38] The frequency of tLESRs is also increased by assuming an upright posture.[33,39] The vagal afferent mechanoreceptors in the gastric cardia then project to the nucleus tractus solitarii in the brainstem and subsequently to the dorsal motor nuclei of the vagus. Finally, dorsal motor nucleus neurons project to inhibitory neurons localized within the myenteric plexus of the distal esophagus. Furthermore, tLESR is an integrated motor response involving not only LES relaxation, but also crural diaphragmatic inhibition and contraction of the costal diaphragm.[32,40] The tLESR reflex is abolished by vagotomy.[32] Recently, animal and human experiments have demonstrated that tLESRs can be inhibited by gamma aminobutyric acid receptor type B agonists (such as baclofen), suggesting a potential new approach to the treatment of GERD.[41-44]

LES (Intrinsic Sphincter) Hypotension

Gastroesophageal reflux disease can occur in the context of diminished LES pressure either by strain-induced or free reflux. Strain-induced reflux occurs when a hypotensive LES is overcome and "blown open" in association with an abrupt increase of intraabdominal pressure.[45] Manometric data suggest that this rarely occurs

when the LES pressure is >10 mm Hg[45,46] (Figure 1.3). It is also a rare occurrence in patients without hiatus hernia.[30] Free reflux is characterized by a decrease in intraesophageal pH without an identifiable change in either intragastric pressure or LES pressure. Episodes of free reflux are observed only when the LES pressure is within 0–4 mm Hg of intragastric pressure. A wide-open or patulous hiatus will predispose to this free reflux as both the intrinsic and extrinsic sphincter are compromised.

A puzzling clinical observation, and one that supports the importance of tLESRs, is that only a minority of patients with GERD have a fasting LES pressure value of <10 mm Hg.[47] This observation can also be reconciled when one considers the dynamic nature of LES pressure. The isolated fasting measurement of LES pressure is probably useful only for identifying patients with a grossly hypotensive sphincter; individuals constantly susceptible to stress and free reflux. However, there is probably a larger population of patients susceptible to strain-induced or free reflux when their LES pressure periodically decreases as a result of specific foods, drugs, or habits (Table 1.1).

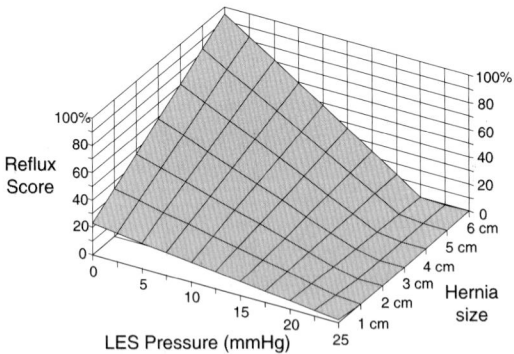

Figure 1.3. Model of the relationship between the LES pressure, size of hernia, and the susceptibility to gastroesophageal reflux induced by provocative straining maneuvers as reflected by the reflux score on the *z* axis. The overall equation of the model is: reflux score = 22.64 + 12.05 (hernia size) − 0.83 (LES pressure) − 0.65 (LES pressure × hernia size). The hernia size is in centimeters, and the LES pressure is in millimeters of mercury. The multiple correlation coefficient of this equation for the 50-subject data set was 0.86 (R^2 = .75). Thus, the susceptibility to stress reflux is dependent on the interaction of the instantaneous value of LES pressure and the size of the hiatus hernia. (Reprinted with permission from Sloan et al.[45])

The Diaphragmatic Sphincter and Hiatus Hernia

Physiological studies by Mittal et al.[48] have clearly demonstrated that the augmentation of EGJ pressure observed during a multitude of activities associated with transient increases in intraabdominal pressure is attributable to contraction of the crural diaphragm. With hiatus hernia, crural diaphragm function is potentially compromised both by its axial displacement[49] and potentially by atrophy consequent from dilatation of the hiatus.[50] The impact of hiatus hernia on reflux elicited by straining maneuvers was demonstrated in studies in normal volunteers compared to GERD patients with and without hiatus hernia.[45] Of several physiological and anatomical variables tested, the size of hiatus hernia was shown to have the highest correlation with the susceptibility to strain-induced reflux. The implication of this observation is that patients with hiatus hernia exhibit progressive impairment of the diaphragmatic component of EGJ function proportional to the extent of axial herniation.[49]

Another effect that hiatus hernia exerts on the anti-reflux barrier is to diminish the intraluminal pressure within the EGJ. Relevant animal experiments revealed that simulating the effect of hiatus hernia by severing the phrenoesophageal ligament reduced the LES pressure and that the subsequent repair of the ligament restored the LES pressure to levels similar to baseline.[51] Similarly, manometric studies in humans using a topographic representation of the EGJ high-pressure zone of hiatus hernia patients revealed distinct intrinsic sphincter and hiatal canal pressure components, each of which was of lower magnitude than the EGJ pressure of a comparator group of normal controls.[52] However, simulating reduction of the hernia by repositioning the intrinsic sphincter back within the hiatal canal and arithmetically summing superimposed pressures resulted in calculated EGJ pressures that were practically indistinguishable from those of the control subjects. Along with previous investigations, these data also demonstrated that hiatus hernia reduced the length of the EGJ high-pressure zone.[49] This is likely the result of disruption of the EGJ segment distal to the SCJ attributable to the opposing sling and clasp fibers of the gastric cardia.[22] It is also the likely explanation for the clinical correlation established in a multitude of surgical publications that EGJ competence is inversely related to manometrically defined EGJ length.[53]

Gastroesophageal Flap Valve

In addition to the two sphincters described above, another mechanism of barrier function at the EGJ lies in the positioning of the distal esophagus in the intraabdominal cavity. A flap valve is formed by a musculomucosal fold created by the entry of the esophagus into the stomach along the lesser curvature. Increased intraabdominal or intragastric pressure can decrease the angle of His and compress the subdiaphragmatic portion of the esophagus, thereby preventing reflux during periods of abdominal straining. Although the clinical relevance of this concept has been controversial, several studies have helped bolster its validity. Hill et al.[24] demonstrated the presence of a gastroesophageal pressure gradient in cadavers without a hiatal hernia. They also showed that the ability of the EGJ in cadavers to resist reflux in the face of increased intraabdominal pressure could be increased by surgically accentuating the length of the flap valve. Hill et al. then went on to define a grading scheme based on endoscopic inspection of the gastroesophageal flap valve (Figure 1.1). Two endoscopic studies have reported that this grading scheme correlated with the severity of reflux disease.[24,54] Most recently, an investigation using wireless pH monitoring found a strong correlation between the degree to which individuals are susceptible to exercise-induced reflux and flap valve grade.[55] No such correlation existed with LES pressure. Because exercise-induced reflux is presumably strain induced, this supports the importance of the flap valve as a defensive mechanism.

Mechanical Properties of the Relaxed EGJ

For reflux to occur in the setting of a relaxed or hypotensive sphincter, it is necessary for the relaxed sphincter to open. Recent physiological studies exploring the role of compliance in GERD reported that GERD patients without and particularly with hiatus hernia had increased compliance at the EGJ compared with normal subjects[56] and patients with fundoplication.[57] These experiments utilized a combination of barostat-controlled distention, manometry, and fluoroscopy to directly measure the compliance of the EGJ. Several parameters of EGJ compliance were shown to be increased in hiatus hernia patients with GERD: 1) the EGJ opened at lower distention pressure, 2) the relaxed EGJ opened at distention pressures that were at or near resting intragastric pressure, and 3) for a given distention pressure the EGJ opened about 0.5 cm wider. Still significant, but lesser compliance related changes were demonstrated in the non-hernia GERD patients (Figure 1.4). These alterations of EGJ mechanics are likely secondary to a disrupted, distensible crural aperture and may be the root causes of the physiological aberrations associated with GERD.

Increased EGJ compliance may help explain why patients with hiatus hernia have a distinct mechanistic reflux profile compared with patients without hiatus hernia.[30] Anatomical alterations, such as hiatal hernia, dilatation of the diaphragmatic hiatus, and disruption of the gastroesophageal flap valve may alter the elastic characteristics of the hiatus such that this factor

is no longer protective in preventing gastroesophageal reflux. In that setting, reflux no longer requires "two hits" to the EGJ because the extrinsic sphincteric mechanism is chronically disrupted. Thus, the only prerequisite for reflux becomes LES relaxation, be that in the setting of swallow-induced relaxation, tLESR, or a period of prolonged LES hypotension.

Increased compliance may also help explain why GERD patients may be more likely to sustain acid reflux in association with tLESRs compared with asymptomatic subjects. In an experiment that sought to quantify this difference, normal subjects exhibited acid reflux with 40–50% of tLESRs compared with 60–70% in patients with GERD.[33] This difference may be the result of increased EGJ compliance and its effect on trans-EGJ flow.

$$\text{Trans-EGJ flow} = (\Delta P \times R^4)/(C \times L \times \eta).$$

In the above flow equation, flow is directly proportional to EGJ diameter to the fourth power and inversely proportional to the length of the narrowed segment and the viscosity of the gas or liquid traversing the segment. Should tLESRs occur in the context of an EGJ with

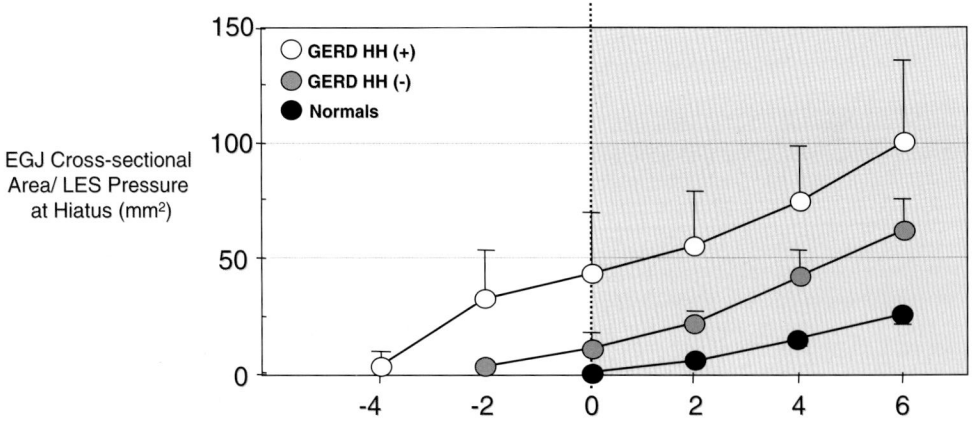

Figure 1.4. Esophagogastric junction cross-sectional area as a function of distention pressure. Cross-sectional area at intrabag pressures >0 mm Hg was significantly increased in the non-hiatus hernia (NHH) GERD patients compared with normal subjects ($P < .0001$) and in the hiatus hernia (HH) patients compared with the NHH patients ($P < .005$). At pressures ≤0 mm Hg, the EGJ cross-sectional area of HH GERD patients was significantly greater than both the NHH GERD patients and normals ($P < .05$). At pressures <0 mm Hg, there was no significant difference between NHH GERD patients and normals. Thus, NHH GERD patients exhibited similar distensile properties to HH patients at pressures greater than intragastric pressure and similar to normal subjects at pressures less than or equal to intragastric pressure. (Reprinted from Pandolfino et al.,[56] Copyright 2003, with permission from the American Gastroenterological Association.)

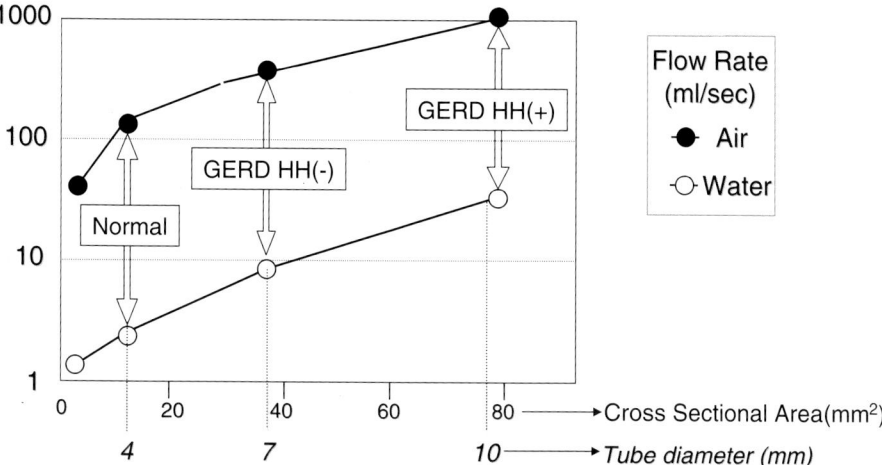

Figure 1.5. Simulated flow rates of water and air across the EGJ using a hydrostat or barostat and short lengths (1 cm) of polyurethane tubing. The diameter of the tubing used to model each group simulates cross-sectional area observed with distention pressures of 4 mm Hg in the three study groups (normal, GERD without hiatus hernia, GERD with hiatus hernia). Given that 57 mL/s was the greatest flow rate attainable with the barostat, higher air flow rates were extrapolated from liquid flow rates using a liquid/air viscosity ratio of 55 : 1. At cross-sectional areas simulating normal subjects, flow of air is preserved whereas flow of liquid is minimal. In contrast, the flow of liquid is significantly increased in both GERD groups.

increased compliance, wider opening diameters will occur under a given set of circumstances and trans-EGJ flow will increase. The impact of this difference in opening diameter is evident in the modeled data illustrating the flow rates of gas and liquid through tubing simulating the aperture size of normal controls and GERD patients with and without hiatus hernia (Figure 5). Note that, because of the reduced opening diameter, the normal EGJ acts as a mechanical filter selectively permitting flow of gas while limiting that of water. Patients without obvious hiatus hernia may still have increased compliance secondary to more subtle defects at the EGJ not readily evident using current radiographic or endoscopic methods of evaluation. These defects may be more akin to minor anatomical variants of the EGJ such as a grade II gastroesophageal flap valve or defects in the LES musculature.

Esophageal Acid Clearance

After an acid reflux event, the duration of time that the esophageal mucosa remains acidified to a pH of <4 is termed the esophageal acid clearance time. Acid clearance begins with peristalsis that empties the refluxed fluid from the esophagus and is completed by titration of the residual acid by swallowed saliva. This was demonstrated in an elegant study using radiolabeled 0.1 N hydrochloric acid.[58] Aspirating saliva from the mouth prolonged acid clearance, suggesting that it was the swallowed saliva rather than peristalsis that restored esophageal pH. It requires approximately 7 mL of saliva to neutralize 1 mL of 0.1 N hydrochloric acid, with 50% of this neutralizing capacity attributable to bicarbonate. The typical rate of salivation is 0.5 mL/min.[58] Thus, in individuals with normal esophageal emptying, maneuvers that increase salivation such as oral lozenges or gum chewing hasten acid clearance whereas hyposalivation prolongs acid clearance. Of note, although salivation virtually ceases during sleep,[59] some acid clearance is still achieved attributable to bicarbonate secretion from esophageal submucosal glands.[60]

Prolongation of esophageal acid clearance among patients with esophagitis was demonstrated along with the initial description of an acid clearance test.[61] Subsequent investigations have demonstrated heterogeneity within the patient population such that about half of the GERD patients had normal clearance values, whereas the other half had prolonged values.[62,63] Ambulatory pH monitoring studies suggest that this heterogeneity is at least partially attributed to hiatus hernia, because this subset of individuals tended to have the most prolonged supine acid clearance.[64] Clinical data also suggest that prolonged acid clearance correlates with both the severity of esophagitis and the presence of Barrett's metaplasia.[65–67] From what we know regarding the mechanisms of acid clearance, the two main potential causes of prolonged esophageal acid clearance are impaired esophageal emptying and impaired salivary function.

Impairments of Esophageal Emptying

Impaired esophageal emptying in reflux disease was inferred by the observation that symptoms of gastroesophageal reflux improve with an upright posture, a maneuver that allows gravity to augment fluid emptying. Subsequently, two mechanisms of impaired esophageal emptying have been identified: peristaltic dysfunction and superimposed reflux associated with nonreducing hiatus hernias. Peristaltic dysfunction in esophagitis has been described by a number of investigators. Of particular significance are failed peristalsis and hypotensive peristaltic contractions (<30 mm Hg) which result in incomplete emptying.[68] As esophagitis increases in severity, so does the incidence of peristaltic dysfunction.[47] More recent investigations of peristaltic function have labeled this "ineffective esophageal motility," defined by the occurrence of >30% of hypotensive or failed contractions.[69] With respect to the reversibility of peristaltic dysfunction, recent studies show no improvement after healing of esophagitis by acid inhibition,[70] or by anti-reflux surgery.[71] Most likely, the acute dysfunction associated with active esophagitis is partially reversible but that associated with stricturing or fibrosis is not.

Hiatus hernia also can impair esophageal emptying. Concurrent pH recording and scintigraphy above the EGJ showed that impaired clearance was caused by reflux of fluid from the hernia sac during swallowing.[72] This observation was subsequently confirmed radiographically in an analysis of esophageal emp-

tying in patients with reducing and nonreducing hiatus hernias.[73] The efficacy of emptying was significantly diminished in both hernia groups when compared with normal controls. Emptying was particularly impaired in the nonreducing hiatus hernia patients who exhibited complete emptying with only one-third of test swallows. The patients with nonreducing hernias were the only group that exhibited retrograde flow of fluid from the hernia during deglutitive relaxation, consistent with the scintigraphic studies.

Salivary Function

The final phase of esophageal acid clearance depends on salivation. Just as impaired esophageal emptying prolongs acid clearance, diminished salivary neutralizing capacity has the same effect. Diminished salivation during sleep, for instance, explains why reflux events during sleep or immediately before sleep are associated with markedly prolonged acid clearance times. Similarly, chronic xerostomia is associated with prolonged esophageal acid exposure and esophagitis.[74] However, no systematic difference has been found in the salivary function of GERD patients compared with controls. One group of subjects shown to have prolonged esophageal acid clearance times attributable to hyposalivation is cigarette smokers. Even those without symptoms of reflux disease exhibited acid clearance times 50% longer than those of nonsmokers and the salivary titratable base content was only 60% of the age-matched nonsmokers.[75]

In addition to bicarbonate, saliva contains growth factors that have the potential to enhance mucosal repair. Epidermal growth factor (EGF), produced in submaxillary ductal cells and duodenal Brunner's glands, has been extensively studied.[76] In animal models, EGF has been shown to provide cytoprotection against irritants, enhance the healing of gastroduodenal ulceration, and decrease the permeability of the esophageal mucosa to hydrogen ions.[76–78] However, studies have not shown consistent differences in EGF concentration in esophagitis or Barrett's metaplasia patients,[79,80] making it impossible to implicate perturbations of growth factor secretion in the pathogenesis of GERD.

Summary

Gastroesophageal reflux disease is likely the most prevalent condition afflicting the gastrointestinal tract in the United States with typical estimates finding 14–20% of the adult population afflicted on at least a weekly basis. The most clearly subset of GERD patients have esophagitis wherein excessive exposure of the esophageal epithelium to gastric acid and pepsin results in erosions, ulcers, and potential complications of these. However, most afflicted individuals will not have endoscopic evidence of esophagitis. Paradoxically, as esophagitis has become less of a problem, at least in part because of more effective treatments, the issue of symptom control has become a more substantial one.

From a pathophysiological viewpoint, GERD results from the excessive reflux of gastric contents into the distal esophagus. Under normal conditions, this is prevented as a function of the anti-reflux barrier at the EGJ, the integrity of which is dependent on the delicate interplay of a host of anatomical and physiological factors including the integrity of the LES, tLESRs, and anatomical degradation of the EGJ inclusive of, but not limited to, hiatus hernia. In fact, considerable investigative focus is now aimed at describing the subtle aberrations of the EGJ that may contribute to the root causes of GERD. The net result is of an increased number of reflux events, an increasing diversity of potential mechanisms of reflux, and a diminished ability of the stomach to selectively vent gas as opposed to gas and gastric juice during tLESRs.

Once reflux has occurred, the duration of resultant esophageal acid exposure is determined by the effectiveness of esophageal acid clearance, the dominant determinants of which are peristalsis, salivation, and, again, the anatomical integrity of the EGJ. About half of GERD patients have abnormal acid clearance and the major contributor to this is hiatus hernia. Abnormalities of acid clearance are probably the major determinant of which GERD patients are most prone to developing esophagitis as opposed to symptomatic GERD.

In summary, GERD is a multifactorial process involving both physiological and anatomical abnormalities. These abnormalities exhibit a complicated interplay that degrades the ability of the EGJ to contain gastric juice within the stomach and to effectively clear the esophagus of gastric juice once reflux has occurred.

Acknowledgment. This work was supported by grants RO1 DC00646 (P.J.K.) and K23 DK062170-01 (J.E.P.) from the Public Health Service.

References

1. Nebel OT, Fornes MF, Castell DO. Symptomatic gastroesophageal reflux: incidence and precipitating factors. Am J Dig Dis 1976;21:953–956.
2. Gallup Organization. Gallup survey on heartburn across America, 1988.
3. Locke GR 3rd, Talley NJ, Fett SL, Zinmeister AR, Melton LJ 3rd. Prevalence and clinical spectrum of gastroesophageal reflux: a population-based study in Olmsted County, Minnesota. Gastroenterology 1997; 112:1448–1456.
4. El-Serag HB, Petersen NJ, Carter J, et al. Gastroesophageal reflux among different racial groups in the United States. Gastroenterology 2004;126:1692–1699.
5. DeMeester TR, Wang CI, Wernly JA, et al. Technique, indications, and clinical use of 24 hour esophageal pH monitoring. J Thorac Cardiovasc Surg 1980;79:656–670.
6. Johnsson F, Joelsson B, Gudmundsson K, Greiff L. Symptoms and endoscopic findings in the diagnosis of gastroesophageal reflux disease. Scand J Gastroenterol 1987;22:714–718.
7. Wienbeck M, Barnert J. Epidemiology of reflux disease and reflux esophagitis. Scand J Gastroenterol Suppl 1989; 156:7–13.
8. Cameron AJ, Zinsmeister AR, Ballard DJ, Carney JA. Prevalence of columnar-lined (Barrett's) esophagus: comparison of population-based clinical and autopsy findings. Gastroenterology 1990;99:918–922.
9. Bainbridge ET, Temple JG, Nicholas SP, Newton JR, Boriah V. Symptomatic gastro-oesophageal reflux in pregnancy: a comparative study of white Europeans and Asians in Birmingham. Br J Clin Pract 1983;37:53–57.
10. Sonnenberg A, El-Serag HB. Clinical epidemiology and natural history of gastroesophageal reflux disease. Yale J Biol Med 1999;72:81–92.
11. El-Serag HB, Sonnenberg A. Opposing time trends of peptic ulcer and reflux disease. Gut 1998;43:327–333.
12. El-Serag HB, Sonnenberg A, Jamal MM, Inadomi JM, Crooks LA, Feddersen RM. Corpus gastritis is protective against reflux oesophagitis. Gut 1999;45:181–185.
13. Graham DY. The changing epidemiology of GERD: geography and Helicobacter pylori. Am J Gastroenterol 2003;98:1462–1470.
14. Abe Y, Ohara S, Koike T, et al. The prevalence of Helicobacter pylori infection and the status of gastric acid secretion in patients with Barrett's esophagus in Japan. Am J Gastroenterol 2004;99:1213–1221.
15. Pandolfino JE, Howden CW, Kahrilas PJ. H. pylori and GERD: is less more? Am J Gastroenterol 2004;99: 1222–1225.

16. Dent J, Dodds WJ, Friedman RH, et al. Mechanism of gastroesophageal reflux in recumbent asymptomatic human subjects. J Clin Invest 1980;65:256–267.

17. Goyal RK, Rattan S. Genesis of basal sphincter pressure: effect of tetrodotoxin on lower esophageal sphincter pressure in opossum in vivo. Gastroenterology 1976;71: 62–67.

18. Goyal RK, Rattan S. Nature of the vagal inhibitory innervation to the lower esophageal sphincter. J Clin Invest 1975;55:1119–1126.

19. Yamato S, Saha JK, Goyal RK. Role of nitric oxide in lower esophageal sphincter relaxation to swallowing. Life Sci 1992;50:1263–1272.

20. Richards WG, Sugarbaker DJ. Neuronal control of esophageal function. Chest Surg Clin N Am 1995;5: 157–171.

21. Kahrilas PJ. Anatomy and physiology of the gastroesophageal junction. Gastroenterol Clin North Am 1997; 26:467–486.

22. Liebermann-Meffert D, Allgower M, Schmid P, Blum AL. Muscular equivalent of the lower esophageal sphincter. Gastroenterology 1979;76:31–38.

23. Thor KB, Hill LD, Mercer DD, Kozarek RD. Reappraisal of the flap valve mechanism in the gastroesophageal junction: a study of a new valvuloplasty procedure in cadavers. Acta Chir Scand 1987;153:25–28.

24. Hill LD, Kozarek RA, Kraemer SJ, et al. The gastroesophageal flap valve: in vitro and in vivo observations. Gastrointest Endosc 1996;44:541–547.

25. Mittal VK, Telmos AJ, Cortez JA. Surgical techniques for gastroesophagostomy with the EEA stapler. Int Surg 1985;70:29–32.

26. De Troyer A, Sampson M, Sigrist S, Macklem PT. Action of costal and crural parts of the diaphragm on the rib cage in dog. J Appl Physiol 1982;53:30–39.

27. Altschuler SM, Boyle JT, Nixon TE, Pack AI, Cohen S. Simultaneous reflex inhibition of lower esophageal sphincter and crural diaphragm in cats. Am J Physiol 1985;249:G586–G591.

28. Mittal RK, Fisher M, McCallum RW, Rochester DF, Dent J, Sluss J. Human lower esophageal sphincter pressure response to increased intra-abdominal pressure. Am J Physiol 1990;258:G624–G630.

29. Klein WA, Parkman HP, Dempsey DT, Fisher RS. Sphincterlike thoracoabdominal high pressure zone after esophagogastrectomy. Gastroenterology 1993;105: 1362–1369.

30. van Herwaarden MA, Samsom M, Smout AJ. Excess gastroesophageal reflux in patients with hiatus hernia is caused by mechanisms other than transient LES relaxations. Gastroenterology 2000;119:1439–1446.

31. Holloway RH, Penagini R, Ireland AC. Criteria for objective definition of transient lower esophageal sphincter relaxation. Am J Physiol 1995;268:G128–G133.

32. Mittal RK, Holloway RH, Penagini R, Blackshaw LA, Dent J. Transient lower esophageal sphincter relaxation. Gastroenterology 1995;109:601–610.

33. Sifrim D, Holloway R. Transient lower esophageal sphincter relaxations: how many or how harmful? Am J Gastroenterol 2001;96:2529–2532.

34. Sifrim D, Holloway R, Silny J, et al. Acid, nonacid, and gas reflux in patients with gastroesophageal reflux disease during ambulatory 24-hour pH-impedance recordings. Gastroenterology 2001;120:1588–1598.

35. Wyman JB, Dent J, Heddle R, Dodds WJ, Toouli J, Downton J. Control of belching by the lower oesophageal sphincter. Gut 1990;31:639–646.

36. Kahrilas PJ, Shi G, Manka M, Joehl RJ. Increased frequency of transient lower esophageal sphincter relaxation induced by gastric distention in reflux patients with hiatal hernia. Gastroenterology 2000;118:688–695.

37. Zagorodnyuk VP, Chen BN, Brookes SJ. Intraganglionic laminar endings are mechano-transduction sites of vagal tension receptors in the guinea-pig stomach. J Physiol 2001;534:255–268.

38. Zagorodnyuk VP, Chen BN, Costa M, Brookes SJ. Mechanotransduction by intraganglionic laminar endings of vagal tension receptors in the guinea-pig oesophagus. J Physiol 2003;553:575–587.

39. Martin CJ, Patrikios J, Dent J. Abolition of gas reflux and transient lower esophageal sphincter relaxation by vagal blockade in the dog. Gastroenterology 1986;91:890–896.

40. Martin CJ, Dodds WJ, Liem HH, Dantas RO, Layman RD, Dent J. Diaphragmatic contribution to gastroesophageal competence and reflux in dogs. Am J Physiol 1992;263: G551–G557.

41. Lehmann A, Antonsson M, Bremner-Danielsen M, Flardh M, Hansson-Branden L, Karrberg L. Activation of the GABA(B) receptor inhibits transient lower esophageal sphincter relaxations in dogs. Gastroenterology 1999;117:1147–1154.

42. Lidums I, Lehmann A, Checklin H, Dent J, Holloway RH. Control of transient lower esophageal sphincter relaxations and reflux by the GABA(B) agonist baclofen in normal subjects. Gastroenterology 2000;118:7–13.

43. van Herwaarden MA, Samsom M, Rydholm H, Smout AJ. The effect of baclofen on gastro-oesophageal reflux, lower oesophageal sphincter function and reflux symptoms in patients with reflux disease. Aliment Pharmacol Ther 2002;16:1655–1662.

44. Koek GH, Sifrim D, Lerut T, Janssens J, Tack J. Effect of the GABA(B) agonist baclofen in patients with symptoms and duodeno-gastro-oesophageal reflux refractory to proton pump inhibitors. Gut 2003;52:1397–1402.

45. Sloan S, Rademaker AW, Kahrilas PJ. Determinants of gastroesophageal junction incompetence: hiatal hernia, lower esophageal sphincter, or both? Ann Intern Med 1992;117:977–982.

46. Dent J, Dodds WJ, Hogan WJ, Toouli J. Factors that influence induction of gastroesophageal reflux in normal human subjects. Dig Dis Sci 1988;33:270–275.

47. Kahrilas PJ, Dodds WJ, Hogan WJ, Kern M, Arndorfer RC, Reece A. Esophageal peristaltic dysfunction in peptic esophagitis. Gastroenterology 1986;91:897–904.

48. Mittal RK, Rochester DF, McCallum RW. Effect of the diaphragmatic contraction on lower oesophageal sphincter pressure in man. Gut 1987;28:1564–1568.

49. Kahrilas PJ, Lin S, Chen J, Manka M. The effect of hiatus hernia on gastro-oesophageal junction pressure. Gut 1999;44:476–482.

50. Marchand P. The surgery for hiatus hernia: is vagotomy rational? S Afr Med J 1970;44:35–39.

51. Michelson E, Siegel C. The role of the phrenico-esophageal ligament in the lower esophageal sphincter. Surg Gynecol Obstet 1964;118:1291–1294.

52. Kahrilas PJ, Lin S, Manka M, Shi G, Joehl RJ. Esophagogastric junction pressure topography after fundoplication. Surgery 2000;127:200–208.

53. Stein HJ, DeMeester TR, Naspetti R, Jamieson J, Perry RE. Three-dimensional imaging of the lower esophageal sphincter in gastroesophageal reflux disease. Ann Surg 1991;214:374–383; discussion 383–384.

54. Contractor QQ, Akhtar SS, Contractor TQ. Endoscopic esophagitis and gastroesophageal flap valve. J Clin Gastroenterol 1999;28:233–237.

55. Pandolfino JE, Bianchi L, Lee TJ, Hirano I, Kahrilas PJ. Esophagogastric junction morphology predicts susceptibility to exercise-induced reflux. Am J Gastroenterol 2004;99:1430–1436.

56. Pandolfino JE, Shi G, Trueworthy B, Kahrilas PJ. Esophagogastric junction opening during relaxation distinguishes nonhernia reflux patients, hernia patients, and normal subjects. Gastroenterology 2003;125:1018–1024.

57. Curry J, Shi G, Pandolfino JE, Joehl RJ, Brasseur JG, Kahrilas PJ. Mechanical characteristics of the EGJ after fundoplication compared to normal subjects and GERD patients. Gastroenterology 2001;120:A112.

58. Helm JF. Role of saliva in esophageal function and disease. Dysphagia 1989;4:76–84.

59. Schneyer LH, Pigman W, Hanahan L, Gilmore RW. Rate of flow of human parotid, sublingual, and submaxillary secretions during sleep. J Dent Res 1956;35:109–114.

60. Singh S, Bradley LA, Richter JE. Determinants of oesophageal "alkaline" pH environment in controls and patients with gastro-oesophageal reflux disease. Gut 1993;34:309–316.

61. Borchardt PJ. Employee productivity and gastroesophageal reflux disease: the payer's viewpoint. Am J Gastroenterol 2001;96:S62–S63.

62. Stanciu C, Bennett JR. Oesophageal acid clearing: one factor in the production of reflux oesophagitis. Gut 1974;15:852–857.

63. Dodds WJ, Kahrilas PJ, Dent J, et al. Analysis of spontaneous gastroesophageal reflux and esophageal acid clearance in patients with reflux esophagitis. J Gastrointest Motil 1990;2:79.

64. Johnson LF. Twenty-four-hour pH monitoring in the study of gastroesophageal reflux. J Clin Gastroenterol 1980;2:387–399.

65. Gillen P, Keeling P, Byrne PJ, Hennessy TP. Barrett's oesophagus: pH profile. Br J Surg 1987;74:774–776.

66. Karvelis KC, Drane WE, Johnson DA, Silverman ED. Barrett esophagus: decreased esophageal clearance shown by radionuclide esophageal scintigraphy. Radiology 1987;162:97–99.

67. Singh P, Adamopoulos A, Taylor RH, Colin-Jones DG. Oesophageal motor function before and after healing of oesophagitis. Gut 1992;33:1590–1596.

68. Kahrilas PJ, Dodds WJ, Hogan WJ. Effect of peristaltic dysfunction on esophageal volume clearance. Gastroenterology 1988;94:73–80.

69. Leite LP, Johnston BT, Barrett J, Castell JA, Castell DO. Ineffective esophageal motility (IEM): the primary finding in patients with nonspecific esophageal motility disorder. Dig Dis Sci 1997;42:1859–1865.

70. Timmer R, Breumelhof R, Nadorp JH, Smout AJ. Oesophageal motility and gastro-oesophageal reflux before and after healing of reflux oesophagitis: a study using 24 hour ambulatory pH and pressure monitoring. Gut 1994;35:1519–1522.

71. Rydberg L, Ruth M, Lundell L. Does oesophageal motor function improve with time after successful anti-reflux surgery? Results of a prospective, randomised clinical study. Gut 1997;41:82–86.

72. Mittal RK, Lange RC, McCallum RW. Identification and mechanism of delayed esophageal acid clearance in subjects with hiatus hernia. Gastroenterology 1987;92:130–135.

73. Sloan S, Kahrilas PJ. Impairment of esophageal emptying with hiatal hernia. Gastroenterology 1991;100:596–605.

74. Korsten MA, Rosman AS, Fishbein S, Shlein RD, Goldberg HE, Biener A. Chronic xerostomia increases esophageal acid exposure and is associated with esophageal injury. Am J Med 1991;90:701–706.

75. Kahrilas PJ, Gupta RR. The effect of cigarette smoking on salivation and esophageal acid clearance. J Lab Clin Med 1989;114:431–438.

76. Konturek JW, Bielanski W, Konturek SJ, Bogdal J, Oleksy J. Distribution and release of epidermal growth factor in man. Gut 1989;30:1194–1200.

77. Skoner DP. Growth effects of asthma and asthma therapy. Curr Opin Pulm Med 2002;8:45–49.

78. Sarosiek J, Feng T, McCallum RW. The interrelationship between salivary epidermal growth factor and the functional integrity of the esophageal mucosal barrier in the rat. Am J Med Sci 1991;302:359–363.

79. Maccini DM, Veit BC. Salivary epidermal growth factor in patients with and without acid peptic disease. Am J Gastroenterol 1990;85:1102–1104.

80. Rourk RM, Namiot Z, Sarosiek J, Yu Z, McCallum RW. Impairment of salivary epidermal growth factor secretory response to esophageal mechanical and chemical stimulation in patients with reflux esophagitis. Am J Gastroenterol 1994;89:237–244.

81. Pandolfino JE, Kahrilas PJ. Esophagel motility abnormalities in barrett's esophagus. In: Sharma P, Sampliner RE, eds. Barrett's Esophagus and Esophageal Adenocarcinoma. Malden, MA: Blackwell Science; 2001:35–44.

2

History of Medical and Surgical Anti-Reflux Therapy

Mark K. Ferguson

Humans have no doubt suffered from the symptoms and complications of gastroesophageal reflux disease (GERD) for millennia. However, recognition of a relationship between acid-pepsin and foregut disorders is relatively recent. The powerful digestive and corrosive capability of gastric juices in humans was first extensively described in 1833 by Beaumont[1] as a result of experiments performed on Alexis St. Martin. That reflux of these juices into the esophagus could cause symptoms and result in tissue injury was suspected as early as 1839 by Albers, who, as reported by Tileston,[2] described a peptic ulcer of the esophagus that was similar to a peptic ulcer of the stomach. Periodic reports of peptic esophageal ulcer subsequently appeared, although the existence of this phenomenon was still in doubt in the second half of the 19th century. Quincke's[3] report of three well-documented cases of peptic esophageal ulceration in 1879 put all doubt to rest. Tileston[2] summarized reports of 40 cases of peptic esophageal ulceration extant in the literature before 1906.

One complication of peptic ulceration, esophageal stricture, was described as early as the 15th century, and dilation for stricture was reported in the early 19th century. Endoscopy was in its infancy in the second half of the 19th century, precluding any useful direct viewing of the type or level of a stricture. The determination of the site of a stricture was based on either auscultation as fluid was swallowed, listening for a gurgling or trickling noise at the point of obstruction, or by the passage of bougies.[4]

Possible causes of obstructions included caustic ingestion, malignancy, webs, and, in retrospect, peptic esophagitis, although the latter etiology was rarely, if ever, suspected. In the absence of an antecedent event such as caustic ingestion, the premortem diagnosis of the etiology of esophageal obstruction was rare. By the time a patient expired from obstructive effects of a peptic stricture, the process was so advanced that detection of a relationship between stricture formation and peptic-acid injury was impossible.

The development of upper gastrointestinal endoscopy led to the premortem diagnosis of esophagitis and esophageal ulceration with some frequency. In 1929 Jackson[5] described 88 cases of acute or healed esophageal ulceration identified among 4000 patients with esophageal symptoms. He correctly ascribed the pain of peptic esophageal ulcer to the effects of gastric juices bathing the ulcerated area, and discounted the prevalent notion that peristalsis was the source of esophageal pain.[5] Although Jackson suggested that some of these ulcers may have been caused by gastric reflux, that claim was made strongly in the mid-1930s by Lyall,[6] who described superficial esophagitis in the presence of reflux and deep esophageal ulcers associated with heterotopic mucosa, now known as Barrett's ulcers. More than 100 years after the initial description of peptic esophageal ulceration, the destructive effects of acid-pepsin on the esophagus were clearly documented.[7]

Anatomic problems were not generally recognized in the 19th century as being associated with GERD. In a review of case reports of 88 diaphragmatic hernias published before 1847, Bowditch[8] identified esophageal hiatal hernias as being among the most common. However, all hernias within this subgroup likely were large paraesophageal hernias that had either strangulated or perforated, and none was documented as being associated with symptoms of gastroesophageal reflux.[8] At the beginning of the 20th century, only a few of the hundreds of diaphragmatic hernias that had been reported in the literature had been diagnosed premortem.[9] The discovery of X-rays in 1895 led to the rapid development of their use as a diagnostic tool, and by 1908 contrast radiography was a reliable technique for the diagnosis of hiatal hernia.[10] However, the anatomic deformity and obstructive complications, not symptoms of heartburn, were the primary indication for hiatal hernia repair in the first half of the 20th century.[10,11]

Chronic peptic ulcer of the esophagus was first related to hiatal hernia in the early 1940s and only dietary therapy was recommended.[12] The pathophysiologic mechanism of an ineffective anti-reflux mechanism resulting from hiatal hernia was suggested by Allison[13,14] in 1948, who noted improvement after surgical correction of the hernia in seven patients. The relationship between hiatal hernia-associated dysfunction of the esophagogastric junction and symptoms of heartburn was then conclusively made by Allison[15] in 1951 when he described the syndrome of heartburn, gastric flatulence, and postural regurgitation, and attributed it to reflux esophagitis. The understanding of this relationship ushered in the era of physiologic therapy for GERD.

Early Nonsurgical Therapy

Early therapy for esophageal disorders included the usual compendium of useless and occasionally life-threatening techniques used for a host of different ailments, including emetics, venesection, leeches, cathartics, enemas, opiates, electrolysis, and immersion in a cold bath. Section of constricting diaphragm muscle was proposed by Bowditch[8] for treatment of diaphragmatic hernia, but no surgeon was recorded as being sufficiently adventuresome to undertake such an operation for almost half a century. Similarly, surgery for esophageal stricture or perforated esophageal ulcer was not successfully undertaken until well into the 20th century. In the absence of reliable anesthetic techniques and the ability to artificially ventilate patients, thoracic operations were nearly always doomed to failure. As a result, conservative management, such as esophageal dilation, grew increasingly popular in the 19th century.

Esophageal Dilation

During the early 19th century, dilation therapy for esophageal obstruction was performed by a variety of physicians including urologists, who expanded their practice of dilating urethral strictures to encompass the esophagus. Early dilators included a swallowed bullet attached to a string, bougies made from cloth and wax, a probang (an egg-shaped ivory ball attached to a flexible shaft made from whale baleen), and gum elastic bougies. After some initial enthusiasm, caustic bougies, originally proposed in 1803 by Erasmus Darwin,[16] grandfather of Charles Darwin, were rapidly abandoned because of their propensity to cause inflammation and worsen a stricture. Although bouginage often resulted in days, if not weeks, of relief from dysphagia, the risk was high. Perforation occurred with relative frequency, to the extent that Trousseau[17] remarked that "sooner or later all cases of stricture of the oesophagus die of the bougie."

Dissatisfaction with bougies led to the development of mechanical devices that appeared (and were) dangerous. Fletcher[18] designed an instrument with blades at its tip that could be deployed to lacerate an esophageal stricture after the device had been positioned across the stricture. Other bladed devices for internal esophagotomy were subsequently introduced by Maisonneuve[19] in 1861 and used by Lannelongue[20] in 1868. This method was not very satisfactory in opening strictures and resulted in a high mortality rate.[21,22] Lerche[23] developed an improved device for use during esophagoscopy (Figure 2.1) and reported good results in a few patients in 1910, but the technique failed to generate a following.

Dilators were continuously modified to improve outcomes and lessen the risk of perforation. In 1915, Hertz[24] introduced a flexible

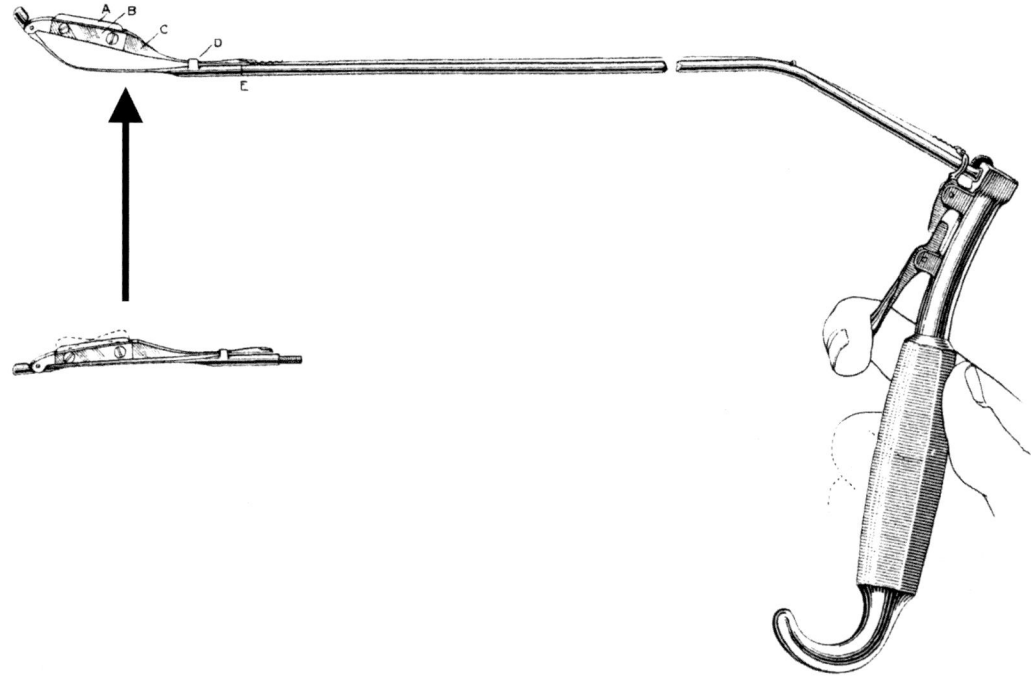

Figure 2.1. This endoluminal device introduced by Lerche in 1910 was designed to be inserted through a rigid esophagoscope with the blade in a holder in a relaxed (straightened) orientation. Pulling on the trigger flexed the blade holder, extending the blade into the esophageal lumen to enable cutting of a short stricture. (Reprinted from Lerche,[23] with permission from the American College of Surgeons.)

weighted rubber bougie, the forerunner of the Maloney dilator, which substantially reduced the risk of perforation. Use of a swallowed thread with a weight attached at the distal end helped avoid errant passage of bougies when used as a guide over which the bougie was passed[25,26] or when attached to either end of a bougie and brought out the mouth and a gastric stoma (Figure 2.2).[27,28] This combination of the string-guided technique and the tapered bougie eventually led to the development of guidewire-aided techniques including the olive (Eder-Puestow) system in the 1950s.[29] These subsequently gave way to the hollow-core polyvinyl bougie (Savary-Gilliard and American Endoscopy) systems that originally became popular in the 1980s.[30] Because of continued concern over the risks associated with forceful dilation of benign strictures, particularly because of the shear forces generated within the esophagus, pneumatic dilators were adopted for use for treating peptic strictures. Their theoretical advantage was the controlled delivery of radial forces that would reduce the risk of esophageal injury. Recent randomized studies have demonstrated that both systems have similar efficacy and are equally safe (Figure 2.3).[31,32]

Esophageal Stents

Stents were first introduced in the management of peptic esophageal stricture in France in the mid-19th century.[17,33] Until the late 19th century, the only effective treatment for an obstructing esophageal stricture was passage of a gum elastic tube that spanned the stricture and protruded through the mouth. The protruding end was so uncomfortable that most patients coughed it out or removed it to relieve the distress.[34] Symonds[35] tailored the tube by cutting off the protruding end of the tube, retaining it in position through use of a loop of silk passed around the patient's ear. This was a popular device for maintaining luminal patency after dilation that probably worked by inducing pressure necrosis.[35]

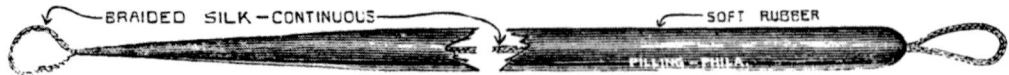

Figure 2.2. Early dilators, such as this string-guided bougie designed by Tucker, were guided by a string that was passed down the mouth, through the esophageal stricture, and out a gastrostomy. The string was left in place between dilations. (Reprinted from Tucker,[28] with permission from Annals Publishing Company.)

The development of endoscopy led to the application of stent technology primarily for malignant esophageal obstruction rather than peptic esophageal stricture, relegating the use of stents for benign esophageal disease to unusual and highly selected cases. Technical developments in stenting in the early 20th century included the use of guides and dilators, which directly led to the introduction of the Souttar tube in the 1920s. This spiral of silver wire was positioned using an introducer, which considerably increased the safety of stent placement.[36] This so-called pulsion-type stent was subsequently modified to include much softer versions made from rubber or silicone. Tapered introducers were adapted to traction-type stents that were drawn down into regions of obstruction through a temporary gastrotomy, including the Mousseau-Barbin and Celestin tubes.[37,38] The introduction of self-expanding

wire-mesh stents in the 1990s revolutionized the use of stents in esophageal obstruction (Figure 2.4). However, their tendency to create inflammation and fibrosis, despite the increasingly nonreactive nature of their component materials, makes them unsuitable for long-term use in peptic esophageal strictures except under unusual circumstances.

Palliative Surgical Therapy

Before endoscopy and radiography were able to delineate the cause of esophageal obstruction, there were few surgical options for its management, all of which were palliative. Gastrostomy was first performed by Sedillot[39] in 1849 as a means for providing nutrition. The first successful use of gastrostomy as an access for retrograde dilation was by von Bergmann in 1883.[40] Cervical esophagostomy was also used in cases of high-grade obstruction as means for expelling saliva but provided no other palliative benefits. Trendelenburg devised a long extension tube for the gastrostomy tube, into which the patient expelled masticated food directly from his mouth and propelled the food into the stomach by blowing into the tube.[41] This idea was subsequently modified so that a cervical esophagostomy tube connected to the gastrostomy tube transmitted swallowed food directly into the stomach via an extracorporeal route (Figure 2.5).[42] This concept was embraced for

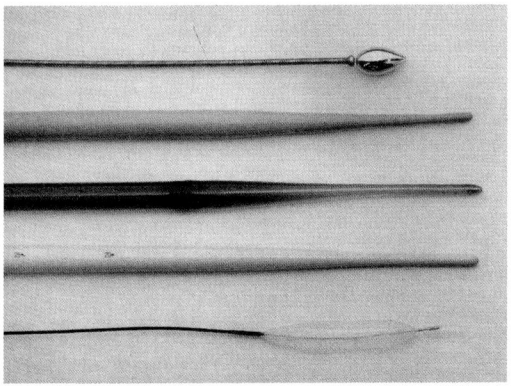

Figure 2.3. Four generations of esophageal dilators. At the top is the olive-tipped (Eder-Puestow) system and below it is a Maloney bougie. The latter dilators were originally filled with mercury to weight them, but now are filled with a tungsten gel. The third and fourth dilators from the top are elements of wire-guided systems, made of polyvinyl chloride. A pneumatic dilator that can be used through the endoscope is pictured at the bottom. (Reprinted from Ferguson M. Chest Surg Clin N Am 1994;4:679, copyright 1994, with permission from Elsevier.)

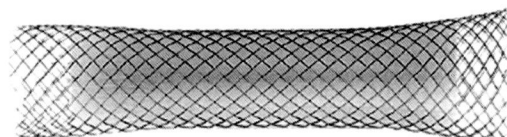

Figure 2.4. Nitinol self-expanding mesh stents are useful for temporary palliation of benign strictures, but the resultant surrounding tissue inflammation can lead to additional scarring if the stent is left in place too long.

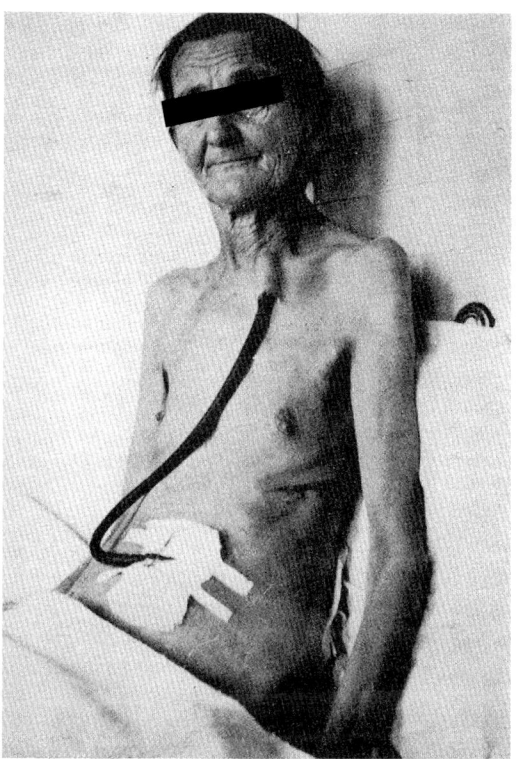

Figure 2.5. This patient underwent the first successful transthoracic esophagectomy for cancer, performed by Franz Torek in New York City in 1913. The patient's alimentary tract continuity was established with an external rubber tube, and reconstruction was never attempted. (Reprinted from Torek,[42] with permission from the American College of Surgeons.)

palliation of esophageal cancer by Akiyama and Hatano[43] and was subsequently introduced for management of failed anti-reflux surgery by Skinner and DeMeester.[44]

Early Surgical Therapy

The first operations performed at least in part for possible gastroesophageal reflux problems were for correction of hiatal hernias, usually giant paraesophageal hernias. Hedblom[11] stated that the first operation for a clinically diagnosed hiatal hernia was by Naumann in 1888, but the stomach could not be reduced into the abdomen and the patient died. By the time of Harrington's[10] report in 1928, successful surgery for hiatal hernia had been accomplished in

dozens of patients. The standard operation included hernia reduction, plication of the hernia orifice, suturing of the formerly herniated stomach to the abdominal wall to help prevent recurrent hernia, and paralysis of the diaphragm by phrenic nerve injury. Large series of operated patients were subsequently reported, although a careful distinction among posttraumatic, esophageal hiatal, and other diaphragmatic hernias was not always carefully observed.[45]

Bypass operations for peptic esophageal stricture were first successfully performed in the early 1900s. Skin tubes were initially constructed for this purpose, but surgeons quickly adopted jejunal interposition, colon interposition, and gastric pull-up operations to bridge the gap between the cervical esophagus and the abdominal gastrointestinal tract. In 1934, Ochsner and Owens[46] summarized the results of all esophageal bypass and reconstructive operations performed until that time for both malignant and benign obstruction. The reconstructive conduit was located in the antesternal or substernal plane, as reconstruction in the bed of the resected esophagus had not been successfully accomplished at that time. In summarizing results in 240 patients, the authors noted several striking features: the mortality of attempted reconstruction/bypass was 37%, the likelihood of completing the reconstruction was barely >50%, and only about 40% of patients were considered to have good functional results. They recommended that such surgery should be used only in cases of impermeable benign stricture. Subsequent experience with esophagectomy and bowel interposition yielded more favorable results, although complication and mortality rates were still high.[47,48]

These less-than-satisfactory results led to direct approaches to peptic esophageal strictures aimed at preservation of esophageal function rather than bypass or resection of the esophagus. Such approaches were made possible by the preoperative diagnosis of a benign stricture enabled by the development of endoscopy, and by the development of endotracheal positive pressure ventilation which permitted elective thoracic surgery. Esophagoplasty for peptic stricture was initially performed by opening the stricture longitudinally and then closing the defect transversely, which had the effect of widening the lumen in the region of the stricture.[49–51] This completely

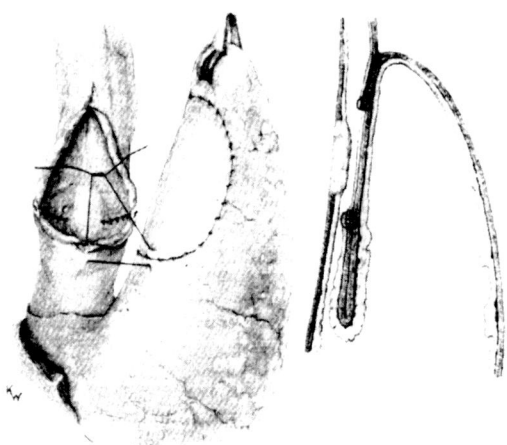

Figure 2.6. One method of treating a nondilatable stricture was to perform a strictureplasty as initially described by Thal in 1965. The stricture was opened lengthwise, partially closed horizontally, and the stomach was brought up and sewn over the open esophageal lumen. The illustrated version used a partial-thickness skin graft as an overlay patch on the gastric serosa to prevent acid erosion through this susceptible tissue, which was a frequent complication of the original version. (Reprinted with permission from Thal.[54])

destroyed the anti-reflux mechanism and created a small iatrogenic hiatal hernia, both of which usually dramatically worsened the patient's reflux problems. As an alternative technique, patch esophagoplasty was introduced as a substitute for closing the longitudinal esophageal defect transversely. Materials used experimentally and clinically for the patch included fascia, skin, dermal grafts, pedicled intercostal muscle, pericardium, diaphragm, and omentum.[52] The introduction of the fundic patch esophagoplasty by Thal et al.[53] simplified the operation and had the additional benefit of reinforcing the anti-reflux mechanism with a partial gastric wrap across the esophagogastric junction (Figure 2.6). Results of the operation were gratifying, with >80% of patients reporting good outcomes.[54,55]

Physiologic Surgical Therapy

Early recognition of the relationship between benign stricture of the esophagus and acid-peptic disease led to gastrectomy as a means for controlling production of acid and pepsin.[56] The

success of this procedure initiated interest in physiologic control of acid reflux as a means to treat peptic stricture, but ultimately as a method for preventing complications of acid reflux. Other operations were devised for managing recalcitrant peptic stricture that included resection of the gastroesophageal junction with primary anastomosis, antrectomy, and Roux-en-Y reconstruction.[57] Modifications of this with and without esophageal resection were subsequently used for recurrent stricture, failed anti-reflux surgery requiring reoperation, and management of alkaline reflux.[58-63]

From the late 1930s to the early 1950s, there was a growing impression that gastroesophageal reflux was related to a failure of the anti-reflux mechanism. Many physicians believed that failure of the anti-reflux mechanism was a result of a hiatus hernia. Allison[15] stated that "the symptoms are those of oesophagitis from the reflux of gastric contents into the oesophagus, due to incompetence of the gastro-oesophageal junction. The cause of the incompetence is a sliding hernia of the stomach through the oesophageal hiatus of the diaphragm into the posterior mediastinum." However, persistent reflux after correction of hiatal hernias simply consisting of plication of the esophageal hiatus, such as the Allison repair, suggested that mechanisms other than hiatal hernia were involved in the pathophysiology of acid reflux disease.[15,64] Barrett[65] was among the first to point out that reconstituting the acute angle at the esophagogastric junction was an important element in correcting reflux problems, as was exposure of a length of esophagus to intraabdominal pressure. Although these mechanisms otherwise were poorly understood in the early 1950s, two eminent surgeons soon were to permanently alter the course of esophageal surgery.

In the 1930s surgery for cryptogenic regurgitation sometimes consisted of resection of the cardia and invagination of the subsequent esophagogastrostomy into folds of the stomach. Good results with this operation led Nissen[66] in 1955 to use the technique of wrapping the stomach around the esophagus, termed fundoplication, as an element of hiatal hernia repair in two patients with severe reflux symptoms (Figure 2.7). Favorable results of this 360-degree wrap in >120 patients subsequently were described in 1961, with success reported in 90–95% of patients.[67] The ability to perform this

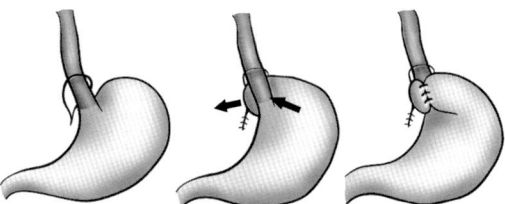

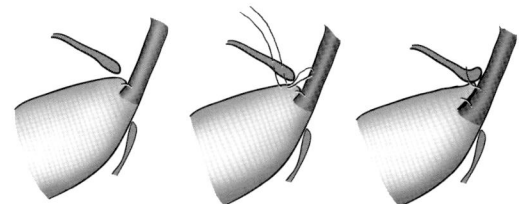

Figure 2.7. The total (Nissen) fundoplication is a 360-degree wrap of gastric fundus around the distal esophagus. After complete distal esophageal and proximal gastric mobilization (including division of the proximal short gastric vessels; left panel), the crura are approximated to close the hiatus to a normal caliber (center panel). The proximal fundus is wrapped posteriorly around the esophagus and a portion of the fundus is brought anterior to the esophagus. The two edges are sutured together to create the fundoplication over a large bougie to calibrate the size of the wrap (right panel).

Figure 2.8. The Belsey Mark IV fundoplication is performed via a thoracic approach. After esophagogastric mobilization, the stomach is sutured to the esophagus 1 cm above the esophagogastric junction encompassing 270 degrees of esophageal circumference (left panel). The second row of sutures is passed first through the diaphragm, then the stomach, and finally the esophagus, and is brought back through those tissues in reverse order in a U-stitch fashion (center panel). When these sutures are tied, the esophagogastric junction and partial wrap superior to it are anchored below the diaphragm (right panel). Crural repair follows completion of the wrap.

operation through abdominal or thoracic incisions, and the intuitive appeal of a total fundoplication, led to its rapid acceptance among surgeons for use in patients with severe gastroesophageal reflux symptoms regardless of whether a hiatal hernia was present.

Beginning in 1949 Belsey began to investigate methods of repairing hiatal hernias and correcting gastroesophageal reflux symptoms. The fourth iteration of his operation, the Belsey Mark IV, consisted of a partial (270-degree) fundoplication performed with two rows of sutures, the latter of which was also brought through the diaphragm to anchor the stomach and the fundoplication within the abdomen (Figure 2.8). This operation was introduced in 1955, and results in >600 patients were reported in 1967 after a median follow-up of almost 5 years.[68] Anatomic correction and symptomatic success were noted in 85% of patients. This represented a milestone in the reporting of surgical treatments, in which long-term and complete follow-up as well as objective evaluation of symptoms were used to assess the outcomes of a new operation. Because of its complexity and the perceived need to perform the procedure exclusively through a thoracotomy incision, the Belsey Mark IV operation never gained quite the following that the total (Nissen) fundoplication did.

At about the same time that Nissen and Belsey were developing their fundoplication operations in Europe, Hill was devising a third type of anti-reflux procedure in the United

States. The posterior gastropexy operation was introduced in 1960, and included a partial fundoplication (180-degree) and a unique technique for anchoring the wrap within the abdomen. The fundoplication was created by using figure-of-8 sutures passed first through the posteromedial region of the gastroesophageal junction, second through the arcuate ligament (the superior portion of the aortic hiatus in the diaphragm), third through the anterior portion of the cardia, and finally through the arcuate ligament again (Figure 2.9). As each suture was tied, the pressure in the lower esophageal sphincter was monitored

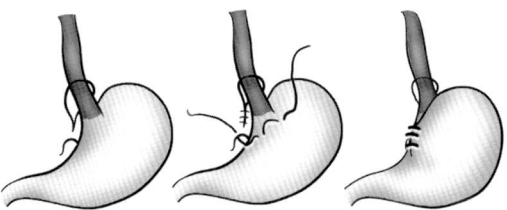

Figure 2.9. The Hill repair is a partial fundoplication that can be performed through a thoracic or abdominal approach. After crural closure and distal esophageal/proximal gastric mobilization (left panel), the median arcuate ligament overlying the aorta is dissected. A heavy suture is placed through the anterior and posterior gastric remnants of the phrenoesophageal ligament and through the median arcuate ligament (center panel). Three similar sutures are placed, one superior and two inferior, to complete the wrap (right panel). The sutures are tied under tension guided by intraoperative manometry.

intraoperatively with manometry to achieve a calibrated sphincter pressure.[69,70] Long-term results in procedures performed by Hill and his protégés were favorable, with good and excellent results in 85–90% of patients.[71] However, the need for intraoperative monitoring of lower esophageal sphincter pressure and the lack of familiarity with the arcuate ligament dissuaded most surgeons from adding this technique to their surgical armamentarium.

Almost simultaneous with the introduction of fundoplication operations, surgical techniques were developed to deal with the problem known as the shortened esophagus. The frequency of its occurrence, and even whether there was such an entity, were (and remain) hotly debated topics. As an example, during the discussion of treatment of short esophagus at the American Surgical Association in 1956, several prominent surgeons all but denied the existence of esophageal shortening.[72] Early references to congenitally shortened esophagus, of which most were either type I (sliding) hiatal hernias without peptic stricture or represented Barrett's changes, fomented confusion in the early days of anti-reflux surgery. In the decades before the introduction of effective acid suppression therapy there no doubt was a higher frequency of severe esophagitis and peptic stricture than is evident currently. Collagen deposited as part of these conditions underwent cicatricial contraction, shortening the esophagus and drawing the cardia into the mediastinum.

Conservative management of the shortened esophagus almost always failed, and, during the 1940s and 1950s, esophageal resection was the mainstay of therapy. In response to this, in 1956 Collis[73] introduced an operation that did "not disorganize the patient's digestive apparatus too much and which [was] easily tolerated by even a frail and aged person." He extended the esophageal tube using the lesser curvature of the stomach, which enabled him to create an acute angle between the gastric fundus and the neoesophagus, a necessary condition of anti-reflux surgery, in his opinion (Figure 2.10). Collis[74] was not enthusiastic about the long-term results of the operation, because reflux symptoms were only partially controlled and 30% of patients had unsatisfactory outcomes. However, realizing the potential of this technique for extending the utility of standard fun-

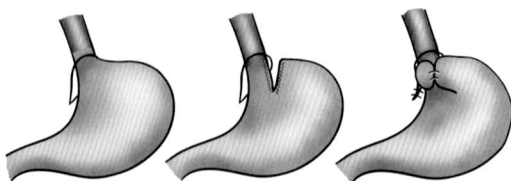

Figure 2.10. A lengthening gastroplasty originally described by Collis is useful when combined with fundoplication for managing the short esophagus. In patients with shortening and a hiatal hernia (left panel) the esophagus and stomach are mobilized. If an adequate length of intraabdominal esophagus cannot be achieved, a lengthening procedure is performed. After inserting a large bougie across the esophagogastric junction, a linear cutting stapler is fired parallel to the lesser gastric curvature alongside the bougie to extend the esophageal tube (center panel). The fundus is then wrapped around this neoesophagus to establish an intraabdominal fundoplication (right panel).

doplication operations, Pearson[75] was the first to combine the Collis gastroplasty with the Belsey Mark IV technique for management of peptic stricture with esophageal shortening. His group subsequently extended the indications for use of this technique to recurrent hiatal hernia, severe esophagitis without stricture, and reflux problems associated with motor disorders.[76] Having experienced less-than-satisfactory outcomes using the Collis-Belsey technique, Orringer and Sloan[77] introduced the Collis-Nissen procedure in 1978. Use of an uncut gastroplasty combined with fundoplication for complicated reflux problems was subsequently reported.[78–80] The conventional and uncut gastroplasties combined with fundoplication are now standard elements of the armamentarium of many surgeons for managing problems of reflux and large hiatal hernia.

Minimally invasive surgical techniques, primarily laparoscopic methods, were introduced for anti-reflux procedures in 1991.[81,82] These techniques rapidly captured the imagination of surgeons and the attention of the public. Within a short time the vast majority of first-time fundoplication procedures were being performed laparoscopically. The low rate of complications and long-term physiologic and quality-of-life outcomes that approach those of open fundoplication surgery have confirmed the initial enthusiastic response to these operations.[83–88] Costs to society are reduced because of the rapid postsurgical recovery experienced by these patients.[89,90] The success has been so impressive that the algorithm of GERD management has changed in the minds of some physicians. Many more patients now undergo laparoscopic fundoplication than would previously have qualified for open fundoplication; in North America and Europe, there has been at least a threefold increase in the frequency of fundoplication operations.[91–93]

Pharmacologic Therapy

Because neither the anatomic nor the chemical source of dyspepsia was determined until the late 19th century, therapy before that time was empiric and often quite imaginative. Recommendations included sedum (stonecrop), chewing green tea, and magnesia. For centuries, relief from dyspepsia was provided by chalk, charcoal, and "slop" diets.[94] At the turn of the 20th century, proprietary medicines were popular, and were offered not only as cures for heartburn but also for impotence and alopecia.[94] Therapy at that time centered on avoidance of acidic foods, otherwise bland diets free of capsaicin, milk, antacids, and elevation of the head of the bed. In addition to their acid-neutralizing effects, antacids were subsequently demonstrated to increase lower esophageal sphincter pressure and decrease gastroesophageal reflux.[95,96] Alginic acid, which reacts with saliva to form a viscous coating that protects the esophagus (and stomach) was shown to have effects on reflux symptoms similar to those of antacids.[97]

The first major medical therapeutic breakthrough came in the 1970s with the identification of two classes of histamine receptors, H_1 and H_2. After testing >700 histamine derivatives, Black et al.[98] identified the first H_2 receptor antagonist, burimamide, in 1972. Although intravenous administration led to inhibition of pentagastrin-stimulated acid secretion in humans, it was not active orally. The second antagonist that was developed, metiamide, was tenfold more potent but was found to cause agranulocytosis and was not suitable for clinical use. The introduction of cimetidine for clinical use led to the eventual introduction of a family of H_2 receptor antagonists (cimetidine, ranitidine, famotidine, nizatidine) available in

both oral and parenteral forms. These compounds reduced basal and stimulated acid production but had no effect on lower esophageal sphincter pressure, esophageal peristalsis, or gastric emptying. They consistently reduced symptoms of heartburn and permitted reduced use of antacids, but significant healing of esophagitis did not reliably occur.[99–101] The development of hyperplasia of gastrin-producing cells during chronic administration of H_2 receptor antagonists led to initial concerns about the possibility of inducing gastric cancer, but more than two decades of experience has allayed these concerns.[102] The H_2 receptor antagonists are now available as nonprescription medications.

By the late 1970s it was recognized that low-amplitude lower esophageal sphincter resting pressure, poor distal esophageal motility, and transient relaxations of the lower esophageal sphincter contributed to reflux frequency and severity. This stimulated interest in the use of prokinetic agents in the management of GERD. Several classes of drugs were assessed, including the dopamine antagonists metoclopramide and domperidone, the acetylcholine receptor agonist bethanechol, the serotonin-4 (5-HT_4) receptor agonist cisapride, and the motilin agonist erythromycin. Metoclopramide was shown to be effective in reducing symptoms of acid reflux by increasing lower esophageal sphincter pressure and by decreasing gastric emptying time. However, no effect on healing of esophagitis was evident.[103,104] Bethanechol was demonstrated to increase resting lower esophageal sphincter pressure resulting in a decrease in acid reflux, and improve esophageal clearance. Some effect on esophageal healing was also identified.[105–108] Overall, these agents produced modest improvement in esophageal motility and gastric emptying, and were similar in efficacy to antacids in relieving reflux symptoms. However, side effects produced by most drugs prevented their widespread acceptance. There were great expectations for cisapride, which demonstrated efficacy similar to H_2 receptor antagonists in relieving reflux symptoms and in healing mild-to-moderate esophagitis.[109–111] Unfortunately, potentially fatal QT interval prolongation and ventricular dysrhythmias caused by cisapride, first reported publicly in 1995, led to its withdrawal from the United States market in 2000.[112] Currently there are no prokinetic agents that are proven effective in managing GERD symptoms.[113]

Intracellular mechanisms of acid production were targeted in the 1980s as therapy for a variety of acid-peptic diseases. Unique to oxyntic cells is gastric hydrogen/potassium adenosine triphosphatase (H^+/K^+-exchanging ATPase), the gastric proton pump that catalyzes the exchange of K^+ for H^+ at the canalicular membrane. A compound, omeprazole, was identified that inhibited (H^+, K^+) ATPase, and was found to inhibit basal and pentagastrin-stimulated acid secretion in humans.[114] The new class of proton pump inhibitors (PPIs) was the most potent inhibitor of gastric acid secretion ever identified. Five PPIs are now labeled by the Food and Drug Administration (FDA): omeprazole, esomeprazole, lansoprazole, rabeprazole, and pantoprazole. The drugs have been associated with relatively few side effects, and are much more effective in controlling symptoms of GERD and in healing esophagitis than any other class of drugs.[115–119] Proton pump inhibitors now are the mainstay of medical therapy for severe GERD.

Endoscopic Therapy

A variety of factors have stimulated advances in endoscopic therapy for GERD. Pharmacologic management lacks complete efficacy, is costly in the long-term, and is associated with considerable compliance issues. In addition, drug therapy currently focuses on suppression of gastric acid production, despite the fact that a number of other substances, including bile constituents, pancreatic enzymes, and pepsin, have been implicated in the pathogenesis of GERD. Finally, control of symptoms is not synonymous with control of reflux, leading to ongoing risks of complications of GERD including the development of Barrett esophagus.

These factors have promoted new investigations into how the mechanical barrier to reflux at the lower esophageal sphincter can be manipulated to minimize GERD. Endoscopic therapies now include sewing/stapling techniques, radiofrequency thermal therapy, and injection/implantable therapies. These treatments are relatively new, and little information exists regarding their short-term utility compared with medical or standard surgical therapy, the long-term outcomes of such therapy, and their cost-effectiveness.

Sewing/stapling techniques were developed beginning in the mid-1980s. Two devices are capable of placing stitches in 3 to 4 locations in a circular or longitudinal pattern beginning 1 cm below the Z line. The purported effect is to plicate the gastroesophageal junction, enhancing the anti-reflux mechanism. The Bard EndoCinch (Bard Endoscopic Technologies, Billerica, MA) endoluminal plication system, which is approved by the FDA, enables the endoscopist to place figure-of-8 sutures, each gathering 1–1.5 cm of tissue. A similar device, the Wilson-Cook Endoscopic Suturing Device (Wilson-Cook Medical, Winston-Salem, NC), enables the placement of mattress sutures without removal of the endoscope, a substantial time savings.[120] A third device, the full-thickness endoscopic plication system (NDO Surgical, Mansfield, MA), enables placement of plicating staples that fold the gastric fundus onto the esophagus in a manner analogous to a fundoplication.

Short-term follow-up of the Endocinch device demonstrated little risk with the procedure, and heart burn symptoms, esophageal acid exposure, and requirements for acid suppression therapy were all improved. However, lower esophageal sphincter length and pressure were not reliably increased by the procedure. Intermediate-term follow-up demonstrated continued improvement in symptoms in many patients, although almost half of the patients either were on their original doses of acid suppression medications or had undergone anti-reflux surgery.[121] Early results with the Endoscopic Suturing Device have been similar, with improvement in basal tone in the lower esophageal sphincter and a decrease in the frequency of transient relaxations of the lower sphincter. However, only modest reductions in gastroesophageal reflux were reported.[120,122] Staple plication of the esophagogastric junction is the simplest of the three techniques and has produced similarly modest results. Reflux symptoms and the need for acid-suppression medications were reduced, but the percentage of patients in whom normalization of esophageal acid exposure occurred was only 30%.[123] Fortunately, it seems that the endoscopic suturing/stapling techniques do not interfere with the performance or outcomes of subsequent fundoplication surgery.[124]

The FDA-approved Stretta System (Curon Medical, Inc., Sunnyvale, CA) consists of a catheter containing four radially oriented extendable electrodes and a control module that generates individually temperature-controlled radiofrequency energy to each of the electrodes. The endoscopic application of radiofrequency energy to generate heat in the region of the lower esophageal sphincter results in contraction of collagen molecules and collagen remodeling over time. Application of energy is performed at 0.5-cm intervals over a distance of 2.5 cm beginning 1 cm above the Z line. The catheter is rotated 45 degrees and energy is reapplied once at each level in the esophagus, yielding a total of 8 treatment spots, whereas two 30-degree rotations provide 12 sites treated at each level in the stomach. The mechanism of action seems to be related to an increase in resting tone and a decrease in the incidence of transient relaxations of the lower sphincter. Early clinical reports indicated that the Stretta procedure decreased esophageal acid exposure, increased lower sphincter pressure, and improved quality of life. Important complications were rarely seen. However, at least 30% of patients continued to require PPIs, and some patients subsequently underwent fundoplication surgery.[125–127]

Implantation therapy for GERD has been explored for more than two decades. Early experience with injection of substances for management of vocal cord dysfunction and urinary incontinence provided evidence that injection of the proper materials was efficacious and well tolerated. Clinical observations that mild stricture formation from gastroesophageal reflux was associated with a reduction in esophageal acid exposure encouraged the use of injectable implantation materials to treat GERD. Requirements for bulking agents include: chemically inert, noncarcinogenic, hypoallergenic, nonimmunogenic, capable of resisting mechanical strain, capable of being sterilized, low viscosity (capable of being injected through a small needle), nonbiodegradable, and persistence at the site of injection. Prior animal and human studies using collagen, Teflon paste, and hylan gel demonstrated that these substances failed to meet the necessary requirements for long-term use in humans, but identified favorable short-term outcomes.[128]

One injectable material has been FDA approved: Enteryx (Enteric Technologies, Foster City, CA) is an injectable solution of 8% ethylene vinyl alcohol copolymer dissolved in dimethyl sulfoxide, the latter of which diffuses away after injection, leaving the precipitated copolymer as a spongy solid in the wall of the gastroesophageal junction. In 2004 two other materials were being clinically tested, including Plexiglas (polymethylmethacrylate) spheres and the Gatekeeper Reflux Repair System (Medtronic, Minneapolis, MN) for injection of a polyacrylonitrile-based hydrogel (Hypan). Early clinical results from studies of these materials indicated that manometric characteristics of the lower sphincter were unchanged but suggested that the incidence of transient relaxation of the sphincter was reduced. Distal esophageal acid exposure was reduced and reflux symptoms were improved, but a substantial percentage of patients continued to require acid suppression therapy.[129–132]

Overall, endoscopic therapies have yet to replace either medical or surgical treatment of GERD. Based on the failure rate of endoscopic therapy experienced thus far in clinical trials, cost-effectiveness analyses suggest that acid suppression therapy is still the most economical treatment option.[133] Although new algorithms are being developed for GERD therapy that incorporate endoscopic treatments for selected patients, additional clinical experience gained in controlled trials is necessary before the role of endoscopic therapies is realized. To this end, a sham-controlled study of Stretta has recently been completed and a similar study of Enteryx injection is planned.[134]

References

1. Beaumont W. The Physiology of Digestion: Experiments on the Gastric Juice. 2nd ed. Burlington, VT: Chauncey Goodrich; 1847:69–94.
2. Tileston W. Peptic ulcer of the oesophagus. Am J Med Sci 1906;132:240–265.
3. Quincke H. Ulcus oesophagi ex digestione. Dtsch Archiv Klin Med 1879;24:72–79.
4. Allbutt TC. On auscultation of the oesophagus. Br Med J 1875;2:420.
5. Jackson C. Peptic ulcer of the esophagus. JAMA 1929; 92:369–372.

6. Lyall A. Chronic peptic ulcer of the oesophagus: a report of eight cases. Br J Surg 1936–1937;24:534–547.

7. Ferguson DJ, Sanchez-Palomera E, Sako Y, et al. Studies on experimental esophagitis. Surgery 1950;28: 1022–1039.

8. Bowditch HI. A treatise on diaphragmatic hernia. Buffalo Med J Monthly Rev 1853;9:65–94.

9. Griffin HZ. The diagnosis of diaphragmatic hernia. Ann Surg 1912;55:388–397.

10. Harrington SW. Diaphragmatic hernia. Arch Surg 1928;16:386–415.

11. Hedblom C. Diaphragmatic hernia. A study of three hundred and seventy-eight cases in which operation was performed. JAMA 1925;85:947–953.

12. Dick RCS, Hurst A. Chronic peptic ulcer of the oesophagus and its association with congenitally short oesophagus and diaphragmatic hernia. Q J Med 1942;35:105–120.

13. Allison PR. Peptic ulcer of the esophagus. J Thorac Surg 1946;15:308–317.

14. Allison PR. Peptic ulcer of the oesophagus. Thorax 1948; 3:20–42.

15. Allison PR. Reflux esophagitis, sliding hiatal hernia, and the anatomy of repair. Surg Gynecol Obstet 1951;92:419–431.

16. Darwin E. Zoonomia; or, the Laws of Organic Life. Part 2. Boston: Thomas and Andrews; 1803:102–103.

17. Trousseau A. Du catheterisme dans le traitement de la dysphagie causee par un retrecissement simple de l'oesophage. Mem Acad R Med 1847;13:600–610.

18. Fletcher R. Medico-Chirurgical Notes and Illustrations. Part I. London: Longman, Ress, Orme, Brown; 1831.

19. Maisonneuve JG. Clinique Chirurgicale. Vol 2. Paris: Savy; 1863–1864:409–416.

20. Lannelongue. Observations avec quelques considerations pour servir a l'histoire de l'oesophagotomie interne. Mem Soc Chir Paris 1868;6:547–560.

21. Mackenzie M. Gastrostomy, oesophagostomy and internal oesophagotomy in the treatment of stricture of the oesophagus. Am J Med Sci 1883;85:420–438.

22. Gross SW. Gastrostomy, oesophagostomy, internal oesophagotomy, combined oesophagotomy, oesophagectomy and retrograde divulsion in the treatment of stricture of the oesophagus. Am J Med Sci 1884;88:58–69.

23. Lerche W. A contribution to the surgery of the oesophagus with report of five cases of cicatricial stricture treated by cutting through the oesophagoscope. Surg Gynecol Obstet 1910;11:345–361.

24. Hertz AF. Achalasia of the cardia. Q J Med 1915;8: 300–308.

25. Mixter SJ. Symposium on surgery of the esophagus: from the standpoint of the general surgeon. Trans Am Laryngol Assoc 1909;31:342–348.

26. Plummer HS. The value of a silk thread as a guide in esophageal technique. Surg Gynecol Obstet 1910;10: 519–523.

27. Dunham T. New instruments for the treatment of esophageal stricture. Ann Surg 1903;37:350–359.

28. Tucker G. Cicatricial stenosis of the esophagus with particular reference to treatment by continuous string retrograde bouginage with the author's bougie. Ann Otol Rhinol Laryngol 1924;33:1180–1223.

29. Puestow KL. Conservative treatment of stenosing diseases of the esophagus. Postgrad Med 1955;18:6–14.

30. Dumon J-F, Meric B, Sivak MV Jr, Fleischer D. A new method of esophageal dilation using Savary-Gilliard bougies. Gastrointest Endosc 1985;6:379–382.

31. Cox JG, Winter RK, Maslin SC, et al. Balloon or bougie dilatation of benign esophageal stricture? Dig Dis Sci 1994;39:776–781.

32. Scolapio JS, Pasha TM, Gostout CJ, et al. A randomized prospective study comparing rigid to balloon dilators for benign esophageal strictures and rings. Gastrointest Endosc 1999;50:13–17.

33. Blandin PF. Retrecissement de l'oesophage traite par dilation temporaire. J Med Chir Pract 1847;18:72–73.

34. Hurt R. The History of Cardiothoracic Surgery from Early Times. New York: The Parthenon Publishing Group; 1996:328.

35. Symonds CJ. A case of malignant stricture of the oesophagus. Trans Clin Soc 1885;18:155–158.

36. Souttar HS. A method of intubating the oesophagus for malignant stricture. Br Med J 1924;1:782–783.

37. Mousseau MM, Forestier JL, Barbin J, Hardy M. Place de l'intubation a demeure dans le traitement palliatif du cancer de l'oesophage. Arch Mal Appareil Digestif 1956;45:208–220.

38. Celestin LR. Permanent intubation in inoperable cancer of the oesophagus and cardia. Ann R Coll Surg Engl 1959;25:165–170.

39. Sedillot. Gaz Med Strasburg 1849;9:366; cited by Mackenzie M. Gastrostomy, oesophagostomy and internal oesophagotomy in the treatment of stricture of the oesophagus. Am J Med Sci 1883;85:420–438.

40. von Bergmann E. Uber operationen am schlundrohre. Dtsch Med Wochenschr 1883;9:605–609, 621–624.

41. Trendelenburg F. Uber einen fall von gastrotomie bei oesophagusstrictur. Arch Klin Chir 1878;22:227–234.

42. Torek F. The first successful case of resection of the thoracic portion of the oesophagus for carcinoma. Surg Gynecol Obstet 1913;16:614–617.

43. Akiyama H, Hatano S. Esophageal cancer: palliative treatment. Jpn J Thorac Surg 1968;21:391–396.

44. Skinner DB, DeMeester TR. Permanent extracorporeal esophagogastric tube for esophageal replacement. Ann Thorac Surg 1976;22:107–111.

45. Sweet RH. Experience with 500 cases of hiatus hernia. A statistical survey. J Thorac Cardiovasc Surg 1962;44: 145–152.

46. Ochsner A, Owens N. Anterothoracic oesophagoplasty for impermeable stricture of the oesophagus. Ann Surg 1934;100:1055–1076.

47. Merindino KA, Thomas GI. The jejunal interposition operation for substitution of the esophagogastric sphincter. Surgery 1958;44:1112–1115.

48. Holt CJ, Large AM. Surgical management of reflux esophagitis. Ann Surg 1961;153:555–562.

49. Sauerbruch F, O'Shaughnessy L. Thoracic Surgery. A Revised and Abridged Edition of Sauerbruch's Die Chirurgie der Brustorgane. London: Edward Arnold; 1937:322.

50. Hale HW Jr, Dapranas T. Reflux esophagitis. Am J Surg 1957;93:228–233.

51. Hayward J. The treatment of fibrous stricture of the oesophagus associated with hiatal hernia. Thorax 1961; 16:45–55.

52. Ferguson MK. Reconstructive Surgery of the Esophagus. Armonk, NY: Futura Publishing; 2002:58.
53. Thal AP, Hatafuku T, Kurtzman R. A new method for reconstruction of the esophagogastric junction. Surg Gynecol Obstet 1965;120:1225–1231.
54. Thal AP. A unified approach to surgical problems of the esophagogastric junction. Ann Surg 1968;168:542–550.
55. Hollenbeck JI, Woodward ER. Treatment of peptic esophageal stricture with combined fundic patch-fundoplication. Ann Surg 1975;182:472–477.
56. Wangensteen OH, Leven NL. Gastric resection for esophagitis and stricture of acid-peptic origin. Surg Gynecol Obstet 1949;88:560–570.
57. Ellis FH Jr, Andersen HA, Clagett OT. Treatment of short esophagus with stricture by esophagogastrectomy and antral excision. Ann Surg 1958;148:526–536.
58. Washer GF, Gear MW, Dowling BL, et al. Randomized prospective trial of Roux-en-Y duodenal diversion versus fundoplication for severe reflux esophagitis. Br J Surg 1984;71:181–184.
59. Washer GF, Gear MW, Dowling BL, et al. Duodenal diversion with vagotomy and antrectomy for severe or recurrent reflux oesophagitis and stricture: an alternative operation at the hiatus. Ann R Coll Surg Engl 1986; 68:222–226.
60. Salo JA, Ala-Kulju KV, Heikkinen LO, Kivilaakso EO. Treatment of severe peptic esophageal stricture with Roux-en-Y partial gastrectomy, vagotomy, and endoscopic dilation. A follow-up study. J Thorac Cardiovasc Surg 1991;101:649–653.
61. Fekete F, Pateron D. What is the place of antrectomy with Roux-en-Y in the treatment of reflux disease? Experience with 83 total duodenal diversions. World J Surg 1992;16:349–354.
62. Ellis FH Jr, Gibb SP. Vagotomy, antrectomy, and Roux-en-Y diversion for complex reoperative gastroesophageal reflux disease. Ann Surg 1994;220:536–543.
63. Deschamps C, Trastek VF, Allen MS, Pairolero PC, Johnson JO, Larson DR. Long-term results after reoperation for failed anti-reflux procedures. J Thorac Cardiovasc Surg 1997;113:545–551.
64. Allison PR. Hiatus hernia: a 20-year retrospective survey. Ann Surg 1973;178:273–276.
65. Barrett NR. Hiatus hernia. Br Med J 1960;2:247–252.
66. Nissen R. Eine einfache Operation zur Beeinflussung der Refluxoesophagitis. Schweiz Med Wochenschr 1956;86:590–592.
67. Nissen R. Gastropexy and "fundoplication" in surgical treatment of hiatal hernia. Am J Dig Dis 1961;6: 954–961.
68. Skinner DB, Belsey RHR. Surgical management of esophageal reflux and hiatus hernia. Long-term results with 1,030 patients. J Thorac Cardiovasc Surg 1967;53: 33–54.
69. Hill LD. An effective operation for hiatal hernia: an eight-year appraisal. Ann Surg 1967;166:681–692.
70. Hill LD. Surgery and gastroesophageal reflux. Gastroenterology 1972;63:183–185.
71. Low DE, Anderson RP, Ilves R, Ricciardelli E, Hill LD. Fifteen- to twenty-year results after the Hill anti-reflux operation. J Thorac Cardiovasc Surg 1989;98:444–450.
72. Burford TH, Lischer CE. Treatment of short esophageal hernia with esophagitis by Finney pyloroplasty. Ann Surg 1956;144:647–652.

73. Collis JL. An operation for hiatus hernia with short esophagus. J Thorac Surg 1957;34:768–778.
74. Collis JL. Gastroplasty. Thorax 1961;16:197–206.
75. Pearson FG, Langer B, Henderson RD. Gastroplasty and Belsey hiatus hernia repair. J Thorac Cardiovasc Surg 1971;61:50–63.
76. Pearson FG, Cooper JD, Nelems JM. Gastroplasty and fundoplication in the management of complex reflux problems. J Thorac Cardiovasc Surg 1978;76:665–672.
77. Orringer MB, Sloan H. Combined Collis-Nissen reconstruction of the esophagogastric junction. Ann Thorac Surg 1978;25:16–21.
78. Demos NJ, Smith N, Williams D. New gastroplasty for strictured short esophagus. NY State J Med 1975;75: 57–59.
79. Bingham JAW. Hiatus hernia repair combined with the construction of an anti-reflux valve in the stomach. Br J Surg 1977;64:460–465.
80. Evangelist FA, Taylor FH, Alford JD. The modified Collis-Nissen operation for control of gastroesophageal reflux. Ann Thorac Surg 1978;26:107–111.
81. Dallemagne B, Weerts JM, Jehaes C, et al. Laparoscopic Nissen fundoplication: preliminary report. Surg Laparosc Endosc 1991;1:138–143.
82. Geagea T. Laparoscopic Nissen's fundoplication: preliminary report on 10 cases. Surg Endosc 1991;5: 170–173.
83. Rantanen TK, Salo JA, Sipponen JT. Fatal and life-threatening complications in anti-reflux surgery: analysis of 5,502 operations. Br J Surg 1999;86:1573–1577.
84. Bais JE, Bartelsman JF, Bonjer HJ, et al. Laparoscopic or conventional Nissen fundoplication for gastro-oesophageal reflux disease: randomised clinical trial. The Netherlands anti-reflux Surgery Study Group. Lancet 2000;355:170–174.
85. Heikkinen TJ, Haukipuro K, Sorasto A, et al. Short-term symptomatic outcome and quality of life after laparoscopic versus open Nissen fundoplication: a prospective randomized trial. Int J Surg Invest 2000;2: 33–39.
86. Carlson MA, Frantzides CT. Complications and results of primary minimally invasive anti-reflux procedures: a review of 10,735 reported cases. J Am Coll Surg 2001; 193:428–439.
87. Chrysos E, Tsiaoussis J, Athanasakis E, et al. Laparoscopic vs open approach for Nissen fundoplication. A comparative study. Surg Endosc 2002;16:1679–1684.
88. Nilsson G, Larsson S, Johnsson F. Randomized clinical trial of laparoscopic versus open fundoplication: evaluation of psychological well-being and changes in everyday life from a patient perspective. Scand J Gastroenterol 2002;37:385–391.
89. Blomqvist AM, Lonroth H, Dalenback J, Lundell L. Laparoscopic of open fundoplication? A complete cost analysis. Surg Endosc 1998;12:1209–1212.
90. Heikkinen TJ, Haukipuro K, Koivukangas P, et al. Comparison of costs between laparoscopic and open Nissen fundoplication: a prospective randomized study with a 3-month followup. J Am Coll Surg 1999;188:368–376.
91. McMahon RL, Mercer CD. National trends in gastroesophageal reflux surgery. Can J Surg 2000;43:48–52.
92. Sandbu R, Haglund U, Arvidsson D, Hallgren T. Anti-reflux surgery in Sweden, 1987–1997: a decade of change. Scand J Gastroenterol 2000;35:345–348.

93. Finlayson SR, Laycock WS, Birkmeyer JD. National trends in utilization and outcomes of anti-reflux surgery. Surg Endosc 2003;17:864–867.

94. Modlin IM, Kidd M, Lye KD. Historical perspectives on the treatment of gastroesophageal reflux disease. Gastrointest Endosc Clin N Am 2003;13:19–55.

95. Higgs RH, Smythe RD, Castell DO. Gastric alkalinization: effect on lower esophageal sphincter pressure and serum gastrin. N Engl J Med 1974;291:486–490.

96. Malmud LS, Fisher RS. Quantitation of gastroesophageal reflux before and after therapy using the gastroesophageal scintiscan. South Med J 1978; 71(suppl 1):10–15.

97. Graham DY, Lanza F, Dorsch ER. Symptomatic reflux esophagitis: a double-blind controlled comparison of antacids and alginate. Curr Ther Res 1977;22:653–658.

98. Black JW, Duncan WAM, Durant CJ, et al. Definition and antagonism of histamine H2-receptors. Nature 1972;236:385–390.

99. Behar J, Brand DL, Brown FC, et al. Cimetidine in the treatment of symptomatic gastroesophageal reflux. A double blind controlled trial. Gastroenterology 1978; 74:441–447.

100. Wesdorp E, Bartelsman J, Pape K, et al. Oral cimetidine in reflux esophagitis: a randomized controlled trial. Gastroenterology 1978;74:821–824.

101. Fiasse R, Hanin C, Lepot A, et al. Controlled trial of cimetidine in reflux esophagitis. Dig Dis Sci 1980;25: 750–755.

102. Colin-Jones DG, Langman MJ, Lawson DH, et al. Post-cimetidine surveillance for up to ten years: incidence of carcinoma of the stomach and esophagus. Q J Med 1991;78:13–19.

103. McCallum RW, Kline MM, Curry N, Sturdevant RAL. Comparative effects of metoclopramide and bethanechol on lower esophageal sphincter pressure in reflux patients. Gastroenterology 1975;68:1114–1118.

104. McCallum RW, Fink SM, Winnan J, Avella J, Callachan C. Metoclopramide in gastroesophageal reflux disease: rationale for use and results of a double-blind trial. Am J Gastroenterol 1984;79:165–172.

105. Farrell RK, Roling GT, Castell DO. Stimulation of the incompetent lower esophageal sphincter: a possible advance in therapy of heartburn. Am J Dig Dis 1973;18: 646–650.

106. Farrell RL, Roling GT, Castell DO. Cholinergic therapy of chronic heartburn. Ann Intern Med 1974;80: 573–576.

107. Miller WN, Ganeshappa KP, Dodds WJ, Hogan WJ, Barresas RF, Arndorfer RC. Effect of bethanechol on gastroesophageal reflux. Am J Dig Dis 1977;22:230–234.

108. Thanik KD, Chey WY, Shah AN, Gutierrez JG. Reflux esophagitis: effect of oral bethanechol on symptoms and endoscopic findings. Ann Intern Med 1980;93: 805–808.

109. Ramirez B, Richter JE. Review article: promotility drugs in the treatment of gastroesophageal reflux disease. Aliment Pharmacol Ther 1993;7:5–20.

110. Barone JA, Jessen LM, Colaizzi JL, Bierman RH. Cisapride: a gastrointestinal prokinetic drug. Ann Pharmacother 1994;28:488–500.

111. Pouderoux P, Kahrilas PJ. A comparative study of cisapride and ranitidine at controlling oesophageal acid exposure in erosive oesophagitis. Aliment Pharmacol Ther 1995;9:661–666.

112. Wysowski DK, Corken A, Gallo-Torres H, et al. Post-marketing reports of QT prolongation and ventricular arrhythmia in association with cisapride and Food and Drug Administration regulatory actions. Am J Gastroenterol 2001;96:1698–1703.

113. van Pinxteren B, Numans ME, Bonis PA, Lau J. Short-term treatment with proton pump inhibitors, H2-receptor antagonists and prokinetics for gastro-esophageal reflux disease symptoms and endoscopy negative reflux disease. Cochrane Database Syst Rev 2001;(4):CD002095.

114. Lind T, Cederberg C, Ekenved G, et al. Effect of omeprazole—a gastric proton pump inhibitor—on pentagastrin stimulated acid secretion in man. Gut 1983;24: 270–276.

115. Havelund T, Laursen LS, Skoubo-Kristensen E, et al. Omeprazole and ranitidine in the treatment of reflux esophagitis: a blind comparative trial. Br Med J 1988; 296:89–92.

116. Jansen JB, Van Oene JC. Standard-dose lansoprazole is more effective than high-dose ranitidine in achieving endoscopic healing and symptom relief in patients with moderately severe reflux esophagitis. The Dutch Lansoprazole Study Group. Aliment Pharmacol Ther 1999;13:1611–1620.

117. Farley A, Wruble LD, Humphries TJ. Rabeprazole versus ranitidine for the treatment of erosive gastroesophageal reflux disease: a double-blind, randomized clinical trial. Rabeprazole Study Group. Am J Gastroenterol 2000;95:1894–1899.

118. van Zyl JH, de K Grundling H, van Rensburg CJ, et al. Efficacy and tolerability of 20 mg pantoprazole versus 300 mg ranitidine in patients with mild reflux-oesophagitis: a randomized double-blind, parallel, and multicentre study. Eur J Gastroenterol Hepatol 2000;12: 197–202.

119. Kovacs TO, Wilcox CM, DeVault K, et al. Comparison of the efficacy of pantoprazole vs. nizatidine in the treatment of erosive esophagitis: a randomized, active-controlled double-blind study. Aliment Pharmcol Ther 2002;16:2043–2052.

120. Rosen M, Ponsky J. Wilson-Cook sewing device; the device, technique, and preclinical studies. Gastrointest Endosc Clin N Am 2003;13:103–108.

121. Rothstein RI, Filipi CJ. Endoscopic suturing for gastroesophageal reflux disease: clinical outcome with the Bard EndoCinch. Gastrointest Endosc Clin N Am 2003;13:89–101.

122. Tam WC, Holloway RH, Dent J, et al. Impact of endoscopic suturing of the gastroesophageal junction on lower esophageal sphincter function and gastroesophageal reflux in patients with reflux disease. Am J Gastroenterol 2004;99:195–202.

123. Pleskow D, Rothstein R, Lo S, et al. Endoscopic full-thickness plication for the treatment of GERD: a multicenter trial. Gastrointest Endosc 2004;59:163–171.

124. Velanovich V, Ben Menachem T. Laparoscopic Nissen fundoplication after failed endoscopic gastroplication. J Laparoendosc Adv Surg Tech A 2002;12:305–308.

125. Triadafilopoulos G, DiBaise JK, Nostrant TT, et al. The Stretta procedure for the treatment of GERD: 6 and 12 month follow-up of the U.S. open label trial. Gastrointest Endosc 2002;55:149–156.

126. Wolfsen HC, Richards WO. The Stretta procedure for the treatment of GERD: a registry of patients. J Laparoendosc Adv Surg Tech A 2002;12:395–402.

127. Richards WO, Houston HL, Torquati A, et al. Paradigm shift in the management of gastroesophageal reflux disease. Ann Surg 2003;237:638–649.

128. Lehman GA. The history and future of implantation therapy for gastroesophageal reflux disease. Gastrointest Endosc Clin N Am 2003;13:157–165.

129. Feretis C, Benakis P, Dimopoulos C, et al. Endoscopic implantation of Plexiglas (PMMA) microspheres for treatment of GERD. Gastrointest Endosc 2001;53: 423–426.

130. Fockens P. Gatekeeper™ reflux repair system: technique, pre-clinical, and clinical experience. Gastrointest Endosc Clin N Am 2003;13:179–189.

131. Johnson DA, Ganz R, Aisenberg J, et al. Endoscopic implantation of enteryx for treatment of GERD: 12-month results of a prospective, multicenter trial. Am J Gastroenterol 2003;98:1921–1930.

132. Louis H, Deviere J. Endoscopic implantation of Enteryx for the treatment of gastroesophageal reflux disease: technique, pre-clinical and clinical experience. Gastrointest Endosc Clin N Am 2003;13:191–200.

133. Harewood GC, Gostout CJ. Cost analysis of endoscopic anti-reflux procedures: endoluminal plication vs. radio-frequency coagulation vs. treatment with a proton pump inhibitor. Gastrointest Endosc 2003;58: 493–499.

134. DiBaise JK. And then there were three—endotherapy for gastroesophageal reflux disease. Am J Gastroenterol 2003;98:1909–1912.

3

Medical Management of GERD: Algorithms and Outcomes

David A. Johnson

Therapeutic efficacy of treatments for gastroesophageal reflux disease (GERD) has been measured using a variety of different endpoints. Across the surgical, endoscopic, and pharmacological treatment interventions for GERD, an attempt has been made to measure the therapeutic effect of these interventions by both objective and subjective means. This has included objective measures such as the effect a treatment has on esophageal sphincter pressure, intraesophageal acid exposure, and endoscopic esophagitis. Subjective measures of effect have included symptom response as assessed by questionnaires, symptom severity scales, physician assessment, and quality-of-life impact. Despite the innumerable studies reporting various treatment interventions for GERD, overall there is a general lack of use of standardized methodology that would allow comparison of the relative success achieved between the various therapies. Furthermore, there is a striking lack of use of validated instruments to accurately assess treatment effect in many of these studies. This review focuses on the questions that should be raised by clinicians in order for them to apply an evidence-based evaluation of the outcomes achieved in these GERD intervention trials.

Background

Gastroesophageal reflux disease is a multifaceted disease defined by consensus as chronic symptoms or mucosal damage produced by the abnormal reflux of gastric contents into the esophagus.[1] Heartburn and regurgitation are the primary associated symptoms of GERD that prompt most patients to seek some form of therapy. There is, however, at present an expanded compendium of associated "extraesophageal manifestations" of GERD including cough, wheezing, atypical chest pain, and hoarseness—among the growing list of associated pulmonary, otolaryngological presentations. Sleep disturbance attributed to GERD is another prevalent association that has also recently become apparent.[2,3]

There have been numerous clinical studies focusing on the patient response to various therapeutic interventions for GERD. Recently, reports on the results of interventions for GERD have also focused on which of the many available therapies might be preferable. Clearly, there are several factors that would weigh into the ultimate decision as to the best therapy in an individual patient with GERD. The clinical outcome would be one factor, but these results would also need to be tempered with the risk/benefit of each of the therapeutic management strategies. Before the question of treatment preference can be considered, a critical question emerges: By which criteria do we hold these therapies ultimately accountable? Is it the subjective assessment of the outcome of symptoms or rather should it be objective findings such as the results of an endoscopy, manometry, or pH monitoring? Furthermore, how can these outcomes be accurately compared across the options of surgical, endoscopic, and medical therapies?

It is difficult to assess the optimal therapy for GERD by measuring treatment outcomes seeking to compare the three therapeutic approaches to GERD intervention—surgical, medical, and endoscopic. The majority of these trials of therapy have had several issues that limit the extrapolation of the reported data. These include:

1. Lack of standardization of the inclusion/exclusion criteria
2. The therapeutic outcomes are not clearly defined "a priori"
3. Rarely are power calculations done to justify the study primary objectives
4. Rarely are validated measures used to assess the primary or secondary outcomes
5. Lack of an appropriate control/sham comparison group to provide comparison outcome with no active treatment intervention.

Additionally, for most of the surgical, medical, and endoscopic anti-reflux trials, variable efficacy endpoints have been targeted. These endpoints include:

1. Esophageal pH monitoring
2. Esophageal manometry
3. Endoscopic identification of esophagitis
4. Patient symptom response
5. Quality-of-life assessment
6. Quantification of medication usage

The purpose of this review is to discuss the effectiveness of the medical therapies for GERD. Although the focus here is on the medical interventions, this discussion is intended to help clinicians critically evaluate trials of surgical and endoscopic therapies for GERD as well.

Lifestyle/Diet Modifications

Traditionally, the cornerstone of the medical management of GERD consisted largely of efforts to modify the patient's lifestyle and diet. Specific lifestyle modifications included elevation of the head of the bed, restriction of alcohol and smoking, dietary therapy, weight loss, and avoidance of lying down soon after a meal, especially at night.[4] The primary reason for dietary modifications such as those noted above was related to the effect certain foods and meals in general had on the lower esophageal sphincter pressure (LESP) or the direct irritative effects of certain foods on the esophageal mucosa. Although it is clear that avoidance of offending foods may decrease sporadic GERD symptoms, there has been no controlled trial data to support that these specific lifestyle modifications are effective in patients with typical and more frequent GERD symptoms. Other lifestyle interventions such as sleeping with the left side down (compared with right side down, prone, or supine) have been shown to decrease esophageal acid exposure both in the postprandial and nocturnal sleeping periods.[5] This is likely the result of a decrease in transient lower esophageal sphincter relaxations (tLESRs).[6] The premise behind the recommendation of avoiding lying down within 3 hours of a meal is based on the fact that gastric distension will increase tLESRs and thereby promote GERD. One relatively simple lifestyle modification that may affect symptoms of GERD is to slow meal ingestion time.[7] Presumably by avoidance of "gulping" food, there is a decrease in concomitant aerophagia, which further increases gastric distension and thereby tLESRs and reflux.

Antacids

Antacids are most often used either by patients that self-direct their treatment with the use of over-the-counter therapy or by those that use them to supplement other antisecretory therapy. Both antacids and alginic acid have been shown to be more effective than placebo in the relief of heartburn.[8] Antacid combined with alginic acid has been shown to be superior to antacid alone in controlling GERD symptoms.[9] In general, however, the studies have shown no significant benefit of antacids over placebo for either long-term symptom control or healing of esophagitis.[8]

Antacids as a class of therapy have the potential for significant side effects when used on a chronic and regular basis. Magnesium containing antacids may cause diarrhea and should be avoided in patients with heart failure, renal insufficiency, and late trimester pregnancy. Aluminum-containing antacids may cause constipation and should also be avoided in patients with chronic renal insufficiency.

Overall, antacids have a marginal benefit as a therapy for GERD. They have no role as primary therapy in a patient with known erosive esophagitis. Antacids may offer some benefit to the patient with rare and episodic heartburn in which case they do have the benefit of providing rapid but unfortunately temporary symptom relief.

Promotility Agents

In the treatment of GERD, prokinetic agents are used with the intent to increase LESP, accelerate gastric emptying, and/or augment esophageal peristalsis. All prokinetic agents (bethanechol, metoclopramide, domperidone, cisapride) have demonstrated some symptom benefit in GERD. However, efficacy data supporting the use of these agents as a treatment for GERD largely comes from small, poorly designed studies, typically without a placebo control comparison.[10]

Bethanechol is a direct-acting muscarinic receptor agonist resulting in cholinergic stimulation. Early studies with this compound demonstrated a mild effect on LESP and improved esophageal peristalsis, and small studies (without placebo) have suggested a symptomatic benefit for GERD.[11] However, the dose of bethanechol that was used in order to be effective was also associated with significant side effects, which precludes any role for bethanechol as a current option for managing GERD symptoms and it is mentioned only as a historical point.

Metoclopramide is a centrally acting dopamine antagonist that crosses the blood–brain barrier. Although symptomatic improvement of GERD has been demonstrated in some studies, placebo-controlled studies have not shown a consistent benefit of this agent versus placebo.[11] Antidopaminergic side effects are common with metoclopramide use—occurring in 20–30% of patients. The most serious side effect is tardive dyskinesia, which may be an irreversible complication of treatment in some individuals.

Domperidone is a dopamine antagonist that, unlike metoclopramide, does not cross the blood–brain barrier. Additionally, this agent rarely causes extrapyramidal side effects. It is not commercially available as a branded product in the United States although some local pharmacies will compound this agent when asked to do so. Domperidone efficacy data for GERD have not been convincing. The largest study with this agent was a comparative trial of domperidone and ranitidine, without a placebo control.[12] Some of the placebo-controlled studies have suggested no benefit for this agent.[11] The major adverse event seen with domperidone use is gynecomastia caused by stimulation of prolactin release and this finding is seen in 10–15% of patients.

Cisapride acts locally to facilitate the release of acetylcholine from postganglionic neurons of the myenteric plexus. There are limited data demonstrating an increase in smooth muscle contractility and LESP with cisapride. This agent was approved for use in the United States only for the indication of "nocturnal heartburn." When compared with histamine-2-receptor antagonists (H2RAs), the healing data for esophagitis were comparable.[11] Additionally, this agent was demonstrated to be better than placebo in improving GERD symptoms.[11] The cardiac issues associated with QT prolongation and ventricular arrhythmias have precluded continued use of this agent in clinical practice.

Tegaserod is a selective partial 5HT4 agonist that has a profound promotility effect throughout the gastrointestinal tract. To date, this drug has only been extensively evaluated as a treatment for irritable bowel syndrome with constipation. Controlled clinical trials evaluating the use of this agent in GERD are soon to be underway.

Combination therapy using promotility agents combined with antisecretory therapy has been a popular management strategy, in particular among primary care physicians. Despite this "popularity" as a clinical therapy for GERD, there are scant data to support this management approach. The best clinical study involved the comparative evaluation of ranitidine, cisapride, ranitidine plus cisapride, omeprazole, and omeprazole plus cisapride.[13] This study showed an advantage of combination therapy over a ranitidine- or cisapride-alone strategy but not over an omeprazole-alone strategy. Hence, given a lack of supporting evidence confirming the utility of this clinical approach, combination therapy as a general approach for treating GERD should be discouraged. However, there may be some role for combination therapy in those patients with gastroparesis and/or functional dyspepsia and associated GERD symptoms.

H2-Receptor Antagonists

These agents competitively and reversibly inhibit gastric acid secretion by blocking the histamine receptor on the parietal cell and perhaps other effector cells as well. There are four available agents—cimetidine, ranitidine, famotidine, and nizatidine. These compounds have been shown to be effective in relieving mild-to-moderate GERD symptoms as well as preventing postprandial GERD symptoms. A review of 20 randomized controlled trials, however, showed only five studies that demonstrated a significant improvement in symptom control over placebo.[14] These agents have also been shown to be effective in controlled clinical trials assessing the healing erosive esophagitis. The efficacy for healing, however, has been particularly poor for severe esophagitis. All comparative trials to date have shown that H2RAs are substantially inferior to proton pump inhibitor (PPI) therapy for healing of erosive esophagitis or in controlling GERD symptoms. This is in part related to the diminished effect versus the PPIs that H2RAs have on gastric acid secretion as well as the tachyphylaxis, or pharmacological tolerance, that has been reported as a consequence of continued administration of these agents. It is likely that tolerance develops as a down-regulation of the H2 receptors.

Proton Pump Inhibitors

Proton pump inhibitors are currently the most effective medical treatment for GERD. These compounds profoundly suppress acid secretion through the inhibition of H^+, K^+ adenosine triphosphatase, the proton pump of the parietal cell, and the site responsible for acid production. All PPIs are substituted benzimidazoles and are prodrugs, which must be activated in the presence of acid in order to inhibit the proton pump. Unlike the H2RAs, PPIs block acid production regardless of the method of cell stimulation, thus providing a greater degree of acid suppression for a longer duration of time. This superior pharmacological effect translates into a higher efficacy rate in GERD symptom relief and healing of esophagitis. Conventional healing rates with the first four PPIs—omeprazole, lansoprazole, rabeprazole, and pantoprazole—have demonstrated that a once-daily morning dose of a PPI will provide relief of symptoms and healing of erosive esophagitis in approximately 80% of patients.[8] Healing rates increase further when therapy is extended another 4–8 weeks. Supporting this estimate of treatment effect with PPIs is a quantitative systematic review of the comparative efficacy of PPIs and H2RAs that analyzed 23 reports comprising 5118 patients.[15] The overall healing was 78% for the PPIs and 44% with H2RAs at week 8. This translated to a relative risk of 1.7 [confidence interval (CI) 1.6–1.8], and number needed to treat (NNT) was 3 (CI 2.8–3.6) for PPIs compared with the H2RAs. As with H2RAs, however, the healing rates with PPI therapy correlate inversely with the severity of esophagitis. Incremental dosing of the PPI has not been shown to increase healing or symptom response—at least when the dose is doubled but still given once a day. There are no studies of esophageal healing that have evaluated the effects of a twice-daily (BID) PPI dosing regimen. Conceptually this clinical approach should improve outcomes given the augmentation of gastric pH effect seen with BID dosing.[16] Esomeprazole, the S isomer of omeprazole, has demonstrated superior pH effect versus the other PPIs and this has correlated with clinical data indicating improved clinical outcomes when this PPI is used versus lansoprazole, pantoprazole, and omeprazole, notably healing of erosive esophagitis and symptom resolution.[17] Previously, there had been few comparisons between individual PPIs that used acceptable evidence-based approaches for analysis. What data that were available showed few differences between the original four PPIs. For instance, a meta-analysis that compared omeprazole with lansoprazole found no significant difference in the healing rates between these PPIs and reported a NNT of 67.[18] More recent studies involving comparison of esomeprazole to the first-generation PPIs have shown clear superiority for healing—in particular for the more severe grades of esophagitis (Los Angeles grades C and D). The NNT for the more severe grades of esophagitis has ranged from 5 to 10 in the trials comparing esomeprazole to omeprazole, lansoprazole, and pantoprazole.[17] Superior symptom resolution was also evident in these same trials.

Nocturnal Acid Breakthrough (PPI Plus H2RA)

Studies evaluating gastric pH using continuous intragastric pH monitoring have demonstrated a curious physiological and pharmacological phenomenon known as nocturnal acid breakthrough (NAB). In these studies, the majority of subjects who were taking a PPI BID still developed an intragastric acidity level of a pH <4 for at least 1 continuous hour in the overnight period of monitoring.[19] This decrease in pH began to be evident 6–7 hours after the second (PM) dosing of the PPI. This is not the result of PPI resistance. Additionally, NAB is a class effect that is seen with all of the PPIs and is evident in healthy subjects and GERD patients alike. Curiously, the addition of an H2RA at bedtime in addition to the BID dose of PPI has been shown to be effective for ameliorating this phenomenon, but not a third bedtime dose of a PPI. The clinical importance of this physiological and pharmacological observation has not been determined and has clearly been overestimated by some, as there have been no studies that demonstrate the concordance of NAB with a particular GERD presentation or symptom manifestation. Nor has there been any benefit from treatment intervention using an H2RA as additive therapy to a BID PPI dose. Furthermore, as with other observations involving extended use of H2RAs, there is a tachyphylaxis and a subsequent waning of benefit seen as early as 7 days after instituting use with this class of drugs.[20] The clinical significance of NAB would seem to be small at best. Perhaps in patients for whom maximal acid inhibition remains problematic, e.g., Barrett's esophagus (BE), there may a theoretical advantage although the durability of such a response remains questionable.

Maintenance of Remission

Because GERD is a chronic medical disorder, most patients will relapse once antisecretory medication is discontinued. Maintenance of remission frequently requires the same dose of medication necessary to effectively induce healing, although maintenance strategies typically try to go to the next lowest dose below that which controlled GERD symptoms or effected healing. Although H2RAs are only approved for the short-term use of GERD, there is also evidence that maintenance therapy with these agents will decrease the relapse of esophagitis somewhat, but they are nearly as effective as PPIs in this regard. Consistent with the superiority of PPIs over the H2RAs as acute GERD therapy, there is a similar superiority demonstrated in comparative maintenance trials.[21] Relapse rates are higher for H2RAs dependent in part on the baseline grade of esophagitis before initial treatment. Additionally, PPIs have been shown to be superior versus H2RAs in the prevention of stricture recurrence and need for repeat esophageal dilation.[22–24] High dose and/or long-term use of PPIs also has been shown to be extremely safe and effective.[25] The differences in the individual PPIs in efficacy of maintaining remission are unclear but a recent comparative trial of esomeprazole and lansoprazole showed a relapse rate of 41% for lansoprazole 15 mg/d compared with 24% for esomeprazole 20 mg/d for those patients with moderate/severe esophagitis (Los Angeles grades C and D).[26]

Barrett's Esophagus

The primary objective in the treatment of GERD in patients with BE is to control GERD symptoms. It seems that in these patients there is a diminished esophageal symptom response to esophageal acid exposure because of the presence of the columnar epithelium in the tubular esophagus. This metaplastic epithelial change has been shown to mute the normal sensory response to acid exposure. The mainstay of the therapy of BE has been PPIs. However, it must be noted that long-term potent acid suppression using PPIs has not been shown to effectively and reliably induce a regression of BE metaplasia.

Reepithelialization with squamous islands of tissue overgrowing the BE metaplasia has been demonstrated with PPI use but complete and predictable reversal has never been demonstrated with pharmacological therapy alone.[27-30]

The primary clinical concern with BE remains the increased cancer risk associated with this disorder. There is theoretical concern that continued acid exposure magnifies this risk and conversely there is indirect evidence that suggests that potent acid suppressive therapy might decrease the cancer risk. There are several molecular and biological reasons supporting this concept. First the cyclooxygenase-2 pathway is believed to have an important role in several carcinogenic pathways, in particular that for esophageal cancer because this pathway has an important role in the cell proliferation and inhibition of apoptosis.[31] In ex vivo studies, pulses of acid cause an increase in cyclooxygenase-2 expression.[32] Additionally, acid pulses have been shown to induce cellular proliferation as well as lipid peroxidation and these changes further contribute to chromosomal damage.[33] Effective suppression of Barrett's acid exposure with PPI therapy has been shown to be effective in in vitro studies in the reduction of these markers of molecular instability and cancer risk. These data provide a theoretic reason to justify potent acid suppression for patients with BE, especially those already with neoplasia (dysplasia) and further increased cancer risk.[34] Furthermore, there is recent epidemiological evidence that also suggests that PPI therapy is associated with a significant reduction in the risk of developing dysplasia with a hazard ratio of 0.25 (95% CI 0.13–0.47).[35] Although these data are intriguing and certainly support the in vitro data, more studies are required before we know for certain whether intensive acid suppression with PPIs decreases cancer risk in patients with BE. It is important to note that anti-reflux surgical studies have also not shown a reduction in risk of dysplasia or adenocarcinoma in Barrett's patients treated in this manner.[36,37]

Extraesophageal GERD

The majority of data regarding healing and symptom relief of GERD have been generated from clinical trials of patients with heartburn and erosive esophagitis. There are very few well-designed trials of medical therapy for patients with extraesophageal GERD-related disease (asthma, cough, noncardiac chest pain, laryngitis). A few uncontrolled trials have demonstrated superiority of PPIs for reducing respiratory symptoms thought related to GERD in patients with GERD-related symptoms but these data also indicate that there has been a need for higher doses and more prolonged therapy with PPIs to achieve adequate symptom relief.[38] Medical therapies for reflux-related asthma have also shown improvement in asthma symptom scores, medication use, and quality-of-life measures, but not improvement in pulmonary function testing.[39] Interestingly, a meta-analysis of the surgical anti-reflux trial data has demonstrated the same lack of improvement of this GERD therapy on pulmonary function results.[40]

Consensus opinion suggests that patients with GERD-related extraesophageal disease should be treated with a twice-daily PPI for 8–16 weeks as an initial course of therapy. This is based on the goal of eliminating even minor amounts of esophageal acid exposure, because even modest amounts of acid may be enough to precipitate symptoms or mucosal injury. Many authors would suggest that even longer treatment intervals are needed to ensure an optimal response, particularly in patients with reflux laryngitis. Although data are lacking, some authorities recommend a 3- to 6-month response time for some difficult-to-treat patients with reflux-related otolaryngological disease. Overall, the response of the extraesophageal disease manifestations of GERD to medical therapy has been variable and less predictable than the healing data. This is likely attributable to the fact that extraesophageal disease manifestations of GERD are often the result of multiple factors—acid reflux being only one of these. Elimination of esophageal acid exposure may not resolve the presenting symptom, e.g., hoarseness, if there are persistent contributing factors such as voice strain, repetitive throat clearing, or postnasal drip. Surgical anti-reflux therapy has also demonstrated variable results in improving the outcomes of extraesophageal GERD. The best predictor of the success of anti-reflux surgery for these extraesophageal symptoms has been a previous response to medical therapy with a PPI.[41]

Measuring Esophageal pH As an Outcome of Anti-Reflux Therapy

The technology to monitor the presence of acid in the esophagus has made this endpoint a logical outcome for assessment of a therapy of GERD. Esophageal pH monitoring measures the frequency and duration of acid reflux as well as allows one to correlate the temporal events with a specific symptom related to GERD.

As part of the analysis of esophageal pH recordings, an esophageal pH <4 has been set as the threshold/standard for defining a reflux event. This cutoff limit of pH <4 is an arbitrary choice but somewhat justified related to physiological and clinical/observational data. First, studies have demonstrated that pepsin, a proteolytic enzyme, is inactivated at a pH > 4.[1] Second, patients with symptomatic reflux events typically relate symptoms at a pH <4.[42,43]

Although esophageal pH testing is not considered a necessary test in the evaluation of patients with classic GERD, it does provide an objective measure of the degree of acid reflux. There are several types of pH electrodes suitable for intraesophageal use. The traditional approach has involved the use of a tube passed transnasally into the esophagus. Data are then accumulated via a direct-contact communication to a data logger worn by the patient. Differences exist between the monopolar electrodes that require an external reference electrode versus the combination electrodes with a built-in reference, because the former is more susceptible to artifact. Recently, a new wireless/tubeless intraesophageal pH device has also been introduced.[44] This device accumulates pH data via a capsule that is attached to the esophageal wall. The pH data are transmitted via radiofrequency to a data recorder worn by the patient. This technique differs from the more conventional pH monitoring by circumventing the problems encountered with conventional transnasal tube monitoring. These problems include limitations on physical activity and diet that may be imposed by the "tube" technique of monitoring.

The optimal duration of ambulatory monitoring has been a subject of much debate. Some investigators have reported that shorter-term monitoring is adequate when particular attention is placed on the postprandial period.[45,46] However, evidence subsequently has shown that a 24-hour period of monitoring is diagnostically superior to a shorter time interval.[46] Although the 24-hour period of monitoring is regarded as the current method of choice, a 16-hour study from 4 PM until 8 AM has been shown to provide accurate information and improved patient tolerance.[46,47] The ability of the "tubeless" Bravo technique to allow for 48 hours of pH monitoring is conceptually attractive, because it does not increase the discomfort of the patient while still providing an extended period of monitoring.[44]

In analyzing pH studies, it is important to note the potential of the acidity and buffering capacity of meals and beverages consumed during the period of monitoring to affect the pH recorded. Additionally, the duration of the periods of upright and supine positioning and physical activity can affect acid reflux exposure times.[47,48] Although standardization of food intake and activity is recommended, it is virtually impossible to accomplish this outside of a controlled inpatient setting. Thus, in clinical trials involving pH monitoring as a primary assessment endpoint of a therapy, there is a potential for bias given the inability to standardize these influences between patients, or even in the same patient who returns for sequential testing. The natural intrasubject variability in intraesophageal acid exposure in patients with GERD has shown that reproducibility of pH monitoring is only "good" or "satisfactory" with a concordance of approximately 77% for detecting pH < 4.[49-51] Some authors have reported even more variation with a variance by a factor of threefold.[51] Additionally, in a study in which patients were investigated 6 weeks apart under identical inpatient monitoring conditions, 6 of 22 patients had a normal total reflux time but other evidence of pathological GERD.[52] In another study, two pH monitors were positioned at the same location within the esophagus, yet there was a discrepancy in the readings in 2 of the 10 patients studied.[53] This difference was notable enough that it would have resulted in a change in the clinical diagnosis of GERD dependent on which probe data was selected for analysis.

Given that the usual definition of abnormal amount of acid reflux is based on a total time pH < 4, it would make sense that the target for monitoring response of a GERD therapy would be the restoration of normal esophageal acid exposure to a "normal" range. This normalization of pH as a target of a successful outcome of a GERD therapy has been used most often in surgical trials. It is clear, however, that normalization of pH does not occur in all patients who have successful outcomes as assessed by clinical criteria. This is the case irrespective of the GERD therapeutic intervention—surgical, endoscopic, and/or medical.

The question arises, therefore, whether normalization of pH, although an attractive outcome, is really necessary. To justify use of normalization of esophageal acid exposure as a relevant clinical endpoint, there also should be a correlation with a clinical endpoint such as improvement in esophageal healing or GERD-related symptoms or prevention of complications such as stricture, BE, or esophageal cancer.

When intraesophageal pH monitoring has been used as an objective target to assess a response to GERD medical therapy, it generally focused on decreasing the total time pH < 4. This objective has been driven primarily by the observation that there is a direct correlation between control of intragastric pH with increased healing rates of erosive esophagitis.

For treatment of BE, there is even a better scientific rationale for more aggressive acid suppression, especially normalization of esophageal pH. Patients with BE have been shown to have greater intraesophageal acid exposure than patients with uncomplicated GERD and successful elimination of symptoms does not ensure adequate control of acid reflux in patients with BE.[54-56] In one study, compared with patients with GERD, patients with BE were more likely to have higher degree of pathological acid reflux despite PPI therapy (DeMeester score 50.5 ± 8.2 vs 31.4 ± 4.6; $P = .03$) and less intragastric acid suppression (percent total; pH < 4; 53.9 ± 2.7 vs 39.9 ± 2.6; $P = .0004$).[57]

Measuring Esophageal Motility and LESP As an Outcome of Anti-Reflux Therapy

Hypotension of the lower esophageal sphincter is recognized as a key factor in the pathogenesis of GERD. The prevalence of low LESP increases with the severity of esophagitis.[58] A large body of information indicates, however, that it is transient lower esophageal sphincter pressure relaxations of the LES (tLESRs) that is the major mechanism for reflux of acid into the both for normal individuals as well as those with GERD.[59,60]

Prokinetics (metoclopramide, cisapride, erythromycin) have not demonstrated any clinically significant effect on LESP.[61] Given that the benefit of PPI therapy is mediated through acid inhibition rather than an effect on LESP, this outcome has never been a primary endpoint for any of the acid suppressive therapies.

Endoscopic Assessment Endpoints As an Outcome of Anti-Reflux Therapy

Endoscopy allows for the identification of GERD-related mucosal damage. This is evident primarily by the demonstration of erosive changes or complications such as stricture or BE. Endoscopic assessment of esophagitis is a very objective parameter that can be followed sequentially to assess disease response to a specific therapeutic intervention. Although erosive esophagitis is easily recognized, there are many diagnostic instruments that have attempted to stratify the severity of erosive damage.

Unfortunately, only 35–57% of patients with symptomatic GERD will have evidence of erosive esophagitis or BE.[62-64] Several other issues are critical when evaluating endoscopic outcomes of a GERD therapy:

1. Was a validated instrument used to assess the grade of esophagitis? Despite the high prevalence of erosive esophagitis in clinical studies, there has only been a recent effort to use a validated instrument for the assessment of disease severity as it relates to the extent of erosions. To date, the Los Angeles grading system is the only validated instrument for the grading of erosive esophagitis.[65] Although the severity of erosive esophagitis has been correlated with the extent of acid reflux in these patients, the extent of erosive damage has not been shown to correlate with the frequency or severity of heartburn or regurgitation.[65]

2. What was the stage of medical therapy at the time of the assessment by endoscopy? If patients were on medical therapy at the time of entry (or had only been off medical therapy for a relatively short while), the potential exists for an underestimate of the true severity of baseline esophagitis. Studies have demonstrated that most of the patients with erosive esophagitis will relapse within 3 months after discontinuance of a PPI.[66] It would seem logical and appropriate, thereby, that patients should be off medical therapy for a minimum of 3 months to accurately define their "baseline" grade of esophagitis before entry into a study.

3. Were the endoscopic findings scored by investigators that were blinded to the stage of the treatment intervention (pre- or post-procedure)?

4. Was intention-to-treat analysis done for all patients who were treated?

There have been many medical trials in which outcome was the endoscopic relapse of esophagitis during maintenance medical therapy.[61] In contradistinction to the surgical and endoscopic trials, most of these studies have attempted to characterize baseline and follow-up endoscopic data and to use intention-to-treat analysis. The vast majority of these recent trials involved a placebo comparison to PPI in patients with erosive esophagitis. Erosive esophagitis relapse at 6 months ranged from 7 to 15% for most of the studies.[61] One trial by Lauritsen et al.[25] highlighted the superiority of esomeprazole when compared with lansoprazole therapy in a 6-month maintenance trial of patients with healed erosive esophagitis. In contrast to the other PPI maintenance studies, this study showed a relapse difference between two active therapies. Of particular note was the difference in relapse rates based on the baseline severity of esophagitis. The data were also analyzed for response based on the entry-level grade of esophagitis. For those patients with Los Angeles grades A and B, the relapse rate was 15% for esomeprazole versus 23% for lansoprazole ($P < .01$). For those with more severe esophagitis grades C and D, these differences were more pronounced: 24% for esomeprazole and 41% for lansoprazole. This study highlights the high relapse rate for more severe grades of esophagitis even while on a potent medical maintenance therapy. The symptom relapse rate

in this study was 22% for esomeprazole and 29% for lansoprazole ($P < .01$), notably less than the esophagitis relapse.

Symptom Assessment As an Outcome of Anti-Reflux Therapy

Reflux disease is associated with a number of symptoms, but in GERD treatment studies, the major focus has been on the effect of an intervention on heartburn and regurgitation. Although heartburn is probably the best characterized symptom of GERD, there is no universally accepted definition of heartburn. This becomes of particular importance, because heartburn has been the major enrollment criterion for most of the GERD therapy trials. A definition of heartburn as "a burning feeling rising from the stomach or lower chest towards the neck" has led to an improved recognition of this symptom indicating GERD.[67] Many patients, however, do not construe heartburn and "retrosternal burning" to be synonymous.[67]

The majority of trials have graded clinical heartburn using a severity scale such as a Likert scale or a visual analog scale. The reproducibility and responsiveness of these scales have been fairly good in the assessment of upper gastrointestinal disease.[68] It has been shown, however, that when these scales are used for serial assessments, the sensitivity of the assessment is enhanced if patients see their previous scores.[69]

The patient assessment of heartburn frequency typically records the number of days with heartburn over the last week or month. Although heartburn frequency has often been used in GERD intervention trials, it is rarely a primary objective defining treatment success. More recently, complete absence of heartburn has been a declared objective for some studies. Furthermore, rapid symptom relief of symptoms has also been a treatment outcome and the more rapid onset of gastric acid suppression may be of particular importance in patients with symptomatic GERD.[69]

Gastroesophageal reflux disease therapy trials have used various endpoints in monitoring response to treatment.[70–74] These range from endpoints of study medication providing "adequate" control, symptomatic improvement, or to complete absence of heartburn over the last

7 days of assessment. In clinical trials, the complete absence of symptoms provides a reproducible endpoint that allows comparison between studies. The value of the absence of heartburn as the optimal target for a therapeutic trial is further supported by the positive impact this outcome has on quality of life.[70,75]

Although patient satisfaction with symptom response would be an intuitively appropriate measure for assessing treatment response, there are a number of potential problems with this approach including: response and acquiescence bias, use of single-item questions, and the lack of evidence of a correlation with the extent of symptom reduction.

Symptoms as assessed by diary records are likely the best way to accurately evaluate symptoms and avoid a potential for recall bias. This type of recording technique captures daily fluctuation in symptoms and allows for a more accurate assessment over the course of treatment. There are some burdens imposed to the patient, however, which may limit the usefulness of this assessment. This imposes some potential for nonadherence to the collection protocol and a potential for "hoarding" of the information, that is, a rapid attempt at recollection of the missing days of data immediately before return for the study visit. Additionally, there is a potential for an adaptation or conditioning of response over sequential periods of assessment and scoring. This may also introduce another potential for bias in a study.

There are limited data on the validity of a physician assessment of the effect of a response to treatment. Although there is a variable correlation, it seems this is primarily in patients reporting mild disease.[68] A significant potential exists for reporting bias especially if the treating physician is involved in the assessment or the evaluating physician is not blinded to the treatment.

Quality-of-Life Assessment As an Outcome of Anti-Reflux Therapy

Health-related quality-of-life (HRQOL) assessment is defined as the functional effect of the illness as perceived by the patient. Health-related quality-of-life assessment has been utilized in recent trials assessing GERD outcomes.[76-78] There are several generic as well as disease-specific instruments that have been utilized in these studies, including the SF-36, psychological general-well-being index (PGWBI), quality of life in reflux and dyspepsia (QOLRAD), and gastrointestinal quality-of-life index (GIQLI), among others. These HRQOL endpoints, however, are subject to the individual thresholds of the patient. If these assessments are used as primary outcomes to assess GERD therapy, they are subject to the variances in the patient expectations for disease management. This may be an issue especially if there is not a control arm in the scientific design of the study. It is clear that disease severity correlates with HRQOL and does contribute to a negative effect on both work productivity and absenteeism. There are, however, cultural and situational variances in patient willingness to go to work when they do not feel well. Absenteeism thereby may not be an accurate outcome measure, in particular in the United States. Work productivity assessment may be a more reasonable measure, provided validated instruments are used to assess this accurately.

In contrast to both the surgical and endoscopic anti-reflux trials, the recent medical trials (primarily involving the use of PPIs) have consistently utilized a GERD HRQOL instrument. Proton pump inhibitor use as a rule has consistently improved the HRQOL, although it is clear that QOL is not normalized until heartburn resolution is achieved.[71,79] This correlation of QOL and symptoms is an important advance in the effort to draw corollaries between the different GERD outcomes.

Medication Use As an Outcome of Anti-Reflux Therapy

A decrease in use of antisecretory or acid-buffering medication would seem to be an important endpoint for a therapeutic intervention for GERD. Recognizably, medication use is somewhat dependent on patient expectations and habit of use. This underscores the need for placebo-controlled studies when using this as an endpoint. The clinical trials of medical therapy for GERD have been relatively conscientious in the capture of data involving ancillary medication use. Most of the more recent trials have accounted for the use of antacids that are provided to the patient as "rescue medication." This type of medication accounting does not, however, account for off-protocol medication use of other over-the-counter medications (H2RA, PPI). Study treatment bias, however, is for the most part precluded by the appropriate use of blinded studies involving a placebo control group. The potential problem of capturing an accurate assessment of ancillary medication use is a bigger issue in light of the expanded availability of over-the-counter antisecretory medications.

Conclusions

Medical therapy has been extremely "successful" in treatment of the symptoms and complications of GERD. Recognizably, the methods to assess treatment outcomes for GERD have been extremely variable among surgical, endoscopic, and medical therapies for this disorder. Comparison between or even within classes of treatments (surgical, endoscopic, medical) cannot be accurately assessed without standardization of patient demographics, scientific design, and treatment assessment. This is likely achievable and best done only in a direct comparison with a randomized prospective blinded trial. Treatment outcome comparison between trials without this study design is inappropriate.

Medical therapy offers a distinct advantage as it relates to risk versus the other endoscopic and surgical therapeutic strategies for GERD. Clearly, medical therapy has been shown to be the safest and most cost-effective therapy compared with surgery and the more limited data with the endoscopic therapies. True "medical failures" are rare and these patients should be thoroughly evaluated before considering an endoscopic or surgical anti-reflux therapy option.

Despite continued improvements in the ability to suppress acid via even more potent PPIs, there remain, however, opportunities for improvement. These would be in the arena of accelerating the onset of action so that PPIs could provide more rapid symptom relief especially when taken in response to a given symptom episode. Additionally, approximately 10–20% of patients do not respond to standard PPI dosing. Improvements in more potent and prolonged acid control will offer potential advantages in particular for those with more severe esophagitis, as well as the patients with BE or extraesophageal complications. Forthcoming advances with the development of medications that provide further enhancements for reducing gastric acid secretion will make the medical approach even more appealing, even for the most difficult-to-treat patients with GERD.

References

1. Tuttle SG, Rufin F, Bettarello A. The physiology of heartburn. Ann Intern Med 1961;55:292–300.
2. Orr W. Sleep issues in gastroesophageal reflux disease: beyond simple heartburn control. Rev Gastroenterol Disord 2003;3(suppl 4):S22–S29.
3. Orr W. Sleep and gastroesophageal reflux disease: a wake-up call. Rev Gastroenterol Disord 2004;4(suppl 4): S25–S32.
4. Katzka D, Castell DO. Lifestyle modifications. In: Castell DO, Richter JE, eds. The Esophagus. Boston: Little Brown and Co.; 1995:505–514.
5. Katz LC, Just R, Castell DO. Body position affects recumbent postprandial reflux. J Clin Gastroenterol 1994; 18:280–284.
6. Van Herwaarden MA, Katzka DA, Smout AJ, Samsom M, Gideon M, Castell DO. Effect of different recumbent positions on postprandial reflux in normal subjects. Am J Gastroenterol 2000;95:2731–2735.
7. Wildi SM, Tutuian R, Castell DO. The influence of rapid food intake on postprandial reflux: studies in healthy volunteers. Am J Gastroenterol 2004;99:1645–1651.
8. Katz PO. Medical management of GERD. In: Castell DO, Richter J, eds. The Esophagus. Philadelphia: Lippincott Williams & Wilkins; 2004:460–479.
9. Klinkenberg-Knol EC, Festen HPM. Pharmacological management of gastro-oesophageal reflux disease. Drugs 1995;49:695–710.
10. Mittal RK. Pathophysiology of gastroesophageal reflux disease: motility factors. In: Castell DO, Richter J, eds. The Esophagus. Philadelphia: Lippincott Williams & Wilkins; 2004:407–420.
11. Ramirez B, Richter JE. Review article: promotility drugs in the treatment of gastro-oesophageal reflux disease. Aliment Pharmacol Ther 1993;7:5–20.
12. Blackwell JN, Heading RC, Fettes MR. Effects of Domperidone on Lower Oesophageal Sphincter Pressure and Gastroesophageal Reflux in Patients with Peptic Esophagitis. Progress with Domperidone. International Congress and Symposium Series. Vol 36. London: Royal Society of Medicine Press; 1981:57–66.
13. Vigneri S, Temini R, Leandro G, et al. A comparison of five maintenance therapies for reflux esophagitis. N Engl J Med 1995;333:1106–1111.

14. Sontag SJ. Rolling review: gastro-oesophageal reflux disease. Aliment Pharmacol Ther 1993;7:293–312.
15. Chiba, et al. Gastroenterology 1996.
16. Johnson DA, Ryan M, Wootton, et al. Comparative study of esomeprazole and lansoprazole for intragastric pH analysis in patients with symptoms of gastroesophageal reflux disease. Gut 2004;56:113.
17. Johnson DA. Evidence-based assessment of the efficacy of esomeprazole for the healing of erosive esophagitis. Expert Rev Pharmacoeconomics Outcomes Res 2004; 4(4):371–382.
18. Sharma VK, Leontiadis GI, Howden CW. Meta-analysis of randomized controlled trials comparing standard clinical doses of omeprazole and lansoprazole in erosive esophagitis. Aliment Pharmacol Ther 2001;15:227–231.
19. Peghini PL, Katz PO, Bracy NA, et al. Nocturnal recovery of gastric acid secretion with twice daily dosing of proton pump inhibitors. Am J Gastroenterol 1998; 93:763–767.
20. Fackler WK, Ours TM, Vaezi MF, et al. Long-term effect of H2RA therapy on nocturnal gastric acid breakthrough. Gastroenterology 2002;122:625–632.
21. Maton P. Efficacy and safety of GERD pharmacotherapy. In: Richter JE, ed. Healing Horizons in Acid Reflux Disease. Cleveland: Cleveland Clinic Foundation; 2003: 183–212.
22. Smith PM, Kerr GD, Cockel R, et al. A comparison of omeprazole and ranitidine in the prevention of recurrence of benign esophageal stricture. Restore Investigator Group. Gastroenterology 1994;197:1312–1318.
23. Swarbrick ET, Gough AL, Foster CS, Christian J, Garrett AD, Langworthy CH. Prevention of recurrence of esophageal stricture: a comparison of lansoprazole and high dose ranitidine. Eur J Gastroenterol Hepatol 1996; 8:431–438.
24. Marks RD, Richter JE, Rizzo J, et al. Omeprazole vs H2 receptor antagonist in treating patients with peptic stricture and esophagitis. Gastroenterology 1994;106: 907–915.
25. Lauritsen K, Deviere J, Bigard MA, et al. Esomeprazole 20 mg and lansoprazole 15 mg in maintaining healed reflux oesophagitis. Aliment Pharmacol Ther 2003;17: 333–341.
26. Klinkenberg-Knol EC, Nelis F, Dent J, et al. Long term omeprazole treatment in resistant gastroesophageal reflux disease: efficacy, safety and influence on gastric mucosa. Gastroenterology 2000;118:661–669.
27. Sampliner RE. Effect of up to 3 yrs of high-dose lansoprazole on Barrett's esophagus. Am J Gastroenterol 1994; 89:1844–1848.
28. Peters FT, Ganesh S, Kuipers EJ, et al. Endoscopic regression of Barrett's oesophagus during omeprazole treatment: a randomized double blind study. Gut 1999;45: 485–494.
29. Sampliner RE, Camargo L, Fass R. Impact of esophageal acid exposure on the endoscopic reversal of Barrett's esophagus. Am J Gastroenterol 2002;97:270–272.
30. Sharma P, Sampliner RE, Carmargo E. Normalization of esophageal pH with high dose proton pump inhibitor therapy does not result in regression of Barrett's esophagus. Am J Gastroenterol 1997;92:582–585.
31. Morris CD, Armstrong GR, Bigley G, et al. Cyclooxygenase-2 expression in the Barrett's metaplasia-dysplasia-adenocarcinoma sequence. Am J Gastroenterol 2001; 96:990–996.

32. Shirvani VN, Ouatu-Lascar R, Kaur BS, et al. Cyclooxygenase 2 expression in Barrett's esophagus and adenocarcinoma: ex vivo induction by bile salts and acid exposure. Gastroenterology 2000;118:487–496.
33. Ouatu-Lascar R, Fitzgerald RC, Triadafilopoulos G. Differentiation and proliferation in Barrett's esophagus and the effects of acid suppression. Gastroenterology 1999;117:327–335.
34. Shirvani VN, Ouatu-Lascar R, Kaur BS, et al. Cyclooxygenase 2 expression by bile salts and acid exposure. Gastroenterology 2000;118(3):487–496.
35. El-Serag HB, Aguiree TV, Davis S, et al. Proton pump inhibitors are associated with reduced incidence of dysplasia in Barrett's esophagus. Am J Gastroenterol 2004; 99:1877–1883.
36. Spechler SJ, Lee E, Ahnen D, et al. Long-term outcome of medical and surgical therapies for gastroesophageal reflux disease: follow-up of a randomized controlled trial. JAMA 2001;285:2331–2338.
37. Parrilla P, Martinez de Haro LF, Ortiz A, et al. Long-term results of a randomized perspective study comparing medical and surgical treatment of Barrett's esophagus. Ann Surg 2003;237:291–298.
38. Harding S, Richter JE, Guzzo MR, et al. Asthma and gastroesophageal reflux: acid suppressive therapy improves asthma outcome. Am J Med 1996;100:395–405.
39. Field SK, Sutherland LR. Does medical anti-reflux therapy improve asthma in asthmatics with gastrooesophageal reflux? Chest 1998;114:275–283.
40. Field SK, Gelfand GA, McFadden SD. The effects of antireflux surgery on asthmatics with gastroesophageal reflux. Chest 1999;116:766–774.
41. So JB, Zeitels SM, Rattner DW. Outcomes of atypical symptoms attributed to gastroesophageal reflux treated by laparoscopic fundoplication. Surgery 1998;124:28–32.
42. Weusten B, Smout AJPM. Ambulatory monitoring of esophageal pH and pressure. In: Castell DO, Richter J, eds. The Esophagus. Philadelphia: Lippincott Williams & Wilkins; 2004:135–164.
43. Kahrilas PJ, Quigley EM. Clinical esophageal pH monitoring: a technical review of practice guideline development. Gastroenterology 1996;110:1982–1986.
44. Pandolfino JE, Richer JE, Ours T, et al. Ambulatory esophageal pH monitoring using a wireless system. Am J Gastroenterol 2003;98(4):740–749.
45. Grande L, Pujol A, Ros E, et al. Intraesophageal pH monitoring after breakfast and lunch in gastroesophageal reflux disease. J Clin Gastroenterol 1988;10: 373–376.
46. Jorgensen F, Elsborg L, Hessse B. The diagnostic value of computerized short term esophageal pH monitoring in suspected gastroesophageal reflux. Scand J Gastroenterol 1988;23:363–367.
47. Bianchi Porro G, Pace F. Comparison of three methods of intraesophageal pH recording in the diagnosis of gastroesophageal reflux. Scand J Gastroenterol 1988;23: 363–367.
48. Clark CS, Kraus BB, Sinclair J, et al. Gastroesophageal reflux induced by exercise in healthy volunteers. JAMA 1989;261:3599–3601.
49. Johnsson F, Joelsson B. Reproducibility of ambulatory esophageal pH monitoring in the diagnosis of gastroesophageal pH monitoring. Gut 1988;33:1127–1133.
50. Schindlbeck NE, Heinrich C, Konig A, Dendorfer A, Pace F, Muller-Lissner SA. Optimal thresholds, sensitivity, and

specificity of long-term pH-metry for the detection of gastroesophageal reflux disease. Gastroenterology 1987; 93:85–90.

51. Wang H, Beck IT, Paterson WG. Reproducibility and physiologic characteristics of 24-hour ambulatory esophageal manometry/pH-metry. Am J Gastroenterol 1996;91:493–497.

52. Vandeplas Y, Helven R, Goyvaerts H, Sacre L. Reproducibility of continuous 24 hour oesophageal pH monitoring in infants and children. Gut 1990;31:374–377.

53. Murphy DW, Yuan Y, Castell DO. Does the intraesophageal pH probe accurately detect acid reflux? Simultaneous recording with two pH probes in humans. Dig Dis Sci 1989;34:649–656.

54. Katzka DA, Castell DO. Successful elimination of reflux symptoms does not ensure adequate control of acid reflux in Barrett's esophagus. Am J Gastroenterol 1994; 89:989–991.

55. Ouatu-Lascar R, Triadafilopoulos G. Complete elimination of reflux symptoms does not guarantee normalization of intraesophageal acid reflux in patients with Barrett's esophagus. Am J Gastroenterol 1998;93: 711–716.

56. Fass R, Sampliner RE, Malagon IB, et al. Failure of oesophageal acid control in candidates for Barrett's oesophagus reversal on a very high dose of proton pump inhibitor. Aliment Pharmacol Ther 2000;14:597–602.

57. Gerson LB, Bopariai V, Ullah N, Triadafilopoulos G. Oesophageal and gastric pH profiles in patients with gastro-oesophageal reflux disease and Barrett's oesophagus treated with proton pump inhibitors. Aliment Pharmacol Ther 2004;20:637–643.

58. Lundell LR. Surgical treatment of gastroesophageal reflux disease. In: Castell DO, Richter JE, eds. The Esophagus. Philadelphia: Lippincottt Williams & Wilkins; 2004:564–571.

59. Dent J, Holloway RH, Toouli J, et al. Mechanisms of lower esophageal sphincter incompetence in patients with symptomatic gastroesophageal reflux. Gut 1988;29: 1020–1024.

60. Mittal RK, Holloway RH, Penagini R, et al. Transient lower esophageal sphincter relaxation. Gastroenterology 1995;109:601–606.

61. Maton P. Efficacy and safety of GERD pharmacotherapy. In: Richter JE, ed. Healing Horizons in Acid Reflux Disease. Cleveland: Cleveland Clinic Foundation; 2003: 183–212.

62. Younes Z, Johnson DA. Diagnostic evaluation in gastroesophageal reflux disease. Gastroenterol Clin North Am 1999;28:809–830.

63. Winters C, Spurling TJ, Chobanian SJ, et al. Barrett's esophagus: a prevalent complication of gastroe-

sophageal reflux disease. Gastroenterology 1987;92: 118–124.

64. DeVault KR, Castell DO. Updated guidelines for the diagnosis and treatment of gastroesphageal reflux disease. Am J Gastroenterol 2005;100(1):190–200.

65. Lundell LR, Dent J, Bennett JR, et al. Endoscopic assessment of oesophagitis: clinical and functional correlates and further validation of the Los Angeles classification. 1997;92:1293–1297.

66. Johnson DA. GERD treatment protocol. In: Richter JE, ed. Healing Horizons in Acid Reflux Disease. Cleveland: Cleveland Clinic Foundation; 2003:247–274.

67. Carlsson R, Dent J, Bolling-Sternevald E, et al. The usefulness of a structured questionnaire in the assessment of symptomatic gastroesophageal reflux disease. Scand J Gastroenterol 1998;33:1023–1029.

68. Bytzer P. Assessment of reflux symptom severity: methodological options and their attributes. Gut 2004; 53(suppl IV):iv28–iv34.

69. Bytzer P. Goals of therapy and guidelines for treatment success in symptomatic gastroesophageal reflux disease patients. Am J Gastroenterol 2003;98(suppl): S31–S39.

70. Guyatt G, Berman LB, Townsend M, et al. Should study subjects see their previous responses? J Chronic Dis 1985;38:1003–1007.

71. Revicki DA, Crawley JA, Zodet MW, et al. Complete resolution of heartburn symptoms and health related quality of life in patients with gastro-oesophageal reflux disease. Aliment Pharmacol Ther 1999;13:1621–1630.

72. Junghard O, Wiklund IK. A comparison of patient and clinician ratings of heartburn. Gastroenterology 2003; 124(4 suppl 1):A541.

73. McColl E. Best practice in symptom assessment: a review. Gut 2004;53(suppl 53 IV):iv49–iv54.

74. Sharma N, Donnellan C, Preston C, et al. A systematic review of symptomatic outcomes used in oesophagitis drug therapy trials. Gut 2004;53(suppl IV):58–65.

75. McColl E. Best practice in symptom assessment: a review. Gut 2004;53(suppl IV):49–54.

76. Irvine EJ. Quality of life assessment in gastro-oesophageal reflux disease. Gut 2004;53(suppl IV): iv35–iv39.

77. Fernando HC, Aschauer PR, Rosenblatt M, et al. Quality of life after anti-reflux surgery compared with non-operative management of severe gastro-esophageal reflux disease. J Am Coll Surg 2002;194:23–27.

78. Velanovich V. Using quality-of-life measurements to predict patient satisfaction outcomes for anti-reflux surgery. Arch Surg 2004;139(6):621–625.

79. Irvine EJ. Quality of life assessment in gastro-oesophageal reflux disease. Gut 2004;53(suppl IV): 35–39.

4

Complications of GERD: Esophagitis, Stricture, Barrett's, and Cancer

John A. Bonino and Prateek Sharma

Gastroesophageal reflux disease (GERD) has become a very prevalent disorder in the United States and the Western hemisphere. It has been estimated that as many as 44% of adults in the United States experience GERD symptoms described as heartburn at least once a month.[1] In addition, as many as 10% of adults in the United States experience daily heartburn.[2] The true prevalence of reflux disease may be largely underestimated when taking into account "atypical" manifestations of the disease as well as those patients who self-medicate.[3,4] Unfortunately, many of these atypical manifestations often go unrecognized, and may take the form of ear-nose-throat, pulmonary, or laryngeal manifestations such as laryngitis, sinusitis, asthma, bronchitis, chronic cough, chest pain, and halitosis.[4] A study by Harding and colleagues[5] showed that among those patients studied with a diagnosis of asthma and who denied reflux symptoms, >29% had abnormal esophageal pH studies. Irwin and Richter,[6] when evaluating the causes of chronic cough, suggested that anywhere from 7 to 40% of cases of patients with chronic cough may be related to gastroesophageal reflux.

Although studies in subjects undergoing upper endoscopy demonstrated that between 30–70% of those with reflux symptoms demonstrate "nonerosive" disease, many others may experience a wide range of complications.[7,8] These complications may include erosive esophagitis, stricture, Barrett's esophagus, and esophageal neoplasia.

Erosive Esophagitis

Erosive esophagitis, or breaks in the esophageal mucosa, represents one of the common manifestations of chronic reflux disease. Histologically, erosive esophagitis is defined as superficial necrotic defects that do not penetrate the muscularis mucosae, whereas esophageal ulcerations are described by a deeper invasion through the muscularis mucosae and into the submucosa.[2] Several classifications have attempted to grade the severity of esophagitis as observed at the time of upper endoscopy. One such classification system, the Los Angeles classification (Table 4.1) grades the esophageal change from A to D, depending on the severity and extent of erosions determined during endoscopy.

Prevalence

Although the exact population prevalence of erosive esophagitis is not known, it is estimated to vary from 0.7 to 1.2% regardless of symptoms of heartburn.[9] This was recently demonstrated in a cross-sectional study performed to explore the complications of GERD in 11,691 patients undergoing endoscopic evaluation. Of these, esophagitis was diagnosed in 1633 patients, with an overall prevalence of 14% (61% men, 39% women).[10] However, in those patients with reflux symptoms, approximately 40–60% may have endoscopic evidence of esophageal

Table 4.1. Los Angeles classification of esophagitis.

Grade A	≥1 mucosal break confined to folds, no >5 mm
Grade B	≥1 mucosal break >5 mm confined to folds but not continuous between tops of folds
Grade C	Mucosal breaks that are NOT circumferential, but are continuous between the tops of two or more mucosal folds
Grade D	Circumferential mucosal breaks

erosions.[11] It is unclear if the prevalence of reflux symptoms and erosive esophagitis is increasing. Some studies have in fact noted a decrease in the frequency of erosive esophagitis. Todd and colleagues[12] reported results from an endoscopic database in Tayside, Scotland over a 15-year period. A significant decrease in the prevalence of esophagitis was discovered, contrasting sharply with an increase in the incidence of Barrett's esophagus during the same time interval.[12]

The prevalence of erosive esophagitis may also differ in various ethnic and racial populations indicating that host factors may have an important role in the pathogenesis of this complication of GERD. El-Serag and colleagues[13] reported the differences in gastroesophageal reflux between different racial groups in the United States and used logistical regression analysis (controlling for several variables) to find an association between various racial groups and GERD. Among 496 individuals who completed a GERD questionnaire, and 215 who had an endoscopy, the age-adjusted prevalence of heartburn was similar among all racial groups studied (whites, blacks, and hispanics). Of note, however, black patients had a significantly lower risk of esophagitis (adjusted odds ratio 0.22–0.46). Thus, although the prevalence of GERD symptoms may be similar between blacks and whites, blacks seem less likely to have endoscopic evidence of esophagitis.[13]

In another study, among a mix of 1985 Chinese, Malaysian, and Indian patients, only 6% had evidence of erosive esophagitis (majority with mild esophagitis). Males seemed to have a higher incidence of esophagitis compared with females, as did those of Indian decent and the presence of hiatal hernia also seemed to increase the chances of finding erosive esophagitis.[14] In a study from Taiwan, Yeh and colleagues[15] evaluated 464 patients with upper gastrointestinal symptoms and 66 (14.5%) of these patients were found to have erosive esophagitis. In addition, a male-to-female pre-ponderance of 3.1:1 was witnessed and disease severity was also found to increase with age, particularly in individuals in their 60s and 70s.[15]

Pathogenesis and Risk Factors

The pathological reflux of gastric and duodenal contents into the esophagus disrupts the normal protective environment. This refluxed material consists not only of acid and pepsin, but also bile and pancreatic juices which contribute to epithelial damage and possibly even to Barrett's metaplasia. The degree and extent of this damage is directly correlated with the type, timing, and duration of the refluxate, but inversely correlated with the speed of esophageal acid clearance and esophageal mucosal resistance.[16,17]

Much controversy surrounding the pathogenesis of erosive esophagitis centers around the concept of disease progression. It has been theorized by some investigators that erosive esophagitis represents a continuum to more complex gastroesophageal complications.[18] This continuum would include natural progression from nonerosive esophageal disease to erosive esophageal disease to Barrett's and possible esophageal adenocarcinoma.[18] Data to the contrary, however, exist as well. A group of 35,725 patients with erosive esophagitis were identified from a database, including some with concurrent ulcerations or strictures and had a follow-up of >4 years. In the group with esophagitis but without stricture or ulcers, no patient had disease progression or developed further esophageal complications.[19,20]

Collen and associates[20] have suggested that older individuals are at an increased risk for the development of erosive esophagitis. These investigators studied 228 consecutive patients with reflux symptoms who underwent upper endoscopy and reported that patients older than 60 years had increased risk for complications of chronic reflux such as erosive esophagitis, and that this risk increased with every decade of life above age 30.[21] A study by Johnson and

Fennerty[11] echoed this sentiment. Of 11,945 patients studied, only 12% of those <21 years were found to have erosive esophagitis, compared with 37% of those >70 years. It was also found that although heartburn was a good indicator for the presence of severe esophagitis in the elderly, they presented more often with respiratory symptoms or even dysphagia.[11]

Why do only some GERD patients develop erosive esophagitis whereas others do not? Although the exact reasons for this are unclear, a number of factors have been recently identified that may contribute to the development of erosive esophagitis. Most recently, investigators have focused on lower esophageal sphincter pressure, presence of a hiatal hernia, impaired esophageal clearance of refluxed material (decreased peristalsis), and presence of bile reflux, to name a few.[22] To date, there has not been a consistently observed difference in rates of esophagitis between males and females, although it seems that the risk may be slightly higher in males. Esophageal ulcerations have also been found to be more common in Caucasians than other races.[23] Investigators have questioned whether Western influences, particularly changes in diet and social habits, may have led to the increased incidence of reflux complications in the Asian subcontinent.

Symptoms

Although the majority of patients with erosive esophagitis experience typical symptoms of esophageal reflux (i.e., heartburn, regurgitation), symptoms do not seem to necessarily predict the presence of erosive esophagitis in GERD patients. A study by Sonnenberg and colleagues[24] revealed that duration, frequency, and severity of heartburn symptoms did not correlate with esophagitis. It was shown that, in fact, there was a large degree of overlap in the severity and frequency of symptoms between patients with erosive esophagitis and nonerosive reflux.[24]

Another study evaluated a total of 644 GERD outpatients who underwent an endoscopy, followed by esophageal manometry, and 24-hour pH monitoring. Analysis of resulting data suggested that there was no clear-cut association between the degree of acid reflux and the presence and severity of erosive esophagitis. In addition, the amount of upright or supine acid contact time, frequency of all or only long reflux episodes, and an overall summary score of pH-metry, did not correlate with the severity of erosive esophagitis.[25]

Treatment

Treatment of erosive esophagitis continues to center around the use of acid suppression therapy. Healing appears to be most apparent and successful with the use of proton pump inhibitors (PPIs), with patients treated up to 12 weeks. Chiba et al.[26] demonstrated healing rates approaching 85% [95% confidence interval (CI): 79.1–88.1%] with use of these medicines compared with approximately 52% (95% CI: 46.9–56.9%) with histamine antagonists. Healing rates, however, have largely been found to be dependent on the baseline grade of erosive esophagitis. In addition, Holtmann and colleagues[27] have also suggested that patients infected with Helicobacter pylori may actually have better response rates to PPIs in the treatment of erosive esophagitis. Maintenance of healing of erosive esophagitis is also helped by use of PPIs. A study by Lundell and colleagues,[28] among others, followed a group of patients with documented erosive esophagitis after being treated with daily omeprazole therapy. After completion of 8 weeks of PPI therapy, these patients were followed up to 6 months to monitor for relapse of erosive esophagitis. In the absence of acid suppression therapy, it was shown that it was possible for all grades of erosive esophagitis (Los Angeles grade A) to relapse.

Anti-reflux surgery can also be an option for the long-term treatment of erosive esophagitis in some patients. A study by Lundell and colleagues[29] randomized 155 patients to medical therapy (omeprazole) or surgical anti-reflux therapy. Over a 3-year follow-up period, 139 of the medically treated patients, and 129 of the surgically treated were evaluated and compared by symptomatology, 24-hour pH monitoring, and endoscopy. Of the surgically treated group, 97 remained in clinical remission, compared with 77 in the medically treated group (P = 0.0016); however, when dose adjustments were made in the medically treated group (i.e., increasing omeprazole dose), the failure rates between the two types of treatment were not significantly different.

Esophageal (Peptic) Stricture

Another well recognized complication of GERD is esophageal strictures (Figure 4.1). Unlike erosive esophagitis, which may present as a sole complication, strictures frequently are diagnosed along with other complications such as erosive esophagitis. The most common location of the strictures are in the distal esophagus, near the gastroesophageal junction.[23,30]

Pathogenesis and Prevalence

Strictures are complications of deep esophageal ulceration in which fibrous tissue and collagen formation laid down during repair of the ulcer site result in stricture formation.[23,30] Stricture formation, in the case of peptic strictures, is initiated by an insult to the esophageal epithelium (i.e., acid reflux). During the healing process, collagen and scar tissue production cause esophageal narrowing.[12] Unfortunately, as many as 10% of patients who seek medical attention for gastroesophageal reflux disease can have esophageal strictures.[31]

Risk Factors

Although gastroesophageal reflux is thought to contribute to a significant percentage of esophageal strictures (>70%), caustic ingestion,

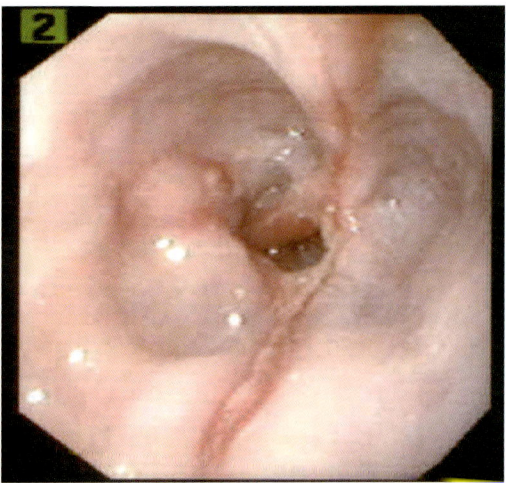

Figure 4.1. An endoscopic view of an esophageal stricture before dilation therapy.

radiation, and infectious esophagitis are other know etiologies to be considered in the appropriate setting.[30–32] As with erosive esophagitis, peptic strictures seem to be more common in men than women, and most prevalent in the sixth to seventh decades of life.[32–34] As would be expected, hiatal hernia seems to increase one's risk for esophageal stricture and hiatus hernia is found in as many as 85% of individuals with peptic esophageal stricture.[35]

Symptoms

Symptoms of esophageal stricture may vary, but typically consist of dysphagia for solid foods that slowly progresses over time.[23] Patients usually experience little to no weight loss as opposed to patients with malignant strictures. Odynophagia may also be present in a number of individuals with esophageal stricture. Although almost all patients present with dysphagia, a significant percentage may also have heartburn (approximately 70%) and regurgitation (approximately 40%).[36] In up to 25% of individuals with peptic strictures, heartburn symptoms may be absent, whereas in others, heartburn may actually resolve as the stricture progresses to the point of significant esophageal narrowing thereby limiting further reflux, and heartburn may actually recur after dilation.[23]

Treatment

Treatment of esophageal strictures centers around mechanical dilation of the involved lumen. Proton pump inhibitors are also used in these patients to heal esophagitis and to prevent relapse of the stricture. Most recently, studies have indicated that acid suppression therapy with PPIs not only improves dysphagia symptoms but also reduces the need for further esophageal dilation. Smith et al. showed that only 30% of patients required repeat stricture dilation if treated with omeprazole 20 mg daily compared with 46% treated with ranitidine 150 mg twice daily.[37,38] It is now standard practice to maintain individuals who have undergone dilation for peptic strictures on long-term PPIs to reduce the risk of recurrence. Of special mention is the importance of appropriate antibiotic prophylaxis in those individuals at high risk for endocarditis because esophageal dilation procedures for strictures may be associated with bacteremia in 11–45% of cases.[39,40]

Barrett's Esophagus

One of the most controversial and intriguing topics discussed with regard to the complications of chronic reflux is Barrett's esophagus. Barrett's esophagus is a metaplastic change in the esophagus that results in replacement of the normal squamous-lined epithelium with a columnar type. The definition of Barrett's esophagus has continued to evolve over time. During an American Gastroenterological Association workshop in February 2003 (Barrett's Esophagus Chicago Workshop), the definition for Barrett's esophagus was adopted as, "a displacement of the squamocolumnar junction proximal to the gastroesophageal junction with the presence of intestinal metaplasia"[41] (Figure 4.2). Given that intestinal metaplasia is the precursor lesion associated with adenocarcinoma, the goal of this definition was to adequately identify individuals at risk for adenocarcinoma.

Barrett's esophagus, first described in the early 20th century, is a well recognized risk factor for the development of esophageal ade-

nocarcinoma. The importance of this finding is realized when reviewing the increasing incidence of esophageal adenocarcinoma around the world over the past several years.[42,43]

Prevalence

The true prevalence of Barrett's esophagus in the general population is unknown. Several studies, however, quote prevalence rates of 0.9–15% in patients presenting for endoscopy for any indication (i.e., with and without GERD symptoms), whereas the prevalence of Barrett's esophagus in patients with chronic GERD has been reported to be 10–12%.[44–46] A more recent study of subjects who underwent colonoscopy and also agreed to have an upper endoscopy, found an 8.3% prevalence of Barrett's esophagus in individuals with heartburn, and 5.6% in those without heartburn.[47] Thus, the prevalence of Barrett's esophagus in the general population may be much higher than previously estimated.[46]

Pathogenesis and Risk Factors

The esophageal mucosal injury in patients with Barrett's esophagus likely begins with both

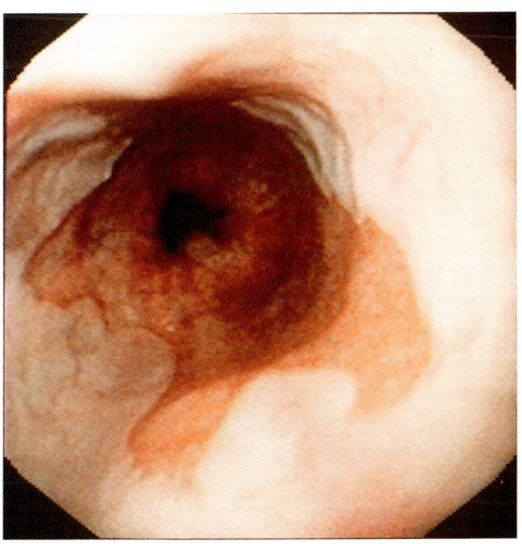 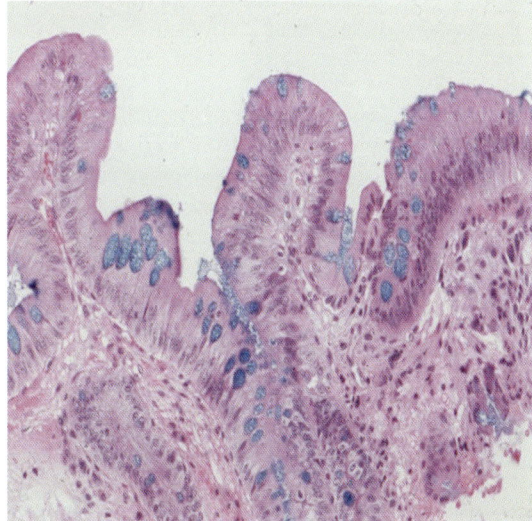

Figure 4.2. Left, Endoscopic evidence of intestinal metaplasia (Barrett's) in the distal segment of the esophagus. Right, A microscopic view of columnar metaplasia of the esophagus. (Reprinted from Sharma P. Recent advances in Barrett's esophagus: short-segment Barrett's esophagus and cardia intestinal metaplasia. Semin Gastrointest Dis 1999;10(3):93–102, Copyright 1999, with permission from Elsevier.)

genetic and environmental triggers that initiate pluripotent stem cells to undergo differentiation resulting in the proliferation of an altered phenotype, in this case intestinal metaplasia.[48] This metaplastic change is an acquired one and results from direct esophageal mucosal injury. In fact, individuals with Barrett's esophagus often have greater esophageal acid exposure based on 24-hour pH monitoring compared with GERD patients without Barrett's.[49] Gaining particular interest recently in the etiology of Barrett's metaplasia is the role of the composition of the refluxate, specifically bile reflux. Animal studies have shown that, although the esophageal mucosa is relatively resistant to reflux of acid alone, the combination of acid with pepsin results in significant mucosal injury.[16,50] In addition, conjugated bile acids, the predominant material in duodenal reflux, also produce esophageal damage at an acidic pH.[16,50] It is likely that important factors such as the composition of the refluxed matter itself, duration of reflux exposure, decreased lower esophageal sphincter tone, increased severity of reflux symptoms, and nighttime reflux symptoms, may increase an individual's risk of Barrett's development.[51] Other recognized risk factors include increasing age, male gender, and Caucasian race (Table 4.2).[3]

Investigators have hypothesized that, once exposure to refluxate occurs, the metaplastic change is secondary to alterations in pluripotent stem cells that are able to undergo a clonal expansion and thus maintain the "abnormal" mucosa.[48] It is also theorized that there must also be a genetic predisposition to this change, because only a small percentage of individuals with chronic gastroesophageal reflux undergo this change and develop Barrett's esophagus.

Table 4.2. Risk factors for development of Barrett's esophagus.

Chronic gastroesophageal reflux
Advanced age
White race
Male gender
Increasing duration of esophagea reflux symptoms
Hiatal hernia

Symptoms

There are no specific symptoms in patients with Barrett's esophagus; they are similar to those in GERD patients without Barrett's. Gerson and colleagues[52] investigated the use of a symptom questionnaire in an attempt to predict those patients with Barrett's esophagus. Symptoms such as heartburn, nocturnal chest pain, or odynophagia were found to be most predictive of Barrett's esophagus. It is also important to recognize, however, that some individuals with Barrett's esophagus may be asymptomatic and not experience any reflux symptoms.[46]

Surveillance

The goal of surveillance endoscopy in patients with Barrett's esophagus is to detect dysplasia and cancer at an early stage, and ultimately to reduce mortality from esophageal adenocarcinoma. To maximize the detection of dysplasia in patients with Barrett's esophagus, most clinicians obtain four quadrant biopsies every 1–2 cm of the endoscopically recognized area of Barrett's. Given that these biopsies are random in nature and sample only a small surface area of the Barrett's segment, a number of new techniques (e.g., magnification endoscopy, spectroscopy, and optical coherence tomography) are being evaluated to increase the yield of detecting dysplastic and cancerous tissue.[53–55] Although these technologies are not yet ready for routine clinical use, they likely will dramatically change how patients with Barrett's esophagus are surveyed in the future.

To date, there have been no prospective trials conducted in patients with Barrett's esophagus that show a survival advantage in those that have undergone endoscopic surveillance compared with those who have not. Several retrospective trials, however, have suggested lower mortality rates in patients enrolled in surveillance programs, indicating that individuals undergoing surveillance are more likely to have adenocarcinoma recognized at an earlier stage resulting in improved survival rates.[56–58] A recent publication described a cost-utility analysis of screening and surveillance for Barrett's esophagus and concluded that screening "high-risk" individuals with GERD symptoms, followed by surveillance of only those

Barrett's esophagus patients with dysplasia, would likely be cost effective.[58] Although current guidelines suggest that patients with Barrett's esophagus undergo surveillance endoscopy based on degree of dysplasia detected during endoscopic biopsy, a recent international workshop was unable to substantiate good evidence to support surveillance for all patients with Barrett's esophagus.[41]

Attempts at identifying a *high risk* group, those at increased risk of transformation of Barrett's esophagus to esophageal adenocarcinoma, perhaps through the use of biological markers of carcinogenesis, may increase the cost effectiveness of surveillance programs. p16 and p53 tumor suppression gene abnormalities (deletions) have generated much interest, and may have predictive utility.[58] Although early phase studies have been promising for p53 tumor suppressor status as a predictor of malignant transformation, there have not yet been good prospective studies confirming these data.

Medical Therapy

Treatment of patients with Barrett's esophagus includes eliminating symptoms of gastroesophageal reflux, and healing of erosive esophagitis and can be accomplished with acid suppressive therapy using PPIs. Some studies indicate, however, that symptomatic control with PPI therapy does not ensure normalization of esophageal pH in as many as 20–30% of patients with Barrett's esophagus.[59] The importance of esophageal reflux control has been proposed by other studies demonstrating that acid reflux predisposes to cellular proliferation by activation of protein kinase regulated pathways that disrupt apoptosis in cell lines exposed to acid.[60] Although there is evidence suggesting that symptom relief and healing of esophagitis can be achieved in patients with Barrett's esophagus, there is very little evidence that acid suppression results in regression of metaplasia or reduces the risk of dysplasia/cancer. The Chicago workshop also concluded that although PPI therapy was most effective in treating patients with Barrett's esophagus medically, neoplasia risk was not significantly altered.[41]

Anti-reflux Surgery

Surgical anti-reflux therapy may also be considered as an alternative to medical therapy in some individuals with Barrett's esophagus; these indications are similar to those in GERD patients without Barrett's esophagus. Although some studies in the surgical literature argue for histological regression in individuals after anti-reflux surgery, cases of high-grade dysplasia and cancer have been reported even after successful anti-reflux surgery. Most recently, a meta-analysis by Corey and colleagues[61] concluded that the risk of esophageal adenocarcinoma was not significantly decreased by surgical anti-reflux procedures.

Endoscopic Therapy

Endoscopic therapies for the treatment of Barrett's esophagus are a more recent, and still largely an investigational, mode of therapy. A variety of endoscopic ablative therapies including thermal, chemical, and mechanical methods have been applied in patients with both dysplastic and nondysplastic Barrett's esophagus. Although the majority of the area of Barrett's esophagus can be replaced by neo-squamous mucosa, persistent metaplastic tissue is often detected underlying the squamous tissue and cases of adenocarcinoma have been reported after "successful" ablation therapy.[62] Other side effects include stricture formation and perforation. Given the low risk of cancer in patients with nondysplastic Barrett's esophagus or even with low-grade dysplasia, endoscopic ablation treatments should not be used outside of study protocols in these patients. In patients with high-grade dyplasia, however, the risk of progression to cancer can be as high as 25–37%.[62] In these patients, aggressive surveillance, early surgical resection, or endoscopic ablation may be considered. A recent randomized trial on the use of photodynamic therapy (PDT) has lent further evidence to this argument. Ackroyd and colleagues[63] followed 36 patients with dysplastic Barrett's who were receiving omeprazole therapy and randomized them to receive PDT or placebo. No dysplasia was found in those treated with PDT compared to 12 (67%) in the placebo arm (p < 0.001). Local endoscopic therapy is thus an advent in the treatment of esophageal neoplasia, and is associated with low morbidity and mortality.

Esophageal Adenocarcinoma

The incidence of esophageal adenocarcinomas has risen rapidly in the United States and western Europe and is now the predominant form of esophageal cancer in these countries.[65,66] The incidence of esophageal adenocarcinoma, in fact, has increased >400% for white males in the United States since the 1970s. It is more common in males than females, with a ratio approaching 3:1.[65,66]

Incidence

The incidence of esophageal adenocarcinoma has increased from 0.4 to 0.7 cases per 100,000 in males in 1975, to 3.2 per 100,000 in 1995.[65,66] Unfortunately, by the time these cancers are diagnosed, they are often incurable; the median survival is 2 years and fewer than 10% survive 5 years. The lifetime risk of developing esophageal cancer ranges from 0.26% for women to 0.33% for men.[65,66] It is estimated that the overall incidence of adenocarcinoma has increased >300% the past 40 years.[42] Although the relative risk of developing adenocarcinoma is increased in patients with Barrett's esophagus, the absolute risk remains low with an annual risk of approximately 0.5%.[67]

Pathogenesis

The evolution of Barrett's esophagus to dysplasia and esophageal adenocarcinoma is proposed to arise from a combination of underlying predilection and specific mutations. Although it is possible for adenocarcinoma to develop without Barrett's esophagus, the majority of these cancer cases are associated with Barrett's esophagus. A clonal evolution is believed to occur early in Barrett's metaplasia following mutations likely as a result of recurrent injury from chronic reflux and a selective survival advantage is gained by this new line of "mutated" cells. The three abnormalities that have been described in Barrett's cells during this clonal evolution include chromosomal aberrations, mutations, and loss of function of a tumor

suppression gene.[68] Loss of heterozygosity is believed to be the single most common mechanism of genetic change in the development of neoplasia. This loss of heterozygosity results in a loss of genetic regions from various chromosomes which may result in loss of regulation of the cell cycle. The loss of suppressor genes (p53 and p16) allows genetically abnormal cells to divide and proliferate, setting the stage for further dysplastic evolution.[68,69]

Experimental studies have demonstrated that exposing cultured intestinal metaplasia to acid for an extended period of time results in an increase in proliferation and expression of proteins inhibiting cell death. One of the antiapoptotic proteins under recent investigation has been cyclooxygenase-2 (COX-2). Cyclooxygenase-2 is induced by cell injury and leads to increased production of prostaglandin E_2.[68] This prostaglandin is known to affect apoptosis, and has generated interest in evaluating COX-2 inhibitors as potential chemopreventive agents. This interest has been further nurtured by recent epidemiological studies showing the possible chemoprotective effects of COX-2 inhibitors in other gastrointestinal malignancies.

Risk Factors

There is a strong and probable causal relationship between GERD symptoms and esophageal adenocarcinoma. A case control study from Sweden showed that among individuals with recurrent symptoms of reflux, the odds ratios were 7.7 for esophageal adenocarcinoma (95% CI: 5.3–11.4).[70] It was also shown that the more frequent, and more severe the symptoms of reflux, the more pronounced the risk of adenocarcinoma.[70] Although Barrett's esophagus is the most widely accepted risk factor for adenocarcinoma, other risk factors exist as well such as tobacco use, increasing age, male gender, diets high in fats and low in fruits and vegetables, and obesity. A recent population-based study showed a strong correlation between increased body mass index (BMI) and esophageal adenocarcinoma; individuals in the highest quarter of BMIs measure had an adjusted odds ratio 7.6 (95% CI: 3.08–15.2) compared with those with the lowest BMIs.[71]

Symptoms

Unfortunately, most individuals with esophageal adenocarcinoma do not present until late in the course of their malignancy. The majority of the patients with adenocarcinoma experience dysphagia, followed by weight loss. Others may present with occult or frank gastrointestinal bleeding or anemia. Lymphadenopathy (Virchow's node), organomegaly, and pleural effusion may be indicators of metastatic spread from primary esophageal malignancy.[72]

Treatment

In the event of a diagnosis of esophageal malignancy, appropriate staging is essential, not only for determining the prognosis, but also for deciding upon appropriate therapy. Current methods of staging follow the TNM classification system. Endoscopy, computed tomography scans, and endoscopic ultrasound are often used to assist in this staging process. Endoscopy allows biopsy and cytological determination to confirm the diagnosis, whereas computed tomography scan and endoscopic ultrasound help in determining the degree of esophageal wall invasion and the presence or absence of metastatic disease.

In general, >50% of patients presenting with esophageal adenocarcinoma have unresectable or metastatic disease at the time of diagnosis, making isolated therapy unlikely.[72] Although localized esophageal cancers may be treated with surgical resection, most likely a combined approach at therapy is effective in most cases. Current approaches often combine preoperative radiotherapy and fluorouracil/cisplatin for maximizing surgical resectability and palliation of symptoms. A survival benefit, however, has not been shown compared with previous therapies when comparing this combination approach. Some use radiotherapy as an alternative to surgical resection in poor surgical candidates, although this seems not to be as effective as other palliative measures such as endoscopic treatment or surgery for symptoms of esophageal obstruction. Additional endoscopic therapies, including expandable stent placement, PDT, and laser are other alterntives.

Given the high rate of mortality and morbidity for early neoplasia in Barrett's esophagus, many investigators have searched for alternatives to radical esophageal resection.[73] Although surgery remains the gold standard for early adenocarcinoma, local therapy with PDT or endoscopic mucosal resection are other options to consider. For patients whose neoplastic lesion is localized to the epithelial layer, lymph node metastasis is unlikely and these patients may be potential candidates for the use of endoscopic therapy.[73] These therapies may replace the columnar metaplastic cells with the native squamous type, but controversy remains on whether this change is permanent, or if the new squamous mucosa just masks deeper areas of metaplasia.[62]

Summary

Esophagitis and esophageal strictures continue to complicate the course of many individuals with reflux symptoms. Much headway has been made, however, with the use of PPIs or antireflux surgery in the acute and maintenance treatment of these conditions. Barrett's esophagus remains a perplexing problem for many clinicians. What is the exact risk of malignant transformation? What interval is appropriate for surveillance of patients with this premalignant stage, and how and when do we treat? A better identification of specific clinical and genetic risk factors for malignant transformation is essential for making surveillance a cost-effective and appropriate way of following these patients. The emergence of more advanced endoscopic therapies may eventually modify the treatment algorithm for individuals with localized intraepithelial neoplasia. Cyclooxygenase-2 inhibition also seems to offer hope for agents that may reduce the risk of progression in individuals with Barrett's esophagus but randomized controlled trials are lacking.

The high prevalence of GERD, yet surprisingly low incidence of Barrett's esophagus and esophageal adenocarcinoma, would suggest that many factors contribute to the progression of reflux to Barrett's to malignancy. Only after a better identification of these factors will more effective treatments aimed at reducing disease progression be realized.

References

1. Shaheen N, Provenzale D. The epidemiology of gastroesophageal reflux disease. Am J MedSci 2003;326(5):264–273.
2. Castell DO, Tutuian R. Barrett's esophagus prevalence and epidemiology. Gastrointest Endosc Clin N Am 2003; 13:227–232.
3. Napierkowski J, Wong RK. Extraesophageal manifestations of GERD. Am J Med Sci 2003;326(5):285–293.
4. Vaezi MF. Extraesophageal manifestations of gastroesophageal reflux disease. Clin Cornerstone 2003;5(4): 32–40.
5. Harding SM, Guzzo MR, Richter JE. The Prevalence of gastroesophageal reflux in asthma patients without reflux symptoms. Am J Respir Crit Care Med 2000;162(1): 34–39.
6. Irwin RS, Richter JE. Gastroesophageal reflux and chronic cough. Am J Gastroenterol 2000;95(8):S9–S14.
7. Voutilainen M, Sipponen P, Mecklin JP, et al. Gastroesophageal reflux disease: prevalence, clinical, endoscopic and histopathological findings in 1,128 consecutive patients referred for endoscopy due to dyspeptic and reflux symptoms. Digestion 2000;61: 6–13.
8. Johansson KE, Ask P, Boeryd B, et al. Oesophagitis, signs of reflux, and gastric acid secretion in patients with symptoms of gastro-oesophageal reflux disease. Scand J Gastroenerol 1986;21:837–847.
9. Johanson JF. Epidemiology of esophageal and supraesophageal reflux injuries. Am J Med 2000;108(suppl 4a): 99S–103S.
10. Loffeld RJLF, van der Putten ABMM. Rising incidence of reflux oesophagitis in patients undergoing upper gastrointestinal endoscopy. Digestion 2003;68:141–144.
11. Johnson DA, Fennerty MB. Heartburn severity underestimates erosive esophagitis severity in elderly patients with gastroesophageal reflux disease. Gastroenterology 2004;126(3):660–664.
12. Todd JA, Johnston DA, Dillon JF. The changing spectrum of gastroesophageal reflux disease. Eur J Cancer Prev 2002;11(3):215–219.
13. El-Serag HB, Mason AC, Petersen N, Key CR. Epidemiological differences between adenocarcinoma of the oesophagus and adenocarcinoma of the gastric cardia in the USA. Gut 2002;50:368–372.
14. Rajendra S, Kutty K, Karim KN. Ethnic differences in the prevalence of endoscopic esophagitis and Barrett's esophagus: the long and short of it all. Dig Dis Sci 2004; 49(2):237–242.
15. Yeh C, Hsu CT, Ho AS, Sampliner RE, Fass R. Erosive esophagitis and Barrett's esophagus in Taiwan: a higher frequency than expected. Dig Dis Sci 1997; 42(4):702–706.
16. Vaezi MF, Richter MF. Role of acid and duodenogastroesophageal reflux in gastroesophageal reflux disease. Gastroenterology 1996;111:1192–1199.
17. Kahrilas PJ. GERD pathogenesis, pathophysiology, and clinical manifestations. Cleve Clin J Med 2003; 70(5):S4–S19.
18. Pace F, Porro GB. Gastroesophageal reflux disease: a typical spectrum of disease (a new conceptual framework is not needed). Am J Gastroenterol 2004;99(5): 946–949.
19. El-Serag HB, Sonnenberg A. Outcome of erosive reflux esophagitis after Nissen fundoplication. Am J Gastroenterol 1999;94(7):1771–1776.
20. Fass R, Ofman JJ. Gastroesophageal reflux disease: should we adopt a new conceptual framework? 2002;97(8):1901–1909.
21. Collen MJ, Abdulian JD, Chen YK. Gastroesophageal reflux disease in the elderly: more severe disease that requires aggressive therapy. Am J Gastroenterol 1995; 90(7):1053–1057.
22. Fennerty MB. The continuum of GERD complications. Cleve Clin J Med 2003;70(5):S33–S50.
23. Kuo W, Kalloo A. Reflux strictures of the esophagus. Gastrointest Endosc Clin N Am 1998;8:273–281.
24. Sonnenberg A, Avidan B, Schnell TG, Sontag SJ. Acid reflux is a poor predictor for severity of erosive reflux esophagitis. Dig Dis Sci 2002;47(11):2565–2573.
25. Venables TL, Newland RD, Patel AC, Hole J, Wilcock C, Turbitt ML. Omeprazole 10 milligrams once daily, omeprazole 20 milligrams once daily, or ranitidine 150 mg twice daily, evaluated as initial therapy for the relief of symptoms of gastro-oesophageal reflux disease in general practice. Scand J Gastroenterol 1997;32(10): 965–973.
26. Chiba N, De Gara CJ, Wilkinson JM, Hunt RH. Speed of healing and symptom relief in grade II to IV gastroesophageal reflux disease: a meta-analysis. Gastroenterology 1997;112(6):1798–1810.
27. Holtmann G, Cain C, Malfertheiner P. Gastric Helicobacter pylori infection accelerates healing of reflux esophagitis during treatment with the proton pump inhibitor pantoprazole. Gastroenterology 1999; 117(1):11–16.
28. Lundell LR, Dent J, Bennett JR, et al. Endoscopic assessment of oesophagitis: clinical and functional correlates and further validation of the Los Angeles classification. Gut 1999;45:172–180.
29. Lundell L, Miettinen P, Myrvold HE, et al. Long-term management of gastro-oesophageal reflux disease with omeprazole or open anti-reflux surgery: results of a prospective, randomized clinical trial. The Nordic GORD Study Group. Eur J Gastroenterol Hepatol 2000; 12(8):879–887.
30. Richter JE. Peptic strictures of the esophagus. Gastroenterol Clin N Am 1999;28:875–891.
31. Marks RD, Shukla M. Diagnosis and management of peptic esophageal strictures. Gastroenterologist 1996;4: 223–237.
32. El-Serag HB, Sonnenber A. Associations between different forms of gastro-oesophageal reflux disease. Gut 1997; 41:594–599.
33. Johanson JF. Epidemiology of esophageal and supraesophageal reflux injuries. Am J Med 2000;108(suppl 4a): 99S–103S.
34. Locke RG. Can symptoms predict endoscopic findings in GERD? Gastrointest Endosc 2003;58(5):661–670.
35. Berstad A, Weberg R, Froyshov Larsen I, et al. Relationship of hiatus hernia to reflux oesophagitis. A prospective study of coincidence, using endoscopy. Scand J Gastroenterol 1986;21(1):55–58.
36. Mazzadi SA, Garcia AO, Salis GB, Chiocca JC. Peptic esophageal stricture: a report from Argentina. Dis Esophagus 2004;17(1):63–66.
37. Spechler SJ. AGA technical review on treatment of patients with dysphagia caused by benign disorders

of the distal esophagus. Gastroenterology 1999;117: 233–254.

38. Smith PM, Kerr GD, Cockel R, et al. A comparison of omeprazole and ranitidine in the prevention of recurrence of benign esophageal stricture. Gastroenterology 1994;107:1312–1318.

39. Nelson DB, Sanderson SJ, Azar MM. Bacteremia with esophageal dilation. Gastrointest Endosc 1998;48:563–567.

40. Botoman VA, Surawicz CM. Bacteremia with gastrointestinal endoscopic procedures. Gastrointest Endosc 1986;33:342–346.

41. Sharma P, McQuaid K, Dent J, Fennerty MB, et al. A critical review of the diagnosis and management of Barrett's esophagus: the AGA Chicago Workshop. Gastroenterology 2004;127(1):310–330.

42. Shaheen NJ, Crosby MA, Bozymski EM, Sandler RS. Is there publication bias in the reporting of cancer risk in Barrett's esophagus? Gastroenterology 2000;119: 333–338.

43. Shaheen N, Ransohoff DF. Gastroesophageal reflux, Barrett esophagus, and esophageal cancer. Scientific review. JAMA 2002;287(15):1972–1979.

44. Koop H. Gastroesophageal reflux disease and Barrett's esophagus. Endoscopy 204;36:103–109.

45. Conio M, Cameron AJ, Romero Y, et at. Secular trends in the epidemiology and outcome of Barrett's oesophagus in Olmsted County, Minnesota. Gut 2001;48:308–309.

46. Rex DK, Cummings OW, Shaw M, et al. Screening for Barrett's esophagus in colonoscopy patients with and without heartburn. Gastroenterology 2003;125: 1670–1677.

47. Sharma P, Sidorenko EI. Are screening and surveillance for Barrett's oesophagus really worthwhile? Gut 2005; 54(suppl 1):i27–i32.

48. Fitzgerald RC, Farthing MJG. The pathogenesis of Barrett's esophagus. Gastrointest Endosc Clin N Am 2003;13(2):233–255.

49. Neumann CS, Cooper BT. 24 Hour ambulatory oesophageal pH monitoring in uncomplicated Barrett's oesophagus. Gut 1994;35:1352–1355.

50. Champion G, Richter JE, Vaezi MF. Duodenogastroesophageal reflux: relationship to pH and importance in Barrett's esophagus. Gastroenterology 1994;107(3): 747–754.

51. Lagergren J, Bergstrom R, Lindgren A, Nyren O. Symptomatic gastroesophageal reflux as a risk factor for esophageal adenocarcinoma. N Engl J Med 1999;340: 825–831.

52. Gerson LB, Edson R, Lavori PW, Triadafilopoulos G. Use of a simple symptom questionnaire to predict Barrett's esophagus in patients with symptoms of gastroesophageal reflux. Am J Gastroenterol 2001;96: 2005–2011.

53. Connor MJ, Sharma P. Chromoendoscopy and magnification endoscopy in Barrett's esophagus. Gastrointest Endosc Clin N Am 2003;13(2):269–277.

54. Richter JE. Duodenogastric reflux-induced esophagitis. Curr Treat Options Gastroenterol 2004;7:53–58.

55. Wong Kee Song LM, Marcon NE. Fluorescence and Raman spectroscopy. Gastrointest Endosc Clin N Am 2003;13(2):279–296.

56. Poneros JM, Nishioka NS. Diagnosis of Barrett's esophagus using optical coherence tomography. Gastrointest Endosc Clin N Am 2003;13(2):309–323.

57. Streitz JM Jr, Andrews CW Jr, Ellis FH Jr. Endoscopic surveillance of Barrett's esophagus. Does it help? J Thorac Cardiovasc Surg 1993;105:383–388.

58. Peters JH, Clark GWB, Ireland AP, et al. Outcome of adenocarcinoma arising in Barrett's esophagus in endoscopically surveyed and nonsurveyed patients. J Gen Thorac Surg 1994;108:813–821.

59. Reid BJ, Blount PL, Rabinovitch PS. Biomarkers in Barrett's esophagus. Gastrointest Endosc Clin N Am 2003;13:369–397.

60. Ouatu-Lascar R, Triadafilopoulos G. Complete elimination of reflux symptoms does not guarantee normalization of intraesophageal acid reflux in patient's with Barrett's esophagus. Am J Gastroenterol 1998; 93(5):711–716.

61. Souza RF, Shewmake K, Terada LS, Spechler SJ. Acid exposure activates the mitogen-activated protein kinase pathways in Barrett's esophagus. Gastroenterology 2002;122:299–307.

62. Corey KE, Schmitz SM, Shaheen NJ. Does a surgical anti-reflux procedure decrease the incidence of esophageal adenocarcinoma in Barrett's esophagus: a meta-analysis. Am J Gastroenterol 2003;98(11): 2310–2314.

63. Photodynamic therapy for dysplastic Barrett's oesophagus: a prospective, double blind, randomised, placebo controlled trial. Gut 2000;47:612–617.

64. Booger JV, Hillegersberg RV, Siersema PD, de Bruin RWF, Tilanus HW. Endoscopic ablation therapy for Barrett's esophagus with high-grade dysplasia: a review. Am J Gastroenterol 1999;94:1153–1158.

65. Sampliner RE and The Practice Parameters Committee of the American College of Gastroenterology. Updated guidelines on the diagnosis, surveillance, and therapy of Barrett's esophagus. Am J Gastroenterol 2002;97: 1888–1895.

66. Shaheen NJ, Wei JT. Epidemiology of esophageal adenocarcinoma. In press.

67. Blot WJ, Devesa SS, Kneller RW, et al. Rising incidence of adenocarcinoma of the esophagus and gastric cardia. JAMA 1991;265:1287–1289.

68. Shaheen NJ, Crosby MA, Bozymski EM, Sandler RS. Is there publication bias in the reporting of cancer risk in Barrett's esophagus? Gastroenterology 2000; 119(2):333–338.

69. Fitzgerald RC, Farthing MJ. The pathogenesis of Barrett's esophagus. Gastrointest Endosc Clin N Am 2003;13:233–255.

70. Reid BJ, Blount PL, Rabinovitch PS. Biomarkers in Barrett's esophagus. Gastrointest Endosc Clin N Am 2003;13:369–397.

71. Lagergren J, Bergstrom R, Lindgren A, Nyren O. Symptomatic gastroesophageal reflux as a risk factor for esophageal adenocarcinoma. N Engl J Med 1999; 340(11):825–831.

72. Lagergren J, Bergstrom R, Nyren O. Association between body mass and adenocarcinoma of the esophagus and gastric cardia. Ann Intern Med 1999;130(11):883–890.

73. Enzinger PC, Mayer RJ. Esophageal cancer. N Engl J Med 2003;349(23):2241–2252.

74. Pech O, May A, Gossner L, et al. Barrett's esophagus: endoscopic resection. Gastrointest Endosc Clin N Am 2003;13(3):505–512.

5

Principles of Successful Surgical Anti-Reflux Procedures

Federico Cuenca-Abente, Brant K. Oelschlager, and Carlos A. Pellegrini

Gastroesophageal reflux disease (GERD) is the most common gastrointestinal disorder in the United States. Although lifestyle changes and medical therapy are the most common forms of therapy, with the advent of laparoscopy, more patients are choosing surgical therapy not only to treat the failures of medical therapy, but as an alternative to it. Surgeons must, therefore, be familiar with the principles of patient selection and with the techniques used to treat this disease.

This chapter discusses the indications (and contraindications) and the work-up of patients suspected of having GERD and consulting for it, and the technique of anti-reflux procedures.

Indications

One of the keys to a good outcome is that the surgical candidate be well selected. The indications are primarily based on two principles: chronicity and severity of GERD in the context of complications and patient preference.[1] As a result, the indications can range from a patient who desires to discontinue antiacid medication[1] to patients with recalcitrant complications (e.g., peptic stricture) despite maximal medical and lifestyle modification. Some of the more common scenarios that involve patients with GERD seeking surgical therapy include the following.

Averse to Lifestyle Changes

To achieve maximum benefit from medical therapy, patients must make certain lifestyle modifications (changes in diet and eating habits, elevation of the head of the bed). These changes are intolerable for some patients, especially young active ones, and thus lead them to seek surgical therapy. In these types of situations, failure of medical therapy is defined by the patient.[1]

Poor Response to Proton Pump Inhibitors

Failure of modern medical treatment to relieve at least some of the patient's symptomatology is one of the most common reasons for surgical referral. Yet, this is described as a poor predictive factor of favorable surgical outcomes.[2] It is important to differentiate from this group those patients who, in fact, initially had a good response to proton pump inhibitors (PPIs) but for whom, over time, the effect of the medication decreased, leading the patient to increase the dose of medication and identifying the disease as being refractory to it. Patients that have never responded to medications, especially those with symptoms not classically associated with GERD such as abdominal pain, bloating, and nausea, are unlikely to benefit from an operation as much as those who initially responded well. Many of these patients may not even have GERD. Extensive testing, even sometimes repeat pH monitoring while the patient is taking medications, may help identify which patients are more likely to respond to surgery.

Patients with Airway Manifestations of GERD

Patients with GERD and related airway symptoms represent a significant management challenge. When compared with patients with typical symptoms, medical therapy is more often ineffective, making surgery a more attractive alternative for these patients.[3] The greater problem is that there is no current diagnostic test to conclusively link GERD and airway symptoms. The gold standard, 24-hour pH monitoring, is helpful, but reflux, although present, may not be the cause of the symptoms. Furthermore, abnormal reflux may be "caused" by pulmonary diseases such as asthma.[4]

Patients with Barrett's Esophagus

Patients with Barrett's esophagus generally have more severe GERD, and thus often seek surgery to relieve symptoms. Surgical therapy is very effective, in our experience, at relieving reflux symptoms,[5] although others have shown slightly less favorable results.[6] We believe that if a technically good operation is performed, excellent results can be obtained in this population.

Moreover, recent data support the fact that Barrett's esophagus regresses after an anti-reflux procedure. Indeed, we reported regression in >50% of patients with short segment (<3 cm) Barrett's esophagus.[5] Hofstetter et al.[7] also reported regression from low-grade dysplasia to nondysplastic Barrett's esophagus in 44% of their patients, and regression of intestinal metaplasia to cardiac mucosa in 14% of cases. Finally, Bowers et al.[8] reported a regression rate of 59% of patients with short segment Barrett's esophagus. For these reasons, surgical therapy should be strongly considered for Barrett's esophagus, especially for young patients with symptomatic reflux.

Contraindications

Morbid Obesity

There is evidence that morbid obesity (body mass index >40) is associated with a higher failure rate, and thus, the presence of marked obesity represents a relative contraindication.[1] Furthermore, there is evidence that a Roux-en-Y gastric bypass provides excellent relief of GERD[9] as well as the health benefits of weight loss. We therefore recommend this approach to morbidly obese patients with severe GERD.[10]

Severe Comorbidities

Anesthetic and perioperative risk due to other medical comorbidities is another relative contraindication. Patient age, in a population-based cohort study, has been shown to be an independent predictor of mortality.[11] The severity of GERD and GERD-related complications should be considered in light of the patient's age and overall risk factors when deciding about the appropriateness of surgical therapy.

Preoperative Evaluation

For a practical description of the preoperative evaluation, we can divide patients into those with typical symptoms (heartburn and regurgitation) and those with atypical ones (airway symptoms, chest pain, etc.). For both groups, we believe an adequate work-up should include upper endoscopy (EGD), manometry, 24-hour esophageal pH monitoring, and upper gastrointestinal series. For those with atypical or airway symptoms, esophageal/pharyngeal pH monitoring and laryngoscopy appear as useful adjunctive tools that help link these manifestations with GERD. Esophageal impedance is becoming recognized as a useful tool to evaluate these patients.

Flexible Endoscopy (EGD)

This test gives the best information regarding the internal anatomy of the foregut. The contour of the cardia has good correlation with its competency as an anti-reflux valve, and is especially important in evaluating the competency in the postoperative setting.[12] Complications of reflux, such as esophagitis and intestinal metaplasia, are diagnosed with endoscopy and can be biopsied appropriately. Endoscopy may identify unexpected findings that may change the surgical strategy, such as unsuspected pathology in the esophagus, stomach, and duodenum. The endoscopic view can also detect the presence of a hiatal or paraesophageal hernia and evaluate the patency of the gastroesophageal valve. Thus, in many instances, it helps to define the severity of the disease as well as the anatomy, both of which have an important role in planning the operation.

Manometry

Esophageal manometry evaluates the peristaltic mechanism of the esophageal body (amplitude and character of peristaltic waves) and the pressure, location, and relaxation of the lower esophageal sphincter (LES). In the past, the results of manometry were used by many surgeons to "tailor" the subsequent fundoplication. Specifically, patients with impaired peristalsis underwent a partial fundoplication, such as a Toupet procedure. We have shown that most patients with defective esophageal peristalsis respond well to a Nissen fundoplication and do not develop postoperative dysphagia.[13] Therefore, we recommend this as the treatment of choice except for those with essentially an aperistaltic esophagus.[13] Others have confirmed our results and these recommendations are becoming accepted by more groups.[14]

Likewise, the finding of other motility disorders such as hypercontractile esophagus (distal esophageal amplitudes >180 mm Hg) and hypertensive LES (>45 mm Hg) in the setting of GERD should not dissuade the surgeon from performing an anti-reflux procedure if the patient's clinical presentation is of GERD (heartburn or regurgitation) and not of a primary motility disorder (dysphagia or chest pain).[15]

Twenty-four-hour pH Esophageal Monitoring

This is the gold standard for the detection and quantification of GERD. At the University of Washington, we, as a matter of routine, simultaneously evaluate both the proximal and distal esophageal acid exposure. Normal pH monitoring should prompt a thorough work-up to rule out other etiologies, because these patients have an inferior result with surgical therapy. This test can also be used to correlate reflux episodes with symptom events, often serving as a confirmation of the clinical association. Finally,

preoperative pH monitoring serves as a baseline by which to compare studies should the patient have recurrent or persistent symptoms after an anti-reflux procedure.[1]

Upper Gastrointestinal Series

This test gives information regarding the anatomy of the esophagus and stomach, as well as the relation between these structures and the hiatus. It may detect a short esophagus, strictures, or a hiatal or paraesophageal hernia, each of which may affect the surgical strategy. The detection of spontaneous reflux during this test usually correlates with abnormal reflux. In general, this test is reserved for those patients in whom an operation is being planned.

Twenty-four-hour Esophageal and Pharyngeal pH Monitoring

We have used pharyngeal pH monitoring to detect acid in the pharynx as an effective proxy for microaspiration.[3,4] The detection of abnormal amounts of pharyngeal reflux (more than one pharyngeal reflux event in 24 hours) is a better predictor of successful medical and surgical therapy than is esophageal pH monitoring.[16,18] Although the positive predictive value of the test is quite good, many patients with reflux-associated respiratory symptoms will have a normal pharyngeal environment during the study period.

Laryngoscopy

Similar to endoscopy of the esophagus, laryngoscopy can identify injury to the larynx caused by acid. Typical findings include erythema, ulcers, swelling, nodules, etc. Unfortunately, these seem to be general markers of injury, and none of these lesions are specific for reflux.[19] Nevertheless, it remains an important test in the evaluation of patients with possible reflux laryngitis.

Impedance

This technology has recently garnered interest in the work-up of patients with GERD. Impedance is the measure of electrical resistance between two electrodes. When multiple pairs of electrodes are placed on a catheter within the esophagus, it is possible to detect the presence of any kind of material within the esophageal lumen and the direction of movement of the material (oral or aboral) can be determined. Thus, impedance has potential to diagnose acid and nonacid reflux as well as esophageal motility disorders. Refluxed material with a pH >4 currently goes undetected when using 24-hour pH monitoring only, yet it may have a significant role in the pathogenesis of GERD, particularly in those patients with poor response to antacid medications, Barrett's esophagus, and respiratory symptoms. Impedance electrodes can also be attached to a pH catheter, thus detecting all episodes of acid and nonacid reflux.

Impedance can also be helpful in the detection of motor disorders. Electrodes added to an otherwise standard manometry catheter can accurately measure the transit of material through the esophagus and determine the clearance of a swallowed bolus, thus providing additional information about the presence of an intrinsic esophageal motility problem. This may ultimately tell us what manometry alone does not: which patients should/should not undergo a complete fundoplication.

Surgical Technique—Nissen Fundoplication

Basic Tenants of Anti-Reflux Procedures

The anti-reflux mechanism is a complex combination of anatomic factors that, if disrupted, may lead to abnormal gastroesophageal reflux. They include: 1) the intrinsic muscle function of the LES; 2) the intraabdominal position of the LES; and 3) the integrity of the collar sling fibers that maintain the angle of His. An effective anti-reflux procedure should address this anatomy, so that the anti-reflux valve is restored to competency.

Several anti-reflux operations have been described (Nissen, Toupet, Hill, Dor, Belsey Mark IV). Although clinical success rates vary among the procedures, all conform to basic principles of successful anti-reflux surgery. These include: 1) establishment of an adequate intraabdominal length of esophagus; 2) appropriate crural closure; 3) anchoring of the esophagogastric junction in the abdomen; and 4) reestablishment of an acute angle of His. Jobe and colleagues[20] recently described the endoscopic characteristics of various fundoplications, and how they adhered to these principles.

Relative Advantages of Different Fundoplications

Nissen fundoplication. This is the most commonly performed fundoplication worldwide. It requires at least 3 cm of intraabdominal esophagus for its creation. It creates a symmetric nipple effect of the cardia. This serves to both augment the intrinsic function of the LES (both increasing resting pressure and decreasing transient relaxation) and recreate the angle of His. Closure of the hiatus by approximating the crura is essential to prevent a recurrent hernia, which can change these anatomic relationships. The Nissen fundoplication is the most commonly performed procedure because it is the easiest to reproduce and adheres to all the principles of an effective anti-reflux procedure.

Collis-Nissen fundoplication. This procedure is used primarily for patients in whom an adequate length of intraabdominal esophagus cannot be obtained. In this case, a neoesophagus is created from the cardia by stapling from the angle of His parallel to the lesser gastric curvature, making a tubular extension of the esophagus along the lesser curve of the stomach. A Nissen is then created around the neoesophagus. In theory, this attempts to adhere to all the principles of a Nissen fundoplication. In practice, the staple line and neoesophagus do not allow for the creation of symmetric valve and nipple effect. This, and presence of acid-secreting cells above the fundoplication, cause it to be inferior to a standard Nissen anti-reflux procedure. However, when a short esophagus exists, it may be the best way to preserve the esophagus and still permit an intraabdominal fundoplication.

Toupet fundoplication. This is the most common "partial" fundoplication performed currently. It is a posterior, approximately 270°, fundoplication. Some surgeons use this procedure routinely, but most use it for patients with impaired esophageal motility. Because it is less than a 360° fundoplication, it does not augment the LES to the degree that a Nissen does, and as a result it generally has less control of reflux than a Nissen. We have abandoned this procedure for most patients, because we found in patients with impaired peristalsis, a Nissen provided better control of GERD without increasing the incidence of dysphagia.[13]

Dor fundoplication. This is an anterior 180° fundoplication. It does not require as much esophageal length, nor does it augment the LES or accentuate the angle of His as much the other fundoplications described. As such, it is rarely used as a primary anti-reflux procedure, and is most often used after a myotomy for achalasia.

Hill fundoplication. This operation is usually referred to as a "cardioplasty," rather than a fundoplication. The operation secures the gastroesophageal junction intraabdominally and tightens the collar sling mechanism. It is a difficult operation to reproduce consistently, thus has few proponents apart from those trained by Lucius Hill, its developer.

We believe that the Nissen fundoplication is the most reproducible fundoplication procedure, has a long track record with exceptional results, and, as we have discussed, can be used for almost all patients. Therefore, we will describe our technique of performing a Nissen fundoplication as an example of how a fundoplication operation adheres to the principles outlined earlier.

Perioperative Considerations

General anesthesia is necessary for this operation. Each patient receives a single dose of broad-spectrum antibiotic. Sequential compression devices are placed to decrease the risk of deep venous thrombosis. A Foley catheter is used to decompress the bladder and monitor urine output during the operation.

We place the patient in low lithotomy position, which allows the surgeon to stand between the patient's legs during the procedure. To secure the patient in steep reverse Trendelenburg position, a seat is fashioned using a beanbag. The monitor is placed over the patient's head so it can be viewed by the whole

operating team. An additional monitor is used to show the anesthesiologist the operative field as he or she is manipulating the esophageal bougie during the operation. The assistant stands on the patient's left side. A self-retaining retractor is secured to the right side of the bed to hold the liver retractor, minimizing the need for a second assistant.

Creation of Pneumoperitoneum and Port Placement

Pneumoperitoneum is established with a Veress needle using the site through which the camera port or left upper quadrant port will be placed (Figure 5.1). An open technique may be used especially if the patient has had a prior operation and adhesions are suspected. We use an optical access port (Visiport™; US Surgical, Norwalk, CT) for the first port because it shows the different layers as one is going through, thus decreasing the chance of bowel or vascular injury and significantly increasing the chance of an immediate diagnosis if they occur. The camera port is placed 2 cm to the left of midline and 10 cm below the costal margin. Diagnostic laparoscopy is performed to exclude injury from entry or other pathology. The upper two ports are used by the surgeon and should form an equilateral triangle with the camera port. This allows the surgeon's instruments to be used at an angle, enabling correct visualization of the tips. The liver retractor and first assistant ports are placed at the level of the camera port in the anterior axillary line.

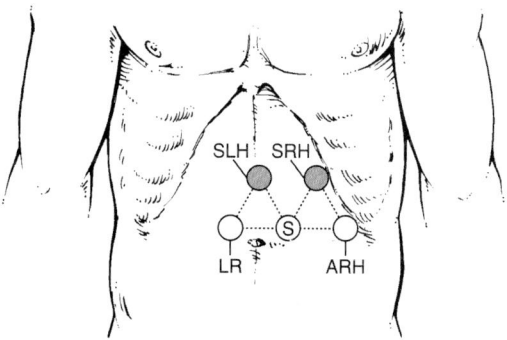

Figure 5.1. Port placement. (Reprinted from Hiatal Hernia and Gastroesophageal Reflux Disease. In: Townsend CM, Beauchamp DR, Evers MB, Mattox KL, eds. Sabiston Textbook of Surgery. 16th ed. 2004:1158, Copyright 2004, with permission from Elsevier.)

Dissection of the Cardia ("Left Crus Approach")

We begin the operation on the left side by dividing the phrenogastric ligament to expose the left crus. This approach minimizes the risk of injury to structures around the gastrohepatic ligament such as the nerve of Latarjet and vena cava in obese patients. This approach also allows for safer division of the short gastric vessels, especially at the superior pole of the spleen.

Division of the Short Gastric Vessels

The fundus is mobilized by dividing the short gastric vessels as this has been shown to result in less dysphagia.[21] A general landmark for the caudal extent of the mobilization is the inferior pole of a normal-sized spleen. Short gastric vessels are subsequently identified and transected with the Autosonic scalpel (Tyco Healthcare, Norwalk, CT), although this can be completed with clips or other energy sources (Figure 5.2). These vessels are divided upward until one reaches the previously dissected left

crus. The vessels to the upper pole of the spleen may be very short and deep, making division very difficult without prior division of the phrenogastric ligament (left crus approach). These last vessels are best exposed by having the assistant retract the posterior wall of the body of the stomach toward the patient's right as the surgeon pulls the posterior wall of the fundus of the stomach anteriorly. A space at the base of the left crus between the lesser sac and our initial dissection along the left crus is created, allowing the more cephalad short gastric vessels to be exposed and divided.

Esophageal Mobilization

After the fundus is free and the left crus completely exposed, the left phrenoesophageal membrane is incised, safely entering the mediastinum between the left crus and esophagus. The dissection is continued anteriorly and superiorly, dividing the peritoneum overlying the anterior aspect of the crus. This line of division is extended down to the base of the right crus. Only now do we divide the gastrohepatic ligament.

Most of the hepatic branches of the vagus and occasional hepatic branch of the left gastric artery can be preserved with this approach. The right phrenoesophageal membrane is divided, exposing the inner edge of the right crus. Another advantage of this technique is that because the decussation of the right and left crus is identified, a posterior esophageal window is created without dissection toward the splenic hilum. A 0.5-in. Penrose drain is placed in this posterior window and secured around the esophagus and two vagi with a clip or suture.

With the assistant tractioning from the Penrose drain, dissection of the intrathoracic esophagus is started. This is done until we achieve an intraabdominal esophageal length of at least 3 cm. Mobilization of the esophagus can usually easily be carried to the carina, and as a result we rarely lack enough intraabdominal esophagus to perform a tension-free repair. Careful attention should be paid to avoiding injury to the anterior and posterior vagal nerves, both pleural surfaces, and the aorta.

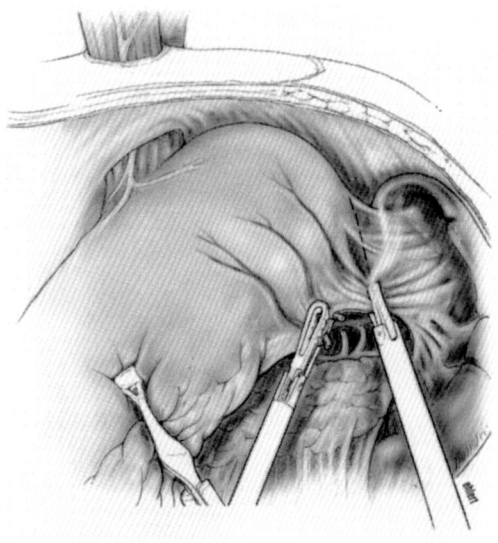

Figure 5.2. Transecting the short gastric vessels. (Reprinted from Hiatal Hernia and Gastroesophageal Reflux Disease. In: Townsend CM, Beauchamp DR, Evers MB, Mattox KL, eds. Sabiston Textbook of Surgery. 16th ed. 2004:755–768, Copyright 2004, with permission from Elsevier.)

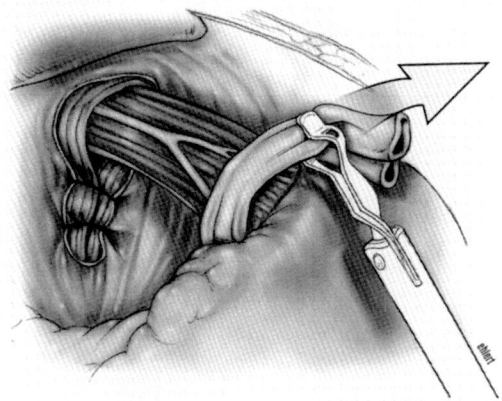

Figure 5.3. Diaphragmatic closure. (Reprinted from Hiatal Hernia and Gastroesophageal Reflux Disease. In: Townsend CM, Beauchamp DR, Evers MB, Mattox KL, eds. Sabiston Textbook of Surgery. 16th ed. 2004:755–768, Copyright 2004, with permission from Elsevier.)

Hiatal Closure

The hiatus is closed posteriorly with simple 2-0 silk stitches placed no more than 5mm apart (Figure 5.3). The hiatal closure is calibrated such that a 52-French bougie fits through the hiatus easily. For large hiatal hernias (type II–IV), we buttress the tenuous closure with a bioprosthesis (Surgisis™; Cook Surgical, Bloomington, IN).[22]

Construction of the Wrap

It is critical to the proper function of the fundoplication that the two flaps of gastric fundus that will wrap the lower end of the esophagus be symmetrical. In other words, it is important that the amount of displacement of the posterior and anterior gastric flaps be the same so that there is no tendency to produce a torque in the esophagus. To achieve this, we first identify a point on the posterior wall of the stomach that is 3cm below the gastroesophageal junction and 2cm away from the greater curvature. We then place a loose stitch to identify this area. This assures that we do not mistakenly grasp the anterior portion or body of the stomach, which is a common error seen in failed fundoplica-

tions.[23] The portion of posterior stomach with the suture is then brought posterior to the esophagus.

A mirror-image portion of the anterior stomach wall (3cm below the gastroesophageal junction and 2cm away from the greater curvature) is grasped with the right hand (the posterior stomach is in the left). This creates a symmetrical fundoplication. Once this is achieved, we check the entire wrap by momentarily undoing it. This is accomplished by passing (and holding) the posterior aspect of the gastric fundus (being held by the left hand) behind the esophagus, back toward the left upper quadrant while the right hand holds the anterior gastric flap. Now the entire wrap can be seen just to the left of the esophagogastric junction, in front of the upper portion of the spleen, and the distance from each point (the left hand grasp and the right hand grasp) to the greater curvature observed and measured once again. The wrap is then restored to its original position around the esophagus and sutured.

The fundoplication is created by suturing these two flaps of gastric fundus with four interrupted stitches of 2-0 silk suture 1cm apart. Care is taken to avoid entrapping the anterior vagal nerve, which is why we do not incorporate a bite of esophagus with these sutures. The fundoplication is created while a 52-French bougie is in place through the gastroesophageal junction and ends up being approximately 3cm long.

Anchoring the Fundoplication

To decrease the likelihood of herniation of the wrap, we anchor it to the diaphragm and esophagus. Two "coronal" sutures are placed, the first from the top of the posterior fundus to the right lateral esophagus and the right crus. A similar suture is placed from the left crus, esophagus and greater curvature. Two additional stitches are placed: the posterior one, fixing the posterior valve to a place in the diaphragm that avoids excessive traction of the stomach, and an anterior one fixing the top of the anterior valve of the fundoplication to the anterior aspect of the hiatus (Figure 5.4).

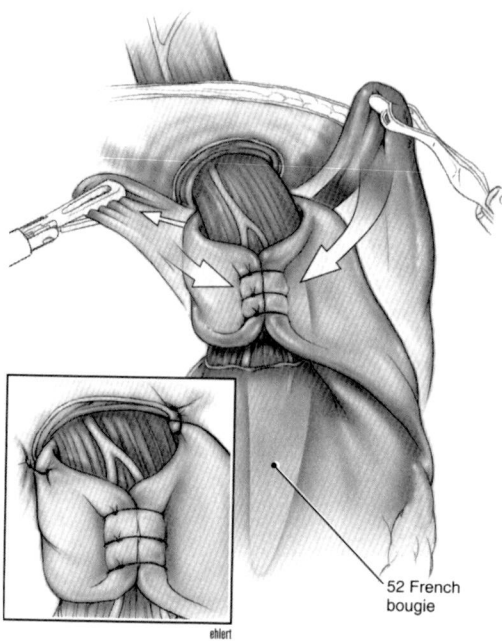
52 French
bougie

ehlert

Figure 5.4. Coronal sutures. (Reprinted from Hiatal Hernia and Gastroesophageal Reflux Disease. In: Townsend CM, Beauchamp DR, Evers MB, Mattox KL, eds. Sabiston Textbook of Surgery. 16th ed. 2004:755–768, Copyright 2004, with permission from Elsevier.)

Conclusion

Laparoscopic anti-reflux surgery, and even open fundoplication operations, are viable alternatives to medical management in the treatment of severe GERD. The key to successful outcomes with this procedure include proper patient selection thorough preoperative evaluation and careful operative technique. The chapter outlines our approach which has resulted in excellent outcomes at the University of Washington.

References

1. Oelschlager BK, Pellegrini CA. Minimally invasive surgery for gastroesophageal reflux disease. J Laparoendosc Adv Surg Tech A 2001;11:341–349.
2. Guilherme MR, Campos MD, Peters JH, et al. Multivariate analysis of factors predicting outcome after laparoscopic Nissen fundoplication. J Gastrointest Surg 1999;3:292–300.
3. Westscher G, Schwab G, Klinger A, et al. Respiratory symptoms in patients with gastroesophageal reflux fol-
lowing medical therapy and following anti-reflux surgery. Am J Surg 1997;174:639–643.
4. Tobin RW, Pope CE II, Pellegrini CA, Emond MJ, Sillery J, Raghu G. Increased prevalence of gastroesophageal reflux in patients with idiopathic pulmonary fibrosis. Am J Respir Crit Care Med 1998;158:1804–1808.
5. Oelschlager BK, Barreca M, Chang L, et al. Clinical and pathologic response of Barrett's esophagus to laparoscopic anti reflux surgery. Ann Surg 2003;238(4): 458–466.
6. Csendes A, Braghetto I, Burdiles P, et al. Long-term results of classic anti-reflux surgery in 152 patients with Barrett's esophagus: clinical, radiologic, endoscopic, manometric, and acid reflux test analysis before and late after operation. Surgery 1998;123:645–657.
7. Hofstetter W, Peters J, DeMeester T, et al. Long-term outcome of anti-reflux surgery in patients with Barrett's esophagus. Ann Surg 2001;234:532–539.
8. Bowers SP, Mattar SG, Smith CD, et al. Clinical and histologic follow-up after anti-reflux surgery for Barrett's esophagus. J Gastrointest Surg 2002;6(4):532–538.
9. Perry Y, Courcoulas AP, Fernando HC, Buenaventura PO, McCaughan JS, Luketich JD. Laparoscopic Roux-en-Y gastric bypass for recalcitrant gastroesophageal reflux disease in morbidly obese patients. JSLS 2004;8:19–23.
10. Perez AR, Moncure AC, Rattner DW. Obesity adversely affects the outcome of anti-reflux operations. Surg Endosc 2001;15:986–989.
11. Flum DR, Koepsell T, Heagerty P, et al. The nationwide frequency of major adverse outcomes in anti-reflux surgery and the role of surgeon experience, 1992–1997. J Am Coll Surg 2002;195:611–618.
12. Jobe BA, Kahrilas PJ, Vernon AH, et al. Endoscopic appraisal of the gastroesophageal valve after anti-reflux surgery. Am J Gastroenterol 2004;99:233–243.
13. Oleynikov D, Eubanks TR, Oelschlager BK, et al. Total fundoplication is the operation of choice for patients with gastroesophageal reflux and defective peristalsis. Surg Endosc 2002;16:909–913.
14. Chrysos E, Tsiaoussis J, Zoras OJ, et al. Laparoscopic surgery for gastroesophageal reflux disease patients with impaired esophageal peristalsis: total or partial fundoplication? J Am Coll Surg 2003;197:8–15.
15. Barreca M, Oelschlager BK, Pellegrini CA. Outcomes of laparoscopic Nissen fundoplication in patients with the "hypercontractile esophagus." Arch Surg 2002;137: 724–729.
16. Eubanks T, Omelanczuk P, Maronian N, et al. Pharyngeal pH measurements in patients with respiratory symptoms prior to and during proton pump inhibitor therapy. Am J Surg 2001;181:466–470.
17. Oelschlager BK, Eubanks T, Oleynikov D, et al. Symptomatic and physiologic outcomes after operative treatment for extraesophageal reflux. Surg Endosc 2002;16(7):1032–1036.
18. Oelschlager B, Pellegrini C. Surgical treatment of respiratory complications associated with gastroesophageal reflux disease. Am J Med 2003;18:72s–77s.
19. Oelschlager BK, Eubanks T, Maronian N, et al. Laryngoscopy and pharyngeal pH are complementary in the diagnosis of gastroesophageal-laryngeal reflux. J Gastrointest Surg 2002;6(2):189–194.
20. Jobe BA, Kahrilas PJ, Vernon AH, et al. Endoscopic appraisal of the gastroesophageal valve after anti-reflux surgery. Am J Gastroenterol 2004;99:233–243.

21. Contini S, Zinicola R, Bertele A, et al. Dysphagia and clinical outcome after laparoscopic Nissen or Rossetti fundoplication: sequential prospective study. World J Surg 2002;26:1106–1111.

22. Oelschlager BK, Barreca M, Chang L, et al. The use of small intestine submucosa in the repair of parae-sophageal hernias: initial observations of a new technique. Am J Surg 2003;186:4–8.

23. Horgan S, Pohl D, Bogetti D, et al. Failed anti-reflux surgery: what have we learned from reoperations? Arch Surg 1999;134:809–815.

6

Acute Complications of Anti-Reflux Surgery

Gianmattia del Genio and Jean-Marie Collard

In the last three decades, surgical procedures for gastroesophageal reflux disease showed significant improvements in outcomes mainly because of standardization of the indications, widespread use of accepted fundoplication techniques, and improved perioperative management. Despite the good results of the currently adopted operations,[1] acute complications of anti-reflux procedures occur and may be life-threatening. Large series with careful long-term follow-up are available and demonstrate recognizable patterns of failure.[2–6] Complications are different in type and frequency in relation to both techniques (e.g., partial vs total fundoplication) and approach (e.g., thoracotomy vs laparotomy). Recently, the evolution toward the use of the laparoscopic approach[7–9] changed the frequency of these untoward events. Some of the complications traditionally associated with open surgery decreased in incidence (e.g., incisional hernia, splenic injury), whereas other specific complications (e.g., intraabdominal hemorrhage, herniation of the wrap into the chest, perforation of the esophagus or stomach, pneumothorax, or pneumomediastinum) occur more frequently after laparoscopic surgery.[10,11]

Because of the high number of anti-reflux procedures performed each year and the lack of any worldwide registry, the exact incidence of acute complications is difficult to estimate. Follow-up studies report a large statistical variation influenced by the relatively small numbers of operations performed in each individual institution. Retrospective surveys of laparo-scopic anti-reflux procedures demonstrate an operative mortality of 0.5%[12] and a morbidity ranging from 4 to 7.3%.[13,14] A nationwide analysis comprehensive of all the serious complications was conducted in Finland between 1987 and 1996, showing a prevalence of 0.8% of life-threatening complications including 0.1% of fatal events.[15] Even though a substantial number of surgical failures do not lead to remedial surgery, another method to estimate the incidence of postoperative complications is to consider the reoperation rate. According to Carlson and Frantzides,[16] the overall reoperation rate reported in the literature for all the primary anti-reflux laparoscopic procedures published between 1993 and 2000 was 2.8%.

In laparoscopic anti-reflux surgery there is a direct correlation between the surgeon's experience and the complication rate[17] with the highest complication rate occurring during the first five cases and declining to a more acceptable level beyond the twentieth procedure.[18] The important role of tutorship is demonstrated by the lower complication rate and shorter operative time during the learning curve of late starters than in the initial experience of pioneers.[18]

This chapter addresses the main acute complications of anti-reflux surgery irrespective of the approach (laparotomy vs laparoscopy vs thoracotomy) and their timing of occurrence (intraoperative vs postoperative). It provides the reader with relevant information, guidelines, and insights that have evolved from study of the surgical literature and from the senior author's personal experience.

Intraoperative Complications

Vascular Injury

Because of the close spatial relationship between the hiatal area and the major vascular structures in the upper abdomen, vascular injuries to major vessels (aorta, vena cava, left hepatic artery, short gastric vessels) may occur during anti-reflux surgery (Table 6.1). Use of an open approach allows the surgeon to put his index finger right on the damaged vessel for immediate control of the bleeding and, subsequently, for easy vascular repair with either a ligature of the vessel (left hepatic artery, short gastric vessels) or a suture of the vascular wall (aorta, vena cava). In contrast, with the laparoscopic approach, immediate control is much more difficult to achieve. For this reason, inex-

Table 6.1. Intraoperative complications and predisposing factors.

Vascular injury
  Direct injury to the aorta, inferior vena cava, left hepatic artery, short gastric vessels, spleen, right ventricle
  Crushing of the liver with the hepatic retractor

Esophageal and gastric tear
  Inaccurate periesophageal dissection
  Excessive cautery
  Inadvertent puncture
  Undue traction
  Blind maneuver (laparoscopy)
  Intraluminal bougie

Vagal injury
  Posterior esophageal dissection
  Removal of the fat pad
  Direct injury to either vagal trunk
  Dense adhesions (reoperative surgery, panesophagitis)
  Complete division of the lesser omentum

Pneumomediastinum (laparoscopy)
  Extended transhiatal mobilization of the esophagus
  High intraabdominal insufflation pressure

Pneumothorax (laparoscopy)
  Inadvertent injury to the pleura
  Panesophagitis
  Esophageal shortening
  Large hiatal hernia

perienced laparoscopists should have the conventional instrumentation opened on a table located in the operating theater, ready to be used at any time. Achieving hemostasis laparoscopically can be a challenging task for the most experienced surgeon even if advanced technologies are readily available (bipolar cautery, ultrasound, argon beam). The use of smooth forceps grasping the damaged vessel is recommended, but injury to either the aorta or inferior vena cava requires immediate conversion to laparotomy. The use of a high-flow insufflator helps to maintain a high intraabdominal pressure while suctioning intraperitoneal blood. Placement of hemostatic clips on the left hepatic or splenic arteries must not totally occlude the vessels because of the potential risk of hepatic or splenic ischemia and necrosis.

In open surgery, injury to the spleen is the most frequent cause of intraoperative bleeding, and is usually related to excessive traction on the greater omentum or stomach. This can necessitate urgent splenectomy if hemostasis cannot be achieved. The incidence of this event has been reduced by the use of minimally invasive surgical techniques. In large series of open anti-reflux procedures the reported splenectomy rate ranged from 1 to 3%,[2,19,20] whereas both the overall incidence of splenic injury and splenectomy rate calculated from >6000 laparoscopic anti-reflux procedures was 0.24 and 0.06%, respectively.[16] Although these data come from specialized centers with high caseload volumes,[21] splenectomy has not been reported in many laparoscopic series exceeding 100 patients.[1] More gentle maneuvers together with the magnification of the image in laparoscopic surgery probably account for the reduced risk of perioperative hemorrhage compared with conventional surgery.[22]

Another cause of intraoperative bleeding during laparoscopic fundoplication is inadvertent laceration of the liver because of excessive pressure exerted by the hepatic retractor on the liver. The small hepatic fracture that is bleeding is usually secured with a compression plug. In case of failure of this technique, a variety of other hemostatic options are available, including argon or bipolar coagulation, biological glue, or collagen-based hemostatic mesh. Overly strong use of the liver retractor may cause myocardial contusion, and cardiac tamponade has been reported caused by laceration of the

right ventricle.[23] Management of these problems is beyond the scope of this chapter.

Esophageal and Gastric Tear

Esophageal perforation during open anti-reflux surgery is very uncommon.[20] Use of a safe method of esophageal dissection helps ensure this low rate of perforation: encircling of the esophagus is performed with the surgeon's index finger passed smoothly from left to right, the fingertip touching the left crus of the diaphragm, the anterior aspect of the aorta, and the right crus successively, rather than the posterior aspect of the esophageal wall itself. In contrast, because of the loss of tactile perception, intraoperative perforation during laparoscopic anti-reflux procedures is more common and may involve either the distal esophagus or gastric fundus.[24] Excessive cautery, inadvertent puncture, undue traction, and incorrect identification of the anatomic planes are the most common mechanisms involved.[25,26] Posterior esophageal perforation attributed to blind dissection of the lower esophagus flush with its outer muscular layer has been reported by several authors.[10,24,27] Perforation of the esophagus or stomach represents the third most frequent intraoperative complication of anti-reflux surgery, occurring in 0.78% of cases.[16] Similar to other complications, the risk of perforation follows a learning curve. Schauer et al.[24] demonstrated that most perforations occur early (first 10 cases) during the course of a surgeon's experience with fundoplication.

An adequate approach to the hiatal area includes starting the dissection just above the hepatic branches of the left vagus nerve within the lesser omentum on the right crus of the diaphragm, which must be clearly identified. Further dissection around the lower esophagus through the mediastinum must be done under careful visual control. The use of a 30° telescope during laparoscopic surgery may be helpful. Conditions predisposing to intraoperative esophageal injury include failure to preoperatively diagnose a short esophagus (Figure 6.1), dense adhesions in relation to severe periesophagitis, and previous hiatal surgery.

Another mechanism involved in intraoperative perforation is the passage of a large-diameter bougie across the gastroesophageal junction. To do this safely, any maneuvers by the

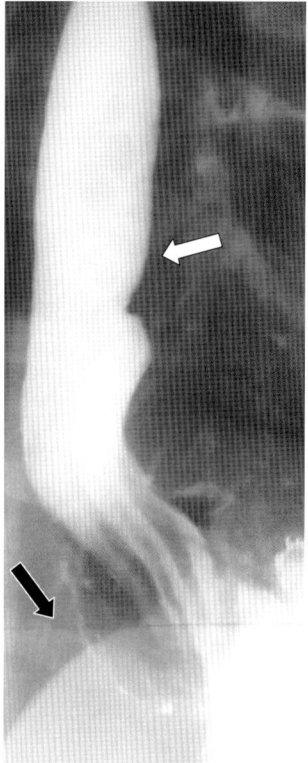

Figure 6.1. Short esophagus with the gastroesophageal junction (white arrow) far away from the diaphragmatic level (black arrow).

anesthetist must be done in perfect coordination with those by the surgeon. This is especially important with the laparoscopic technique because the surgeon is unable to palpate the gastroesophageal junction as the bougie is being passed. In addition, during laparoscopy no traction can be exerted on the lower esophagus when the distal tip of the bougie is thought to have reached the cardia.

Another process involved in some of the reported perforations is the presence of a bougie in the lower esophagus during esophageal dissection.[28] Under these circumstances, the bougie puts the esophageal wall under tension so as to make it more rigid. Most surgeons agree that it is best to insert the calibration bougie just before suturing the fundic wrap after the lower esophagus has been isolated from its crural attachments.[29]

The worst problem is failure of recognition of the tear at the time of the operation. This is especially possible for both posterior esophageal and gastric tears. Any doubtful surgical maneuver requires careful checking of the esophagogastric junction. Either methylene blue injected through the channel of the nasogastric tube lying across the esophagogastric junction or intraoperative upper gastrointestinal endoscopy with transillumination and insufflation are useful adjuncts for detecting even very small transmural tears.[30,31]

When a perforation is discovered intraoperatively, primary repair of the tear in two layers with interrupted stitches is simple and rarely results in postoperative complications. Coverage of the suture line with the fundoplication may help to reinforce the repair.

Vagal Nerve Injury

Circumferential dissection of the lower esophagus exposes the patient to the risk of inadvertent injury to one or both vagus nerves. Anatomic landmarks for recognition of the vagal nerves are the anterior aspect of the esophageal wall for the left (anterior) trunk and the internal aspect of the right crus for the right (posterior) one. These landmarks are particularly relevant in laparoscopy, an approach that precludes blunt encircling of the esophagus with the index finger. In some patients, early decussation of the left trunk results in the presence of several thin fibers that spread over the anterior aspect of the esophageal wall. Circumstances leading to vagal injury are:

- Posterior dissection between the posterior esophageal wall and the right vagus nerve to pass the fundus in between when constructing the wrap (optional surgical step)[19]
- Anterior dissection including the removal of a large fat pad across the cardia
- Incorporation of the left trunk in the suture when anchoring the wrap to the anterior aspect of the esophageal wall
- Direct injury to either vagal trunk with the needle when suturing the wrap
- Dense periesophageal adhesions in repeat operations, as reported by Skinner and Belsey three decades ago[32]
- Division of both the left hepatic artery and the hepatic branches of the left vagus nerve

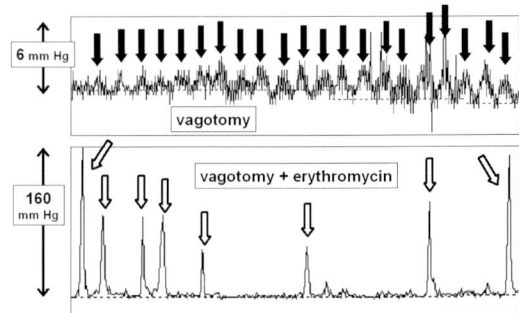

Figure 6.2. Antral manometry tracings showing very low-amplitude contractions after vagotomy (upper tracing, black arrows) and high-amplitude contractions after erythromycin therapy has been started (lower tracing, white arrows).

within the lesser omentum (unnecessary surgical maneuver)

We know that truncal vagotomy disturbs the functioning of all the organs of the digestive system. It impairs fundic relaxation, antral propulsive activity, pyloric relaxation, gallbladder contractility, and possibly results in diarrhea, dumping or gastric stasis, early satiety, increased antral exposure to duodenal contents, and even cholelithiasis.[33–38] Should vagal injury occur, erythromycin therapy (motilin-receptor agonist[39]) should be started as early as possible to enhance the spontaneous motor recovery process that takes place in the myenteric plexus of the gastric wall over time[40] (Figure 6.2). Doing so is likely to minimize the unfortunate side effects of the nerve injury for patients who anticipate improvement in quality of life and digestive comfort by means of an otherwise straightforward functional operation.

Pneumomediastinum and Pneumothorax

An unusual occurrence in conventional open fundoplication surgery, both pneumomediastinum and pneumothorax are new complications that may occur when the anti-reflux procedure is performed laparoscopically. Pneumomediastinum may result from extended transhiatal mobilization of the esophagus in combination with a high intraabdominal insufflation pressure. It is recognized by subcutaneous emphysema that usually develops in the neck. Lowering the insufflation pressure during the procedure may prevent progression of the pneumomediastinum. In most cases, no specific treatment is needed; the pneumomediastinum spontaneously resolves by absorption of the gas within a few hours after the operation.[41]

Pneumothorax may develop in relation to either direct opening of either pleural cavity or diffusion of CO_2 through intact pleura. Factors predisposing to pneumothorax are:

- Periesophagitis with dense adhesions between the esophageal or fundic wall and the pleura
- Inadvertent injury to the pleura caused by technically inadequate lower mediastinal dissection
- Extended mediastinal dissection in the presence of esophageal shortening or in patients with a large type III (paraesophageal) hiatal hernia

Intraoperative pneumothorax must be recognized as early as possible to avoid the development of gas-exchange disturbances. Intraoperative closure of the pleural defect may help stop CO_2 diffusion into the pleural cavity. The most critical maneuver to be done if the patient becomes unstable because of a tension pneumothorax is placement of a large-bore needle or intravenous catheter in the pleural cavity through the anterior aspect of the chest wall. This allows intrathoracic CO_2 to escape from the chest cavity with subsequent reexpansion of the lung parenchyma. Formal evacuation of gas from the pleural cavity must be done at the end of the procedure after release of the pneumoperitoneum. Incomplete pleural evacuation or recurrence of pneumothorax on a chest X-ray taken in the recovery room suggests that the lung parenchyma itself has been injured and requires pleural drainage with a conventional chest tube until a parenchymal seal is achieved.

Acute Postoperative Complications

Gastric and Esophageal Fistula

A fistula may develop from either the esophagus or stomach in the early postoperative course and is usually related to a transmural injury to the esophageal or gastric wall that was not rec-

ognized during the operative procedure (Table 6.2). Reports suggest that such an unfortunate outcome is more likely to occur with the laparoscopic approach than after a conventional anti-reflux operation by laparotomy or thoracotomy.[13,24] Although laparoscopy has been favored because it provides the surgeon with a better view of the operative field, it may also necessitate blind maneuvers, such as those needed for the creation of a large retroesophageal window or by the insertion of the first trocar into the abdomen. Inappropriate use of the coagulating system also may expose the upper gastrointestinal tract to the risk of heat injury.[42] Another cause of postoperative fistula is leakage of an esophageal or gastric suture used for repair of an upper gastrointestinal tear that was recognized intraoperatively. In the same way, excessive tightening of the knots when anchoring the wrap to the lower esopha-

Table 6.2. Postoperative complications and predisposing factors.

Gastric and esophageal fistula
Unrecognized intraoperative tear (blind dissection)
Heat injury to the gastric or esophageal wall
Postoperative leakage from erosion of an esophageal or gastric suture
Excessive tightening of the knots when anchoring the wrap to the esophagus
Excessive tension on the anchoring sites of an intrathoracic fundoplication to the diaphragm
Bleeding
Rebleeding from any intraoperative vascular repair
Injury to the intercostal artery (thoracic approach)
Injury to the epigastric artery (laparoscopic approach)
Slippage of a clip placed on a short gastric vessel
Herniation of the wrap into the chest
Sudden increase in intraabdominal pressure (tumultuous recovery from anesthesia, prostatism, constipation, straining under heavy loads)
Inappropriate approximation of the crura
Large hiatal hernia
Short esophagus
Postoperative gastric distension
Acute dysphagia
Periesophageal dissection
Too tight a crural closure
Too long or too tight a wrap
Excessive scarring of the hiatal sling
Unrecognized esophageal body dysmotility

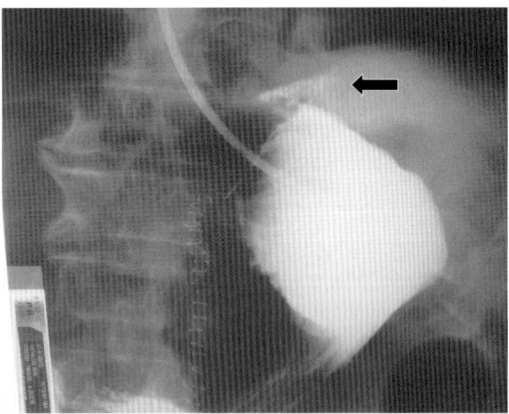

Figure 6.3. Gastric perforation (black arrow) after laparotomic Nissen fundoplication, in relation to too tight a gastroesophagogastric suture.

gus may create local ischemia leading to early postoperative perforation (Figure 6.3). If clinical symptoms such as fever, excessive abdominal pain, or abdominal tenderness develop, a contrast swallow using a water-soluble medium must be performed urgently.

Twenty years ago, use of an intrathoracic Nissen fundoplication for management of short esophagus came into disrepute because of reports of gastric perforation at the anchoring sites of the wrap to the crura.[43–45] Because it is the only anti-reflux procedure that encircles the distal segment of a short esophagus, we modified Nissen's initial technique[46] in an attempt to lower the risk of early postoperative perforation[45,47]:

- The hiatus, already enlarged by the presence of the sliding hernia, is widened further by division of the left crus or performance of a 3-cm diaphragmatic incision radially from the anterior margin of the crural sling.
- The wrap is made as floppy as possible using a rather large amount of gastric tissue.
- To anchor the wrap to the crural sling, the surgeon pushes the left part of the diaphragm down with his left hand, mimicking diaphragmatic contractions that arise on cough, before placing the sutures.

- The nasogastric tube is removed only when bowel activity resumes.

Perforations confined to the immediate vicinity of the digestive wall may be treated conservatively with antibiotics, acid-suppressing medications, evacuation of gastric contents at regular intervals through the nasogastric tube, and total parenteral nutrition.[48] In contrast, noncontained leaks require immediate revision by laparoscopy, laparotomy, or thoracotomy.[48] Laparoscopy must be converted into laparotomy whenever proper repair of the defect cannot be achieved through the minimally invasive approach.

Late recognition of an esophageal or gastric leak may lead to life-threatening peritonitis which could necessitate a procedure as radical as esophagectomy or gastrectomy.[49] Mediastinitis with pleural effusion also may develop from an esophageal injury,[50] especially after extended transhiatal dissection of the esophagus to reduce the gastrointestinal junction below the diaphragm. In such an instance, thoracotomy must be considered if the abdominal approach to the lower esophagus precludes proper suturing of the parietal defect and effective mediastinal drainage.

These complex surgical situations emphasize the fact that anti-reflux surgery must be performed by surgeons experienced with both abdominal and thoracic surgical procedures.

Bleeding

Bleeding in the immediate postoperative period is a rare event that must be suspected in the presence of acute hypotension, tachycardia, contraction of the urinary output, or shock. The absence of intraabdominal drainage may cause a delay in diagnosis and necessitate an urgent, rather than semielective, reoperation. Bleeding may come from an intraoperative vascular repair, any splenic or hepatic injury that rebleeds after hemostasis has apparently been achieved, or from the incision itself, possibly involving an intercostal artery or vein after thoracotomy or the epigastric artery caused by trocar placement for laparoscopy. Watson and colleagues[51] reported on a patient who underwent a laparotomy 6 hours after the initial laparoscopic anti-reflux operation for bleeding caused by slippage of a clip placed on a short gastric vessel. To prevent such a complication, it is wise to apply two hemostatic clips on both sides of the presumed division point of a vessel. This is especially important because such clips can be dislodged while passing the fundus through the retroesophageal window to wrap the lower esophagus.

Herniation of the Wrap into the Chest

Herniation of the fundic wrap into the chest may occur in the early postoperative period, even as early as while the patient awakens from the anesthetic. Various conditions predispose to this unfortunate outcome:

- The physiologic intraabdominal pressure is higher than the one existing in the thorax so that abdominal organs are naturally attracted to the chest through any defect in the diaphragm, the roof of the abdominal cavity.

- A sudden increase in abdominal pressure, as may occur when the patient strains while awakening from anesthesia, may push the freshly constructed wrap through the hiatus, with subsequent breakdown of the crural closure.

- The absence of any crural closure gives even better access to the lower mediastinum, especially in patients operated on for gastroesophageal reflux disease with a hiatal hernia and in whom the fundic wrap has not been anchored to the hiatal sling.

- Postoperative distension, which may occur if a nasogastric tube has not been placed, may put the hiatal repair under stress and account, in part at least, for the acute disruption of the crural sutures.

- In the presence of esophageal shortening, undue traction on the esophageal tube to construct the wrap below the diaphragm also predisposes to early herniation into the chest, which reflects the spontaneous tendency of the short esophagus to go back to its natural location in the lower mediastinum.

- In those patients operated on for a short esophagus, inappropriate anchoring of an intrathoracic Nissen fundoplication[45] to the crural sling predisposes to either further herniation of the stomach or herniation of the splenic flexure of the colon alongside the fundoplication into the chest.[47]

- After discharge home, manual workers should be advised against carrying heavy loads; similarly, patients with prostatism or constipation should be warned not to strain too much when they urinate or have a bowel movement. Each of these conditions increases intraabdominal pressure excessively and can predispose to breakdown of a repair and wrap herniation.

- Herniation of the fundoplication into the chest is more common with the laparoscopic approach than after conventional surgery.[10] Possible reasons for this are excessive cautery of the peritoneal sheet covering the crura and misestimation of the amount of tissue incorporated in bites when approximating the crura with the laparoscopic technique.[52]

Total disruption of the crural closure with herniation of the wrap into the chest may remain totally asymptomatic. Sometimes the fundoplication has sufficient room in the hiatus and has become fixed in the lower mediastinum, creating a situation similar to what is achieved when an intrathoracic fundoplication is constructed around a short esophagus.[46] To be effective in controlling gastroesophageal reflux, a total fundoplication does not necessarily have to be located below the diaphragm; rather, our own experience of intrathoracic Nissen fundoplications when performed for true esophageal shortening indicates that an intrathoracic wrap is at least as effective as an intraabdominal one, with a long-term pH-controlled success rate of 97%.[48]

Partial disruption of the crural closure, together with the absence of spontaneous fixation of the herniated wrap to the lower mediastinal tissue, may result in gastric compression at the diaphragmatic level. This can lead to dysphagia, chest pain, dyspnea, and cardiac dysrhythmia, symptoms that require reoperation to reposition the fundoplication below the diaphragm. Usually, herniation of the wrap into the chest is not the only anatomic abnormality found at reoperation.[37,53] The wrap is often found to have been partially disrupted, sometimes the wrap no longer exists, or the wrap may have slipped onto the gastric body. Patients with these anatomic problems experience recurrence of heartburn, which requires take down of the residual wrap followed by the construction of a proper one around the lower esophagus below the diaphragm.

Acute transhiatal herniation of the wrap through a relatively narrow hiatal sling may result in strangulation of the hernia with gastric necrosis (Figure 6.4). This life-threatening complication requires an emergency operation and may require resection of the fundus or even esophagogastrectomy whenever the gastric wall cannot be sutured after the removal of the necrotic area.

Techniques for preventing herniation of an intraabdominal fundoplication into the chest include the following:

- Proper approximation of the diaphragmatic crura with incorporation of their sturdy peritoneal sheet in the suture
- Anchoring of the wrap to both diaphragmatic crura with nonabsorbable sutures
- Smooth recovery from anesthesia, preventing the patient from excessive coughing
- Placement of a nasogastric tube during the first 12 hours after the operation

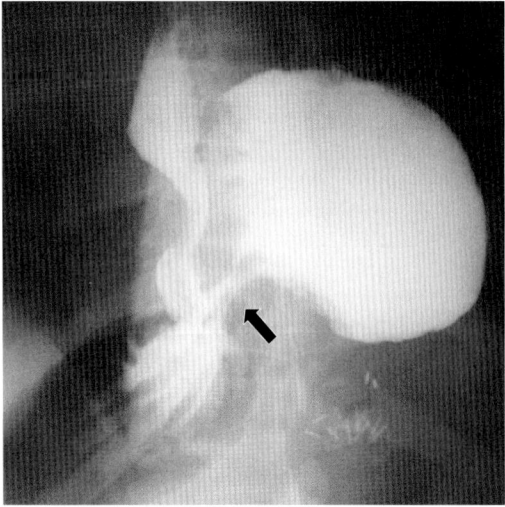

Figure 6.4. Acute herniation and diaphragmatic strangulation (black arrow) of the greater curvature after laparoscopic Nissen fundoplication in relation to postoperative vomiting.

- A 2-month convalescence period for manual workers
- Appropriate management of prostatism and constipation during the early postoperative period
- True esophageal shortening on preoperative barium swallow series must be operated on via thoracotomy[45,46]

Acute Dysphagia

Almost all patients experience some degree of dysphagia after fundoplication surgery. This transient side effect of the procedure usually resolves within a few weeks postoperatively. Transient dysphagia is likely a result of physiologic inflammation that develops in the hiatal region after any dissection of the distal esophagus and gastroesophageal junction, as was demonstrated in the 1980s after proximal gastric vagotomy without fundoplication for duodenal ulcer disease.[54,55] In contrast, severe dysphagia is suggestive of the crural closure being too tight, a wrap that is too long or too tight, unrecognized esophageal body dysmotility, or excessive scarring of the hiatal sling. The latter situation was described by Watson et al.[56] at the beginning of the laparoscopic era in relation to poor hiatal dissection with excessive use of electric coagulation. Acute incarceration of a freshly constructed wrap in the hiatus also may account for the sudden onset of dysphagia postoperatively.

The role of the absence of division of the short gastric vessels in the genesis of esophageal dysphagia is still debated, despite the publication of randomized studies[57–59] that fail to show any significant difference depending on whether the vessels are severed or not. However, large series of remedial operations[60–62] indicate that, in almost all patients who required a reoperative procedure for persistent dysphagia, their short gastric vessels were left intact at the time of the first operation.

The symptom of dysphagia is best assessed by dynamic radiological examination of the esophageal anatomy. An increased diameter of the esophageal tube on barium swallow suggests that, sooner or later, remedial surgery will need to be considered (Figure 6.5). However, normal passage of the liquid medium through the

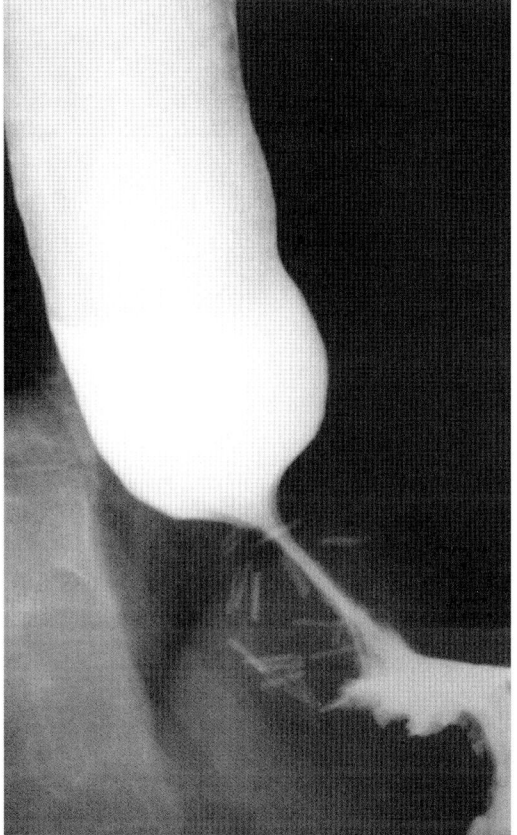

Figure 6.5. Conventional barium swallow study, showing a dilatation of the esophageal body secondary to excessive scarring of the crural sling after laparoscopic Nissen fundoplication.

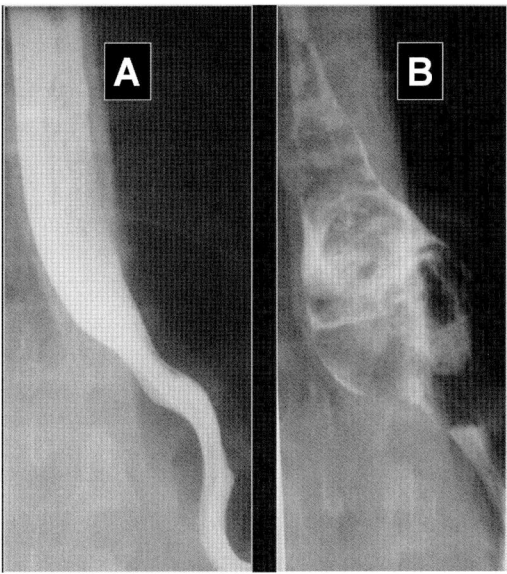

Figure 6.6. A, Conventional barium swallow study in a patient with excessive scarring of the crural sling after laparoscopic Nissen fundoplication, showing a good passage of the medium through the cardia without any enlargement of the esophageal body. B, Marshmallow study in the same patient, showing stasis of the ingested material in the lower esophagus.

cardia with no esophageal dilatation does not exclude an underlying organic problem. Indeed, esophageal stasis in some of these patients may only be revealed by barium-impregnated marshmallow ingestion (Figure 6.6).

Summary

Acute complications of anti-reflux surgery may occur during or after the operation. Intraoperative complications include injury to the upper abdominal vessels, tear of the esophageal or gastric wall, injury to the vagus nerves, pneumothorax, and pneumomediastinum (laparoscopic approach).

Postoperative complications may consist of intraabdominal or intrathoracic bleeding, gastric or esophageal fistula, herniation of the fundoplication into the chest, and acute dysphagia. Experience with both primary and remedial anti-reflux operations together with a good knowledge of the mechanisms that underly these acute complications are the key factors for their prevention and management.

References

1. Catarci M, Gentileschi P, Papi C, et al. Evidence-based appraisal of anti-reflux fundoplication. Ann Surg 2004; 239:325–337.
2. Donahue PE, Samelson S, Nyhus LM, et al. The floppy Nissen fundoplication. Effective long-term control of pathologic reflux. Arch Surg 1985;120:663–668.
3. Lundell L, Abrahamsson H, Ruth M, et al. Long-term results of a prospective randomized comparison of total fundic wrap (Nissen-Rossetti) or semifundoplication (Toupet) for gastro-oesophageal reflux. Br J Surg 1996; 83:830–835.
4. Bammer T, Hinder RA, Klaus A, et al. Five- to eight-year outcome of the first laparoscopic Nissen fundoplications. J Gastrointest Surg 2001;5:42–48.

5. Sandbu R, Khamis H, Gustavsson S, et al. Long-term results of anti-reflux surgery indicate the need for a randomized clinical trial. Br J Surg 2002;89:225–230.

6. Hunter JG, Smith CD, Branum GD, et al. Laparoscopic fundoplication failures: patterns of failure and response to fundoplication revision. Ann Surg 1999;230:595–604; discussion 604–606.

7. Detailed diagnoses and procedures, National Hospital Discharge Survey. www.cdc.gov/nchs.

8. Sandbu R, Haglund U, Arvidsson D, et al. Anti-reflux surgery in Sweden, 1987–1997: a decade of change. Scand J Gastroenterol 2000;35:345–348.

9. Laparoscopic anti-reflux surgery for gastroesophageal reflux disease (GERD). Results of a consensus development conference. Surg Endosc 1997;11:413–426.

10. Watson DI, Jamieson GG. Anti-reflux surgery in the laparoscopic era. Br J Surg 1998;85:1173–1184.

11. Soper NJ, Dunnegan D. Anatomic fundoplication failure after laparoscopic anti-reflux surgery. Ann Surg 1999; 229:669–677.

12. Finlayson SR, Laycock WS, Birkmeyer JD. National trends in utilization and outcomes of anti-reflux surgery. Surg Endosc 2003;17:864–867.

13. Collet D, Cadiere GB. Conversions and complications of laparoscopic treatment of gastroesophageal reflux disease. Formation for the Development of Laparoscopic Surgery for Gastroesophageal Reflux Disease Group. Am J Surg 1995;169:622–626.

14. Zaninotto G, Molena D, Ancona E. A prospective multicenter study on laparoscopic treatment of gastroesophageal reflux disease in Italy: type of surgery, conversions, complications, and early results. Study Group for the Laparoscopic Treatment of Gastroesophageal Reflux Disease of the Italian Society of Endoscopic Surgery (SICE). Surg Endosc 2000;14: 282–288.

15. Rantanen TK, Salo JA, Sipponen JT. Fatal and life-threatening complications in anti-reflux surgery: analysis of 5502 operations. Br J Surg 1999;86:1573–1577.

16. Carlson MA, Frantzides CT. Complications and results of primary minimally invasive anti-reflux procedures: a review of 10,735 reported cases. J Am Coll Surg 2001; 193:428–439.

17. Bowrey DJ, Peters JH. Laparoscopic esophageal surgery. Surg Clin North Am 2000;80:1213–1242.

18. Watson DI, Baigrie RJ, Jamieson GG. A learning curve for laparoscopic fundoplication. Definable, avoidable, or a waste of time? Ann Surg 1996;224:198–203.

19. DeMeester TR, Bonavina L, Albertucci M. Nissen fundoplication for gastro-esophageal reflux disease: evaluation of primary repair in 100 consecutive patients. Ann Surg 1986;204:9–20.

20. Urschel JD. Complications of anti-reflux surgery. Am J Surg 1993;166:68–70.

21. Black N, Johnston A. Volume and outcome in hospital care: evidence, explanations, and implications. Health Serv Manage Res 1990;3:108–114.

22. Hinder RA, Filipi CJ, Wetscher G, et al. Laparoscopic Nissen fundoplication is an effective treatment for gastroesophageal reflux disease. Ann Surg 1994;220: 472–483.

23. Farlo J, Thawgathurai D, Mikhail M, et al. Cardiac tamponade during laparoscopic Nissen fundoplication. Eur J Anaesthesiol 1998;15:246–247.

24. Schauer PR, Meyers WC, Eubanks S, et al. Mechanisms of gastric and esophageal perforations during laparoscopic Nissen fundoplication. Ann Surg 1996;223: 43–52.

25. Ellis FH. Editorial comment on: Mullen JT, Burke EK, Diamond AB. Esophagogastric fistula: a complication of combined operations for esophageal disease. Arch Surg 1975;110:826–828.

26. Gott JP, Polk HC Jr. Repeat operation for failure of anti-reflux procedures. Surg Clin North Am 1991;71: 13–32.

27. Cadiere GB, Himpens J, Bruyns J. How to avoid esophageal perforation while performing laparoscopic dissection of the hiatus. Surg Endosc 1995;9:450–452.

28. Horgan S, Pellegrini CA. Surgical treatment of gastroesophageal reflux disease. Surg Clin North Am 1997;77: 1063–1082.

29. Lowham AS, Filipi CJ, Hinder RA, et al. Mechanisms and avoidance of esophageal perforation by anesthesia personnel during laparoscopic foregut surgery. Surg Endosc 1996;10:979–982.

30. Del Genio A, Izzo G, Maffettone V. The surgical treatment of gastroesophageal reflux (GER). Minerva Chir 1992;47:571–577.

31. Chang L, Oelschlager B, Barreca M, et al. Improving accuracy in identifying the gastroesophageal junction during laparoscopic anti-reflux surgery. Surg Endosc 2003;17:390–393.

32. Skinner DB, Belsey RHR. Surgical management of esophageal reflux and hiatus hernia: long term results with 1030 patients. J Thorac Cardiovasc Surg 1967;53: 33–54.

33. Stadaas JO. Intragastric pressure/volume relationship before and after proximal gastric vagotomy. Scand J Gastroenterol 1975;10:129–134.

34. Bremner CG. Gastric ulceration after a fundoplication operation for gastroesophageal reflux. Surg Gynecol Obstet 1979;148:62–64.

35. Ihasz M, Griffith CA. Gallstones after vagotomy. Am J Surg 1981;141:48–50.

36. Baxter JN, Grime JS, Critchley M, et al. Relationship between gastric emptying of a solid meal and emptying of the gall bladder before and after vagotomy. Gut 1987; 28:855–863.

37. Collard JM, Verstraete L, Otte JB, et al. Clinical, radiological and functional results of remedial anti-reflux operations. Int Surg 1993;78:298–306.

38. Gutschow CA, Collard JM, Romagnoli R, et al. Bile exposure of the denervated stomach as an esophageal substitute. Ann Thorac Surg 2001;71: 1786–1791.

39. Annese V, Janssens J, Vantrappen G, et al. Erythromycin accelerates gastric emptying by inducing antral contractions and improved gastroduodenal coordination. Gastroenterology 1992;102:823–828.

40. Collard JM, Romagnoli R, Otte JB, et al. Erythromycin enhances early postoperative contractility of the denervated whole stomach as an esophageal substitute. Ann Surg 1999;229:337–343.

41. Clements RH, Reddy S, Holzman MD, et al. Incidence and significance of pneumomediastinum after laparoscopic esophageal surgery. Surg Endosc 2000;14: 553–555.

42. Testas P. The danger of and correct procedure in laparo-scopic electrosurgery. In: Steichen FM, Welter R, eds. Minimally Invasive Surgery and New Technology. St. Louis: Quality Medical Publishing; 1994:102–104.

43. Mansour KA, Burton HG, Miller JI Jr, et al. Complica-tions of intrathoracic Nissen fundoplication. Ann Thorac Surg 1981;32:173–178.

44. Richardson JD, Larson GM, Polk HC Jr. Intrathoracic fundoplication for shortened esophagus. Treacherous solution to a challenging problem. Am J Surg 1982;143: 29–35.

45. Collard JM, De Koninck XJ, Otte JB, et al. Intrathoracic Nissen fundoplication: long-term clinical and pH-monitoring evaluation. Ann Thorac Surg 1991;51:34–38.

46. Nissen R, Rossetti M. Die Behandlung Von Hiatush-ernien und Refluxösophagitis Mit Gastropexie und Fundoplicatio. Indikation, Technik und Ergebnisse. Stuttgard: Georg Thieme Verlag; 1959:30–50.

47. Gutschow C, Romagnoli R, Collard JM. What are the indications for an intra-thoracic Nissen fundoplication? What are the drawbacks of this technique? In: Giuli R, Siewert JR, Couturier D, Scarpignato C, eds. Barrett's Esophagus. Paris: John Libbey Eurotext; 2003:498–506.

48. Michel L, Collard JM. Surgical management of the Mallory-Weiss syndrome and oesophageal perforations. In: Morris PJ, Malt RA, eds. Oxford Textbook of Surgery. Oxford, UK: Oxford University Press; 1994:868–873.

49. Bladergroen MR, Lowe JE, Postlethwait RW. Diagnosis and recommended management of esophageal perfora-tion and rupture. Ann Thorac Surg 1986;42:235–239.

50. DeMeester TR. Perforation of the esophagus. Ann Thorac Surg 1986;42:231–232.

51. Watson DI, Pike GK, Baigrie RJ, et al. Prospective double-blind randomized trial of laparoscopic Nissen fundoplication with division and without division of short gastric vessels. Ann Surg 1997;226:642–652.

52. Hainaux B, Sattari A, Coppens E, et al. Intrathoracic migration of the wrap after laparoscopic Nissen fundo-plication: radiologic evaluation. AJR Am J Roentgenol 2002;178:859–862.

53. Collard JM, Verstraete L, Romagnoli R. What are the consequences of herniation of the repair into the chest? Why are they different from the primary intra-thoracic Nissen? In: Giuli R, Galmiche JP, Jamieson GG, Scarpig-nato C, eds. The Esophagogastric Junction. Paris: John Libbey Eurotext; 1998:796–798.

54. Skellenger ME, Jordan PH Jr. Complications of vago-tomy and pyloroplasty. Surg Clin North Am 1983;63: 1167–1180.

55. Guelrud M, Zambrano-Rincones V, Simon C, et al. Dys-phagia and lower esophageal sphincter abnormalities after proximal gastric vagotomy. Am J Surg 1985;149: 232–235.

56. Watson DI, Jamieson GG, Mitchell PC, et al. Stenosis of the esophageal hiatus following laparoscopic fundopli-cation. Arch Surg 1995;130:1014–1016.

57. Luostarinen ME, Isolauri JO. Randomized trial to study the effect of fundic mobilization on long-term results of Nissen fundoplication. Br J Surg 1999;86:614–618.

58. Blomqvist A, Dalenback J, Hagedorn C, et al. Impact of complete gastric fundus mobilization on outcome after laparoscopic total fundoplication. J Gastrointest Surg 2000;4:493–500.

59. O'Boyle CJ, Watson DI, Jamieson GG, et al. Division of short gastric vessels at laparoscopic Nissen fundoplica-tion: a prospective double-blind randomized trial with 5-year follow-up. Ann Surg 2002;235:165–170.

60. Collard JM, Romagnoli R, Kestens PJ. Reoperations for unsatisfactory outcome after laparoscopic anti-reflux surgery. Dis Esophagus 1996;9:56–62.

61. Dallemagne B, Weerts JM, Jehaes C, et al. Causes of fail-ures of laparoscopic anti-reflux operations. Surg Endosc 1996;10:305–310.

62. Hunter JG, Swanstrom L, Waring JP. Dysphagia after laparoscopic anti-reflux surgery. The impact of opera-tive technique. Ann Surg 1996;224:51–57.

7

Persistent Symptoms after Anti-Reflux Surgery and their Management

John G. Hunter and M. Brian Fennerty

Introduction

Since the development of laparoscopic fundo-plication, 14 years ago, many individuals with severe gastroesophageal reflux disease (GERD) have undergone laparoscopic fundoplication to free themselves from medication dependence or side effects, because medical therapy was incompletely effective, to treat extraesophageal reflux symptoms and/or to treat reflux complications including esophageal stricture, aspiration, bleeding, and Barrett's esophagus.

The most popular laparoscopic procedures performed in North America have been the total fundoplication (Nissen fundoplication) and the partial, 270° posterior fundoplication (Toupet fundoplication). In other parts of the world, anterior fundoplication (Dor or Watson fundo-plication) has also been popular. When fundo-plication is performed through a laparotomy or thoracotomy, recurrent symptoms or new troublesome symptoms have been reported in 9–30% of patients.[1,2] Laparoscopic fundoplica-tion has been associated with failure rates ranging from 2 to 17%, depending on how failure is defined.[3,4] The lower failure rates reported for laparoscopic fundoplication may reflect the fact that follow-up for these proce-dures has generally been shorter than that for open anti-reflux surgery.

The taxonomy of failed anti-reflux surgery can be based on symptoms (e.g., heartburn, dys-phagia, gas bloat) or it may be based on the anatomy of failure, using a description of how

the anatomy detected deviates from the ideal. For a surgeon, looking for defects that can be fixed, the anatomic description of failure is preferable. Kenneth DeVault discusses post-operative symptoms that are not related to anatomic fundoplication failure in Chapter 9. The anatomy or failure includes four com-monly described anatomic problems, previously described with open surgery. These problems are: 1) slipped or misplaced fundoplication, 2) disrupted fundoplication, 3) herniated fundo-plication, and 4) fundoplication that is too tight or too long.[5] Laparoscopic fundoplication has been associated with two new anatomic prob-lems, the two-compartment stomach, and the twisted fundoplication.[6]

Evaluation of Patients with New or Recurrent Symptoms of GERD

Early Postoperative Symptoms

The management of patients with new or recurrent GERD symptoms after surgery is dependent on the time of presentation. Early postoperatively (<3 months) the presence of several symptoms is extremely common and no treatment or evaluation is necessary.

The most common of these early postopera-tive symptoms after anti-reflux surgery is dys-phagia. Dysphagia to solids after anti-reflux surgery is nearly universal, and the sensation of liquids "hanging up" is not unusual either. The cause of these symptoms postoperatively is likely multifactorial. Distal esophageal edema is seen universally postoperatively, transient esophageal dysmotility has been demonstrated after anti-reflux surgery, and recently performed fundoplication-related hematomas can also cause temporary outflow obstruction from this section of the esophagus. For all these reasons, we recommend that the patients stay on a full liquid diet for the first 5–7 days after surgery, and then follow a special soft diet for the next 3 weeks. This special diet restricts the intake of large bolus foods such as meats, raw vegetables, and high-gluten-containing items such as cakes and breads. This protocol dramatically reduced the incidence of postoperative symptomatic dysphagia, food impaction, and retching that occur when a regular diet has begun too soon after surgery and the associate phone calls expressing alarm over these symptoms that will be the norm if they occur.

Despite these instructions aimed at minimizing postoperative dysphagia, when patients do complain of early postoperative dysphagia, we then instruct them to return to a liquid diet until swallowing again becomes easy and then they can be readvanced to a soft diet. If a patient has difficulty tolerating a full liquid diet, early intervention may now be necessary. These interventions include esophageal dilatation, and/or placement of a nasoenteric feeding tube. In patients who will not tolerate a nasal tube, we have used percutaneous endoscopic gastrostomy when early postoperative dysphagia became so severe as to cause weight loss or dehydration (Figure 7.1).

Another early postoperative symptom of no great consequence is the development of chest pain or recurrent reflux symptoms. The mechanism(s) related to these symptoms remains unclear. However, during the first 3 months after surgery, the patient should be reassured that it is extremely unlikely that the symptoms reflect recurring gastroesophageal reflux, especially if no postoperative events such as retching have occurred. A simple screening study such as a barium swallow may provide the opportunity to provide a worried patient great reassurance that their fundoplication has not come undone. A trial of proton pump inhibitors (PPIs) is often initiated if the patient returns to their primary care provider, but these PPIs are rarely effective for early postoperative difficulties. The best management of most early postoperative complaints is patience and reassurance, not reoperation or other reflux therapy.

Recurrent GERD Symptoms

When recurrent or new symptoms of gastroesophageal reflux develop in the late postoperative period (>3 months), the symptoms should be investigated. For individuals who develop symptoms identical to those in which they underwent surgery, a trial of PPIs is appropriate. In addition, a barium swallow will demonstrate any new anatomic abnormalities in 90% of patients with anatomic failure.[6] If the barium swallow does not demonstrate any anatomic problems, it is unlikely that the PPIs will be of much benefit. In this case, it is likely that the recurrent symptom is the result of a problem distinct from GERD. Because so-called extraesophageal reflux symptoms (cough, asthma, hoarseness, chest pain, etc.) are so common, it may be difficult to determine which of these symptoms, if any, are related to reflux and which are related to other conditions such as extrinsic asthma, or postnasal drip. It may take the performance of a fundoplication to determine, once and for all, which extraesophageal symptoms are related to reflux and which are not. It seems that extraesophageal symptoms that correlate with reflux events on a 24-hour pH study are more likely to respond to surgery than symptoms that occur with no correlation to reflux events. Frequently we have found that the typical symptoms of reflux (heartburn, dysphagia, regurgitation) will be eliminated by fundoplication but the extraesophageal symptoms in the same patient (sore throat, cough, hoarseness, wheezing) will not be eliminated by surgery. The best preoperative predictors of symptom relief after fundoplication are the presence of typical symptoms, an abnormal preoperative 24-hour pH study with a positive symptom index, and responsiveness to PPIs.

If the barium swallow does not reveal any anatomic abnormalities, and trial of medical therapy fails, further investigation is unlikely to detect problems but should be done anyway. In 10% of patients referred for postoperative reflux symptoms, esophagogastroduodenoscopy (EGD)

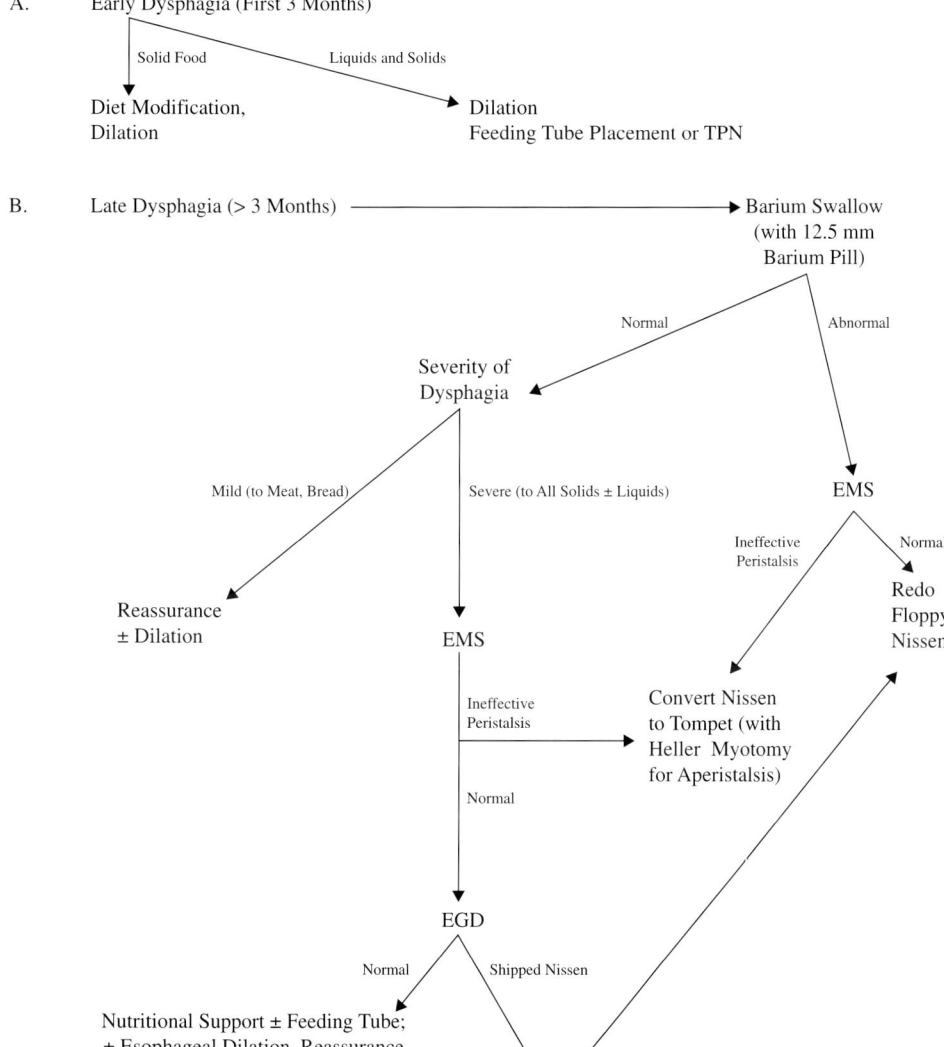

Figure 7.1. Evaluation of the patient with new dysphagia after laparoscopic Nissen fundoplication. TPN, total parenteral nutrition; EGD, esophagogastroduodenoscopy; EMS, esophageal motility study. (Reprinted from Hunter JG. Approach and management of patients with recurrent gastroesophageal reflux disease. J Gastrointest Surg 2001;5(5):451–457, Copyright 2001, with permission from Elsevier.)

revealed an additional anatomic problem that was not detected on barium swallow.[6] The most common anatomic problem discovered by EGD when the barium swallow was normal is a slipped or misplaced fundoplication. Because the gastroesophageal junction may be difficult to define on barium swallow, the EGD is necessary to demonstrate the presence of gastric folds extending through and above the fundoplication narrowing. In addition, the gastric folds may be seen coursing up into the valve, instead of remaining circumferential around the retroflexed scope (Figure 7.2). Also, a partially disrupted fundoplication may only be visible on EGD in a retroflexed position and missed with a barium swallow. This may be best demon-

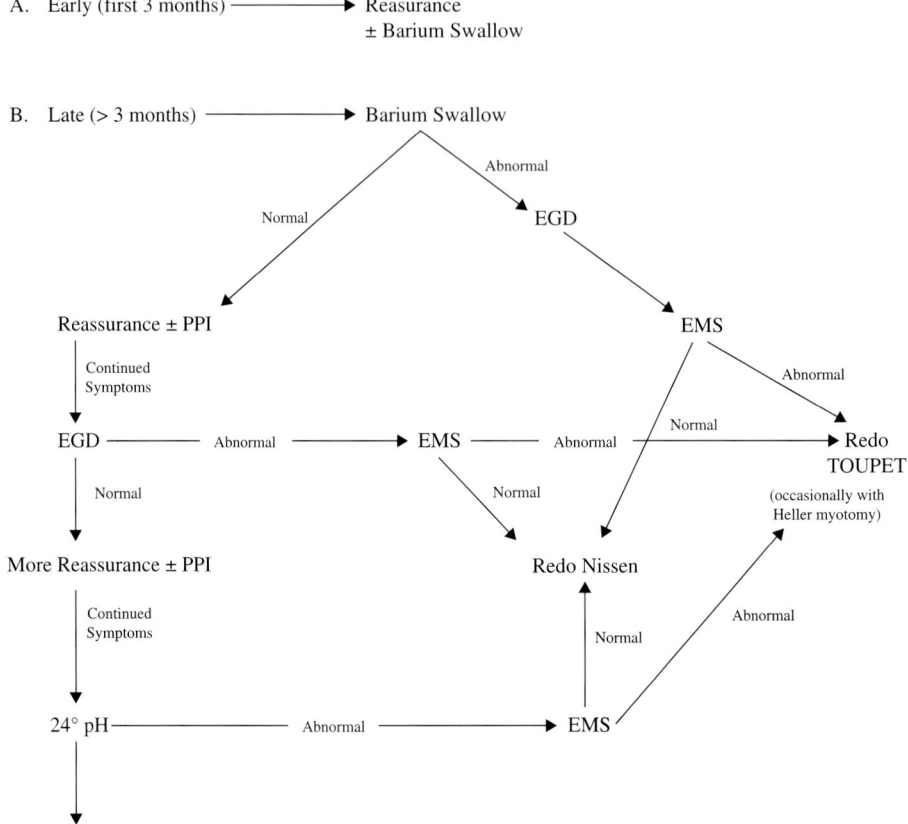

Figure 7.2. Evaluation of the patient with recurrent reflux symptoms after laparoscopic Nissen fundoplication. EGD, esophagogastroduodenoscopy; EMS, esophageal motility study; PPI, proton pump inhibitor. (Reprinted from Hunter JG. Approach and management of patients with recurrent gastroesophageal reflux disease. J Gastrointest Surg 2001;5(5):451–457, Copyright 2001, with permission from Elsevier.)

strated by a patulous gastroesophageal junction (does not hug the retroflexed endoscope), or a portion of the valve that has fallen away from the circumferential wrap. When the results of the EGD are normal and the barium swallow is normal, it is most unusual to find a patient that has a positive 24-hour pH study confirming GERD (Figure 7.3).

Persistent Postoperative Dysphagia

In contrast to the patient with recurrent GERD symptoms, the patient with persistent postoperative dysphagia represents a different problem. The management of the patient with early postoperative dysphagia was discussed above. In the patient with dysphagia persistent for >3

months, we first confirm an anatomic abnormality exists by performing a video barium swallow with a 12.5-mm barium tablet. If the pill passes the gastroesophageal junction readily, there is little that one can do to fix the "problem." Under these circumstances, the dysphagia is usually functional, or may indicate ineffective esophageal peristalsis. Thus, a normal barium swallow should be followed by an esophageal motility study in patients with significant dysphagia. If the barium tablet hangs up at the gastroesophageal junction, the problem is most likely related to the fundoplication itself, or otherwise undetected achalasia or other lower esophageal sphincter motor pathology. For this reason, a motility study is helpful, but only in preparation for a redo oper-

PERSISTENT SYMPTOMS AFTER ANTI-REFLUX SURGERY AND THEIR MANAGEMENT

ation or to detect previously unrecognized pre-operative primary esophageal dysmotility unrelated to the anti-reflux surgery. The decision to reoperate or not must be individualized based on the patient's nutritional status and the severity of the dysphagia. Early elective reoperation should be performed in patients who are confined to liquids after 3 months of watchful waiting, and patients who are losing weight because of persistent dysphagia. However, if solid food dysphagia is mild, dietary restrictions are few, and weight loss is not present, we prefer a conservative course of management for at least 1 year postoperatively. During that year,

>50% of patients will resolve their postoperative dysphagia without any intervention. However, if a barium tablet still hangs up at the distal esophagus 1 year postoperatively, and the patient is still bothered by dietary restrictions, a second operation is usually offered. A third scenario is one in which the barium tablet may or may not hang up, but the barium swallow demonstrates an obvious anatomic difficulty such as a slipped or herniated fundoplication. These patients will usually do best with reoperation and this is what we most often recommend. Although esophageal dilatation may be beneficial for early postoperative dysphagia, it is rarely helpful after

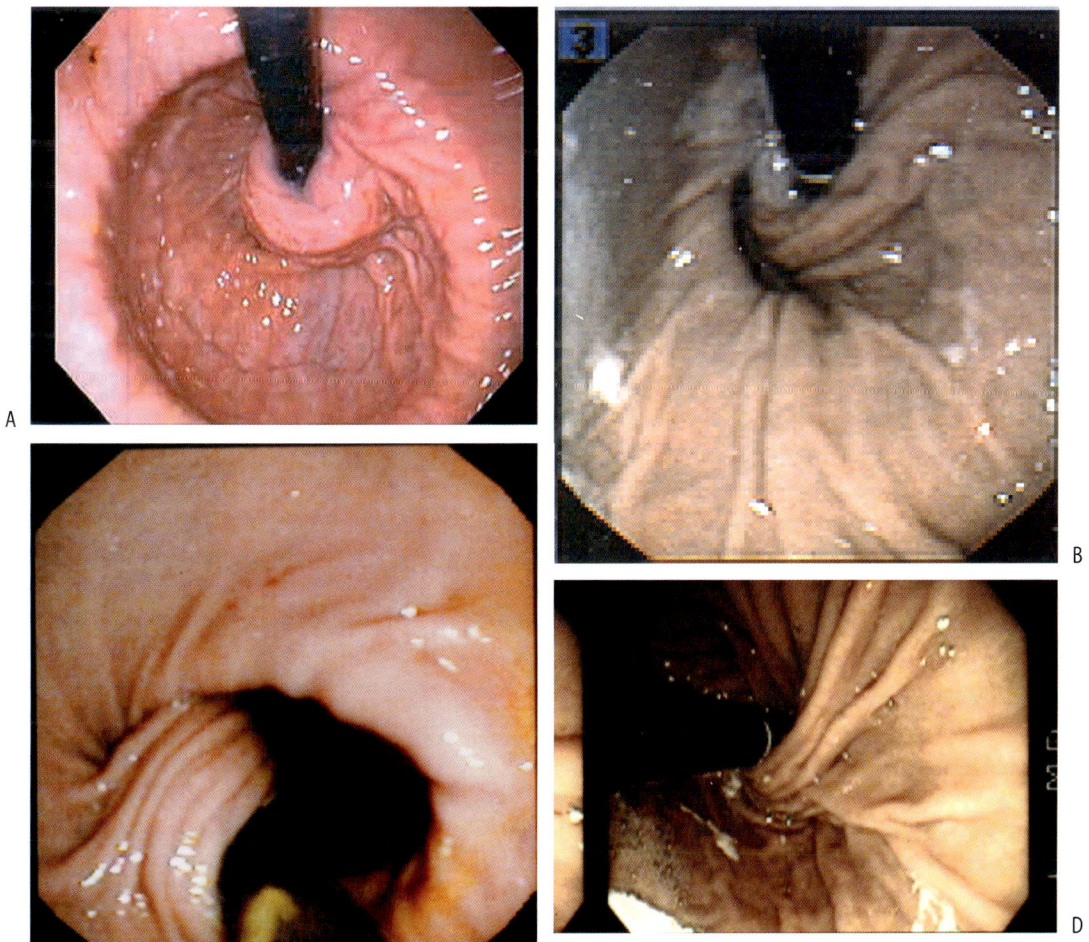

Figure 7.3. A retroflex gastroscope identifies most abnormalities of the fundoplication. A, Retroflexed view of a well-formed Nissen fundoplication. B, A herniated fundoplication. C, A twisted valve in a "two-compartment stomach." D, Partially disrupted fundoplication.

3 months postoperatively, especially if it has been used previously and failed.

Anatomic Failure of Nissen Fundoplication

Fundoplication Herniation

In our early experience, the most frequent anatomic problem we encountered after laparoscopic fundoplication was herniation of the fundoplication across the diaphragm.[6] This has almost always occurred in one of four clinical scenarios. The first situation is the patient who strains or retches in the early postoperative period. Patients often report feeling something "pop" and usually develop chest pain immediately thereafter correlating with herniation of the fundoplication. This is a true surgical emergency. The herniation should be confirmed with water-soluble contrast radiography followed by a rapid return to the operating room for laparoscopic or open reduction of the herniated stomach.

The second situation is the patient who has a similar event but more remote from the time of operation. Although these patients may develop severe acute pain after herniation of the fundoplication, the return of symptoms is usually more insidious, and the time of herniation may be difficult to pinpoint. Under these circumstances, the herniation is more frequently heralded by the symptoms of heartburn, new onset dysphagia, or postprandial chest pain resulting from gas or food distending the mediastinal portion of the herniated fundoplication. These patients should be evaluated with a barium swallow and EGD. Depending on the length of time between the first operation and the development of the hernia, we will perform esophageal motility and/or a gastric emptying study to better define foregut physiology in this postoperative state in planning for a second surgery.

The third situation is even more insidious. In this situation, the patient develops a slow onset of recurrent or new symptoms (chest pain, dysphagia, heartburn) in the absence of a precipitating event. In this scenario, the inciting etiology may be acquired esophageal shortening, rather than a transdiaphragmatic stressor.

In these patients, the indication for the primary operation was more frequently a giant hiatal (paraesophageal) hernia, esophageal stricture, or Barrett's esophagus. In these patients, the herniation likely occurred because of esophageal shortening that was not detected and adequately treated with an esophageal lengthening procedure at the first operation. Elective reoperation should include an esophageal lengthening procedure such as a Collis gastroplasty along with a reinforcement and closure of the esophageal hiatus.

The fourth presentation of fundoplication herniation is those with small herniation who usually remain asymptomatic. In our experience, nearly half of the patients who develop fundoplication herniation will be asymptomatic, especially if the first operation was performed for a paraesophageal hiatal hernia.[7] If a patient with a small asymptomatic recurrent hernia is not anemic, and has no evidence of ulceration in the herniated fundoplication, we recommend a strategy of watchful waiting.

In summary, patients with acute postoperative herniation require an emergency operation, those with "event induced" recurrence should undergo elective reoperation, those with a recurrent secondary to esophageal shortening should undergo Collis gastroplasty and repeat fundoplication, and those with asymptomatic recurrence need not undergo reoperation at all.

Slipped Nissen Fundoplication

Patients with a slipped Nissen represent a difficult challenge. Those with a gastric pouch above the fundoplication will often have symptoms of severe reflux, regurgitation, and dysphagia. Not only is food trapped in this pouch during swallowing, acid-rich refluxate pools in this pouch, immediately below an incompetent sphincter. These patients may develop severe erosive esophagitis, strictures, and even Barrett's esophagus if this problem is not alleviated. It should be no surprise that these patients are extremely grateful when the fundoplication is placed in the correct location on the esophagus. It may be impossible, preoperatively, for the surgeon to determine whether the fundoplication has truly slipped, or whether it was misplaced initially. Reoperation in patients with a misplaced fundoplication often reveals that the mediastinal component of the esophagus, just above the gastroesophageal junction, was never mobilized during the first procedure and there is very adequate esophageal length to place the fundoplication higher up in the correct position. Alternatively, if the fundoplication is truly slipped onto the stomach, especially in patients with advanced esophageal disease, this may indicate a shortened esophagus which will need to be addressed with a gastroplasty. The operative principles will be discussed in another chapter.

Disrupted Fundoplication, Twisted Fundoplication, and the Two-compartment Stomach

The disrupted fundoplication is perhaps easiest to diagnose and repair. The preoperative evaluation of these patients will usually include a 24-hour pH study, esophageal motility testing, barium swallow, and EGD. If the patient has erosive esophagitis on EGD, the pH study may be omitted but it is generally advisable to do a complete physiologic evaluation before reoperating on a patient with a disrupted fundoplication.

Although disrupted fundoplications are well known in the era of open surgery, two new defects were described after the advent of laparoscopic fundoplication. These are the twisted fundoplication and the two-compartment stomach. The twisted fundoplication results when the surgeon fails to mobilize the greater curvature of the stomach from the spleen and diaphragm. This is more frequently the case when the short gastric vessels are not divided. A portion of the anterior wall of the stomach is pulled from the left around the esophagus posteriorly and sutured to another portion of the anterior wall of the stomach which has been pulled from a spot low on the greater curvature. This creates tension at the gastroesophageal junction which can result in a rotation of the distal esophagus and fundoplication to develop a spiral-type deformity seen in retroflexion of the endoscope (Figure 7.3). This deformity is usually associated with symptoms of dysphagia and severe postoperative gas bloat. An esophageal dilator will usually pass through this defect easily, but upon removal of the dilator, the twist will be recreated. Thus,

esophageal dilation has little role in managing this deformity.

Occasionally, individuals who have a spiral deformity because of inadequate fundus mobilization will develop a second problem, which is that of the two-compartment stomach. This occurs because the point on the greater curvature chosen for the left side of the fundoplication, when pulled through the gastroesophageal junction, will create a waste around the mid-stomach. The fundic compartment resides against the posterior left hemidiaphragm in the distal compartment (the atrium) lies below the septation. The proximal compartment is filled preferentially with food and will create early satiety, upper gastric discomfort, nausea, and retching. The twisted valve relaxes poorly and thus retching does not usually result in relief of the gastric distension. These patients are extremely uncomfortable and require urgent operation once the diagnosis is made. Barium swallow and upper endoscopy usually reveal the septated nature of the stomach, and the diagnosis is not difficult.

Bloating, Nausea, and Epigastric Pain

The small group of patients who undergo laparoscopic Nissen fundoplication will be plagued by persistent bloating, nausea, and epigastric pain postoperatively. These patients may be divided into two groups: those with functional problems, discussed by Dr. DeVault in a later chapter, and those with severe gastric emptying which may be a result of inadvertent vagal injury or may be preoperative gastroparesis that was undetected until an operation was performed. The optimal treatment of postoperative nausea involves the use of antiemetics for the first few months. When nausea persists beyond the early postoperative period, an investigation is warranted. Initially, we believed that these symptoms were a result of PPI withdrawal, but found little evidence that proton pump inhibition was of any benefit in treating postoperative nausea. When nausea is persistent postoperatively we recommend an EGD be performed despite this examination usually detecting no explanatory pathology. Symptom-directed therapy is then indicated. An antiemetic cocktail frequently successful in this situation includes ondansetron, Phenergan, and the pro-kinetic agent, metoclopramide. In contrast, when the EGD demonstrates food in the stomach after a 12-hour fast, it is likely that gastroparesis is present. There is probably little need to perform a gastric emptying study in these patients, but we generally perform this study to quantify the amount of gastric retention. This measurement may be useful when compared with gastric emptying studies performed after therapy is initiated. If the gastric emptying cannot be normalized on prokinetic agents, we sometimes recommend that a pyloro-plasty be performed. In addition, we have started using gastric stimulation with an implantable system (Medtronics, Minneapolis, MN) in some of these selected cases. If the patient has lost a significant amount of weight, a feeding jejunostomy can be performed. After these interventions, we prefer to wait at least a year to determine whether gastric emptying will return. If there is no appreciable improvement in symptoms or gastric emptying after a 12-month follow-up period, subtotal gastrectomy with Roux-en-Y gastrojejunostomy may be considered (Figure 7.4). Unfortunately, the results of

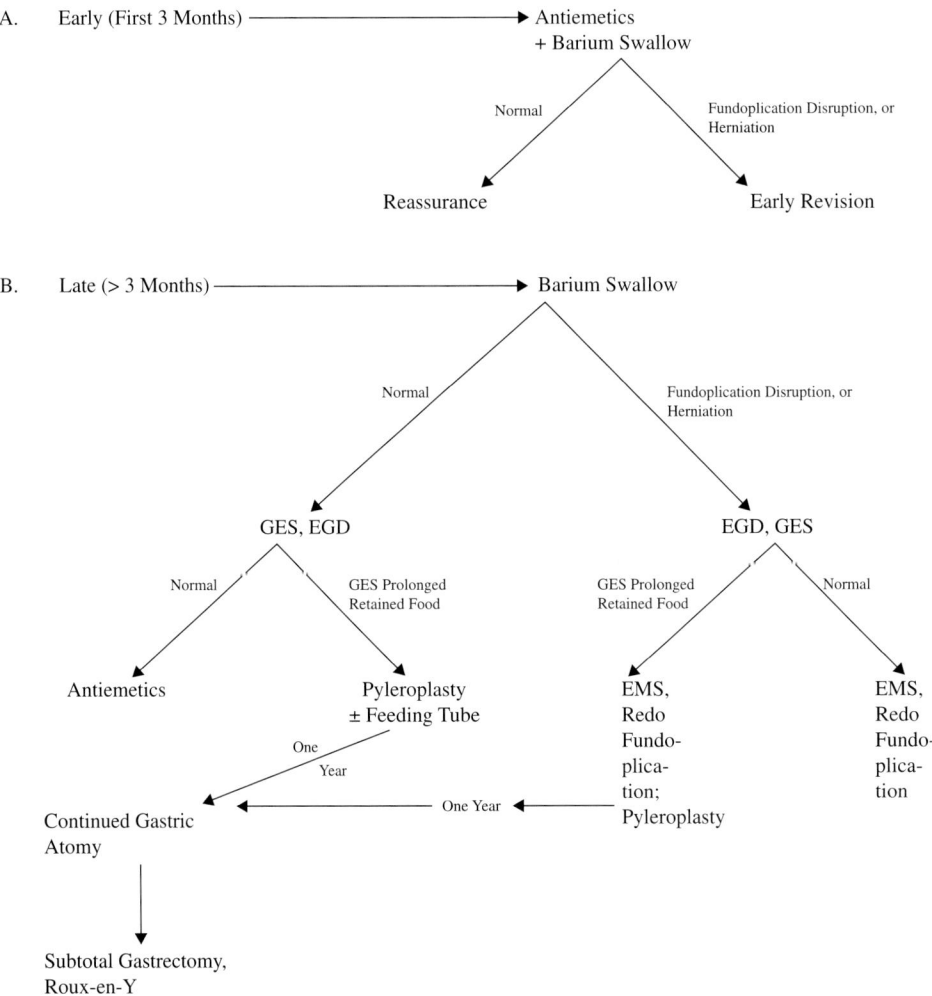

Figure 7.4. Evaluation of the patient with severe bloating, nausea, and retching after laparoscopic Nissen fundoplication. GES, gastric emptying study; EGD, esophagogastroduodenoscopy; EMS, esophageal motility study. (Reprinted from Hunter JG. Approach and management of patients with recurrent gastroesophageal reflux disease. J Gastrointest Surg 2001;5(5):451–457, Copyright 2001, with permission from Elsevier.)

this operation in this patient population are frequently poor.

Reoperation for Fundoplication Failure

Several studies have addressed the performance of reoperative laparoscopic fundoplication.[6,8–11] Some surgeons will attempt to perform all reoperative fundoplications laparoscopically, some will perform all reoperative fundoplications via thoracotomy, and some will perform all redo fundoplications through a laparotomy. We generally tailor our reoperative surgery according to the method used for the previous operation. That is, when the first operation was performed through a thoracotomy or with laparoscopy, the preferred approach is laparoscopic. When the first operation was performed through a laparotomy, our preferred approach is through a laparotomy, because when we approach this latter group through a thoracotomy, the intraabdominal adhesions make redo surgery difficult. When we perform the redo operation after laparotomy with laparoscopy, we have found that intraabdominal adhesions also make the laparoscopic procedure quite lengthy.[6,10] Whether the redo fundoplication is performed laparoscopically or through a laparotomy, the operative principles are the same.

Exposure for Reoperative Laparoscopic Fundoplication

For reoperative surgery, we use the same five-trocar technique that was used for the primary operation. Before one can elevate the left lobe of the liver adequately, adhesions between the fundoplication and the liver must be taken down. It is occasionally necessary to replace the liver retractor several times during the process of this dissection. Adhesiolysis is best performed with electrosurgical scissors, or ultrasonic shears (harmonic scalpel; Ethicon Inc., Cincinnati, OH). The goal of dissection is to identify the diaphragmatic hiatus in its entirety. Similar to a first-time fundoplication, safe dissection is dissection that stays away from the esophagus and stays on the diaphragmatic hiatus. It is usually easiest to approach the diaphragmatic hiatus from the left side of the patient as adhesions between the liver, stomach, and right crus often make the initial approach on the right side more problematic. If the short gastric vessels have been previously mobilized, it is relatively easy to follow the stomach to the left crus of the diaphragm and then follow the left crus down to its base. The right diaphragm is best approached by identifying the caudate lobe of the liver and the gastrohepatic omentum and then proceeding superiorly and to the left until the right crus is identified. If the hepatic branch of the vagus has not been divided during the first operation, it is usually necessary to do so at the second operation to facilitate exposure of the diaphragm. Similarly, if the short gastric vessels were not divided during the first operation, this too needs to be performed during the second procedure. A 360° dissection of the hiatus will allow a Penrose drain to be placed around the esophagus. If the stomach is truly herniated through the hiatus, a longer length of Penrose is passed with which to encircle the herniated stomach. The drain is held in place with endosurgical clips or with an Endoloop. Inferior traction is then placed on the drain to allow the surgeon to reduce the herniated fundoplication back into the abdomen, or to further dissect out the mediastinal esophagus. A herniated stomach may be easily reduced or may require meticulous dissection to free it from the diaphragm and mediastinal structures. Significant mediastinal adhesions are more common when the fundoplication herniates early postoperatively, and may present a formidable technical challenge. It is occasionally necessary to open the diaphragm by dividing the crural arch anteriorly or laterally to gain more working room during this mobilization. It is not unusual for a pneumothorax to develop during such mobilization but generally this is well tolerated. The anesthesiologist may notice some mild desaturation, but usually notices nothing at all. If we detect a pneumothorax, we usually decrease our intraabdominal pressure to approximately 10 mm Hg, and place a red rubber catheter with several additional side holes cut across the diaphragm and into the chest cavity (usually the left chest).

Once the fundoplication has been reduced from the chest, the next step is to completely take down the previous fundoplication. This is performed with sharp dissection by identifying the sutures on the anterior portion of the fundoplication and dividing them sharply. The fundus of the stomach is then peeled to the left and to the right from the midline. The dissection of the left portion of the fundoplication is usually fairly easy, but dissection of the right portion of the fundoplication, off the esophagus, may be more problematic because of extensive adhesions. It is important during the takedown of the fundoplication to identify the anterior and posterior vagus nerves. To prevent injury to these nerves, it is best not to use electrosurgery or harmonic scalpel close to the nerves. Generally, the vagal trunks can be found in the fundoplication. When the posterior vagus nerve is left within the fundoplication, it is usually easy to preserve; however, if it was left outside of the fundoplication, it may be sectioned inadvertently. The anterior vagus nerve is closely adherent to the esophagus, often encased in scar, and may be best preserved by staying away from this region. Once the fundoplication has been entirely taken down, an assessment of intraabdominal length is performed by reapproximating the crura with graspers and letting go of all inferior traction on the gastroesophageal junction. If 2 cm of esophagus remains in the abdomen, without tension, the esophagus is not shortened and a lengthening procedure need not be done. If the gastroesophageal junction springs back to within 2 cm of the closed hiatus, an esophageal lengthening procedure is performed. There are several ways to perform a Collis gastroplasty with minimally invasive techniques.[12–14] Occasionally, patients appear to have adequate intraabdominal length but will have had a twice-herniated fundoplication without known diaphragmatic stressors. Under these circumstances, we advocate performing an esophageal lengthening procedure regardless of the intraoperative measurements.

I am often asked whether a pyloroplasty is indicated when neither vagal nerve can be identified because of previous operations. We generally do not recommend routine pyloroplasty because many vagotomized stomachs will empty reasonably normally and pyloroplasty can then be used selectively in those patients who develop postoperative gastric emptying abnormalities. It has been extremely rare that we have found it necessary to return later to perform pyloroplasty.

Occasionally the need for a second or third revision arises. We have reported that the results of redo fundoplications deteriorate with each successive operation.[6] Whereas success rates for the first operation range between 90–95%, second operations have been successful between 80–90% of the time, and third operations are successful between 50–66% of the time. Because fourth operations are rarely successful at all, some experts suggest that an esophageal resection be performed after three failed fundoplications. Despite this policy, we have performed fewer than five esophageal resections over 10 years for repeated fundoplication failure.

Conclusion

The revolution in laparoscopic anti-reflux surgery has created new and challenging problems for the laparoscopic surgeon, the failed laparoscopic Nissen fundoplication. With thorough preoperative evaluation and meticulous surgical technique, many of these patients may undergo successful reoperation using laparoscopic methods with good or excellent outcome.

References

1. DeMeester TR, Bonivina L, Albertucci M. Nissen fundoplication for gastroesophageal reflux disease: evaluation of primary repair in 100 consecutive patients. Ann Surg 1986;204:9–20.
2. Shirazzi SS, Schulze K, Soper RT. Long-term follow-up for treatment of complicated chronic reflux esophagitis. Arch Surg 1987;122:548–552.
3. Hinder RA, Filipi CJ, Wetscher G, Neary P, DeMeester TR, Perdikis G. Laparoscopic Nissen fundoplication is an effective treatment for gastroesophageal reflux disease. Ann Surg 1994;220:472–483.
4. Cushieri A, Hunter JG, Wolfe B, Swanstrom LL, Hutson W. Multicenter prospective evaluation of laparoscopic anti-reflux surgery. Surg Endosc 1995;7:505–510.
5. Hinder RA, Klingler PJ, Perdikis G, Smith SL. Management of the failed anti-reflux operation. Surg Clin North Am 1997;77:1083–1098.
6. Hunter JG, Smith CD, Branum GD, et al. Laparoscopic fundoplication failures: patterns of failure and response to fundoplication revision. Ann Surg 1999;230:595–606.
7. Watson DI, Jamieson GG, Devitt PG, Mitchell PC, Game PA. Paraesophageal hiatus hernia: an important complication of laparoscopic Nissen fundoplication. Br J Surg 1995;82:521–523.
8. Soper NJ, Dunnegan D. Anatomic fundoplication failure after laparoscopic anti-reflux surgery. Ann Surg 1999; 229:669–677.
9. Curet MJ, Josloff RK, Schoeb O, Zucker KA. Laparoscopic reoperation for failed anti-reflux procedures. Arch Surg 1999;134:559–563.

10. Pointer R, Bammer T, Then P, Kamolz T. Laparoscopic re-fundoplications after failed anti-reflux surgery. Am J Surg 1999;178:541–544.

11. Horgan S, Pohl D, Bogetti D, Eubanks T, Pellegrini C. Failed anti-reflux surgery: what have we learned from reoperations? Arch Surg 1999;134:809–817.

12. Johnson AB, Oddsdottir M, Hunter JG. Laparoscopic Collis gastroplasty and Nissen fundoplication: a new technique for the management of esophageal shortening. Surg Endosc 1998;12:1055–1060.

13. Terry ML, Vernon A, Hunter JG. Stapled-wedge Collis gastroplasty for the shortened esophagus. Am J Surg 2004;188:195–199.

14. Swanstrom LL, Marcus DR, Galloway GQ. Laparoscopic Collis gastroplasty is the treatment of choice for the shortened esophagus. Am J Surg 1996;171(5):477–481.

8

Technical Surgical Failures: Presentation, Etiology, and Evaluation

Carrie A. Sims and David W. Rattner

Approximately 48,000 patients undergo anti-reflux procedures each year in the United States. Although surgery is the most effective treatment for gastroesophageal reflux disease (GERD), anti-reflux operations have reported failure rates between 3–30%. This wide variability reflects differences in operative technique, differences in the length of reported follow-up, and differences in the definitions used to describe failure. For the purposes of this chapter, failure is defined as the development of recurrent or new symptoms after anti-reflux surgery combined with documented pathologic gastroesophageal reflux or anatomic failure. Failures occurring within the first 3 months of surgery are termed early failures and are generally caused by technical errors. Diaphragmatic stressors such as coughing, straining, vomiting, retching, and weight lifting increase the risk of recurrence, especially in the early postoperative period. When failures occur after 3 months, they are termed late failures and a combination of factors may be responsible. The size of the original hiatal hernia, increased intraabdominal pressure, the presence of Barrett's esophagus, and the use of steroids predispose to late failures. This chapter will discuss the evaluation and management of failed fundoplications.

Presenting Symptoms of Failed Anti-Reflux Operations

Patients with GERD often have associated gastrointestinal motility disorders. Because patients have high expectations of anti-reflux surgery, many perceive that residual symptoms represent an indication of fundoplication failure. It is well known, however, that symptoms correlate poorly with the presence of acid reflux after fundoplication. Soper and Dunnegan[1] found that 26% of those undergoing laparoscopic anti-reflux surgery reported postoperative foregut symptoms. After an extensive evaluation, 35% had no demonstrable abnormality and their symptoms resolved without intervention.[1] Galvani et al.[2] studied 124 patients with persistent or recurrent foregut symptoms after laparoscopic fundoplication. Only 39% were found to have acid reflux by 24-hour pH monitoring. Viewed another way, two-thirds of the patients who were taking acid-reducing medications postoperatively were found to have normal 24-hour pH probes studies (the studies were performed off medication).[2] Almost every patient experiences some degree of dysphagia in the early postoperative period. In a review by Perdikis et al.,[3] dysphagia occurred in 20% of the 2453 patients analyzed. Initial dysphagia may be secondary to distal esophageal edema or transient esophageal dysmotility and most patients can be treated expectantly. Given the disparity between symptoms and demonstrable anatomic or physiologic abnormalities, documenting functional status with appropriate testing must be performed before ascribing symptoms after fundoplication to a failed operation.

Patients with failed anti-reflux surgery typically complain of dysphagia, heartburn, vomiting, or a combination of these symptoms.[4] The

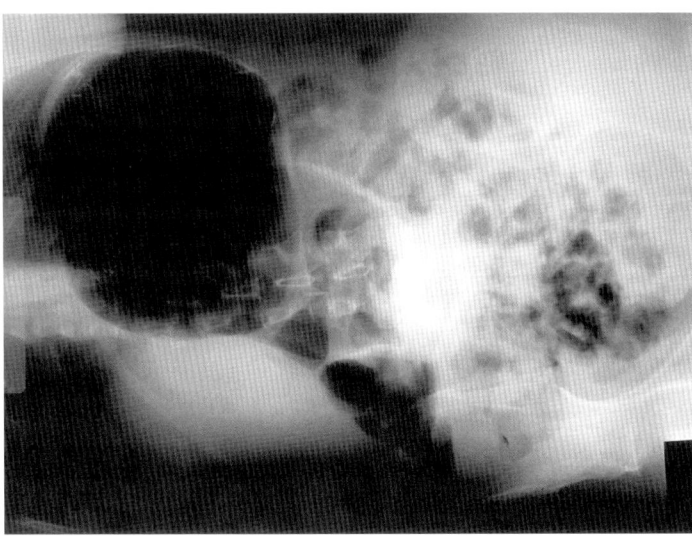

Figure 8.1. Upright abdominal radiograph demonstrating a dilated gas-filled stomach consistent with the gas bloat syndrome.

majority of symptomatic recurrences occur within 2 years.[5] Patients whose dysphagia persists for more than 3 months postoperatively should be suspected of having an anatomic problem. In the early postoperative period, substernal chest pain or discomfort is another common symptom. Although the etiology is not well understood, the pain may be secondary to esophageal spasm, irritation from the esophageal dissection and mobilization, or referred pain from the crural repair. The pain may be described as a dull ache although some patients describe it as heartburn. Usually this, too, can be managed conservatively. Vomiting in the postoperative setting is very abnormal and often signifies disruption of the fundoplication. More ominously, it may be the presenting sign of an incarcerated iatrogenic paraesophageal hernia. If a patient experiences severe chest pain in the setting of retching or straining, the diagnosis of a transhiatal herniation of the wrap should be considered. This is a surgical emergency and a water-soluble contrast study should be done immediately to confirm the diagnosis. If herniation is present, the patient should be returned expeditiously to the operating room for a laparoscopic or open reduction of the herniated stomach.

Whereas dysphagia and heartburn are the most common symptoms after fundoplication, rarely, patients may complain of "gas bloat" characterized by the onset of severe epigastric pain approximately 30 minutes after eating.

Patients with an improperly constructed fundoplication may not be able to easily belch and painful abdominal bloating may arise when swallowed air is "trapped." This is readily diagnosed with a plain film of the abdomen showing a distended gas-filled stomach (Figure 8.1) or in the absence of an X-ray, prompt relief of pain by passage of a nasogastric tube. The "gas bloat syndrome" should be differentiated from the more common complaint of generalized abdominal bloating and increased flatulence as the latter tends to resolve on its own over time.

Methods of Evaluation

Given the poor correlation between symptoms and anatomic failure, a careful and thorough evaluation is warranted. A complete history and physical should be performed with particular attention to the patient's current symptoms. Are the symptoms similar to those experienced before the original surgery? Do symptoms of reflux or dysphagia predominate? Was there a precipitating event? Do antacid medications ameliorate the symptoms? The patient's original operative report should be obtained to clarify the type of fundoplication and extent of dissection. Any prior preoperative radiographs and physiologic test results should also be obtained and reviewed. If the patient's symptoms are identical to their prior symptoms of reflux, a 2-week trial of omeprazole at 40 mg/d should be initiated. Symptoms that completely resolve on this regimen should raise suspicion for recurrent reflux. The patient can be offered a continued course of medical therapy as a reasonable option. Many patients feel so well after successful anti-reflux surgery, however, that they prefer another operation to a lifetime of medical therapy. If the patient does not respond to omeprazole or has symptoms of dysphagia, the work-up should proceed with more invasive monitoring and diagnostic studies in an attempt to elucidate the etiology of their symptoms.

A barium swallow should be the initial diagnostic study in the work-up of any symptomatic patient. This relatively noninvasive, inexpensive study will define the patient's anatomy and help clarify the relationship of the gastroesophageal junction to the hiatus. This study may also demonstrate gastroesophageal reflux and can detect evidence of delayed esophageal emptying. A barium swallow is particularly helpful when the patient presents with symptoms of dysphagia or pain and can help delineate a gross anatomic defect that might explain the patient's symptoms (Figure 8.2). However, the failure to visualize reflux on a barium study does not exclude the possibility that the patient is experiencing pathologic reflux. Because patients may have symptoms consistent with reflux without evidence of gastroesophageal reflux, a 24-hour pH study is important in patients whose anatomy seems to be intact. This functional study confirms the presence of pathologic gastroesophageal reflux. By maintaining a 24-hour diary, the patient's subjective assessment of reflux can be correlated with monitored episodes of reflux. Patients who have "reflux" symptoms, but a normal 24-hour pH study, are likely to have another cause for their symptoms and will not benefit from refundoplication.

Upper gastrointestinal endoscopy should be routinely performed in evaluating patients who are symptomatic after a fundoplication. Endoscopy and barium swallows provide complementary information. In up to 10% of patients, an endoscopy will reveal an anatomic problem not appreciated by a barium swallow.[6] In particular, endoscopic evaluation may reveal a "spiraling" or "twisting" of the wrap that may be missed by standard barium studies (Figure 8.3). Endoscopy also helps assess complications of gastroesophageal reflux such as esophagitis and Barrett's mucosal changes. The degree of

these changes may impact the decision to reoperate or treat medically.

Esophageal manometry should be routinely performed before considering reoperation. Manometry provides an objective means of assessing the location and resting pressure of the lower esophageal sphincter. It can also provide an assessment of the functional status of esophageal peristalsis and sphincter relaxation. Manometric studies are critical when

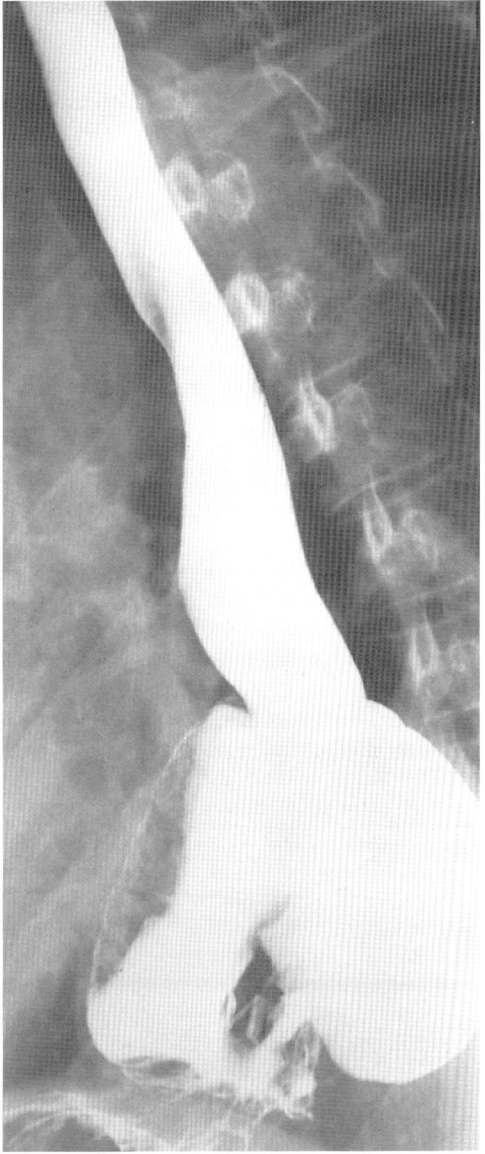

Figure 8.2. A barium swallow demonstrating a slipped Nissen fundoplication.

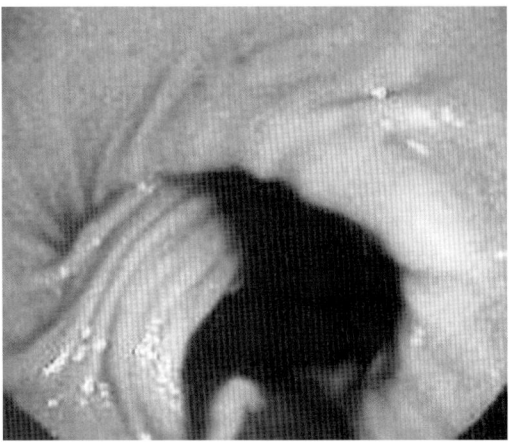

Figure 8.3. A retroflexed endoscopic view of the gastroesophageal junction demonstrating a twisted fundoplication.

evaluating the patient who presents with dysphagia, as these patients may have a previously undiagnosed esophageal motility disorder. It may be particularly difficult to differentiate patients with misdiagnosed achalasia from those whose fundoplication is too tight causing secondary poor esophageal peristaltic function. Moreover, patients who initially had normal esophageal function before surgery may develop secondary achalasia after fundoplication.[7] If reoperative surgery is indicated, the type of fundoplication chosen may depend on the results of esophageal manometry. Patients complaining of dysphagia who are found to have poor esophageal motility probably should not be offered a 360° wrap.

Patients with persistent bloating, nausea, vomiting, abdominal pain, and early satiety should undergo gastric emptying studies. These symptoms may be secondary to previously undiagnosed gastroparesis. An injury to the vagus nerves may also lead to abnormal gastric function with rapid emptying of liquids and delayed emptying of solids. If gastroparesis is detected, the success rate of a reoperation is lower and a pyloroplasty should be performed.

Potential Causes of Failure

Regardless of the surgical nuances, failed anti-reflux operations can be analyzed and subdivided into three distinct anatomic regions.

Failure can occur at the esophageal, wrap, or crural level, although there may be overlapping or concurrent issues. Before the wide adoption of laparoscopic techniques, wrap disruption was the most common mode of failure. In the laparoscopic era, the most common cause of failure is herniation of the wrap through the diaphragmatic hiatus.

The construction of a fundoplication (particularly a 360° fundoplication) may unmask previously unrecognized esophageal dysmotility or misdiagnosed achalasia leading to severe postoperative dysphagia. Chronic inflammation can also contribute to esophageal failure. Both Barrett's esophagus and severe esophageal reflux are associated with chronic esophageal inflammation. Chronic inflammation results in fibrosis, foreshortening, esophageal dysmotility, and poor acid clearance. Poor acid clearance in turn contributes to more esophageal irritation and the vicious cycle is propagated. Over time, the esophagus may become significantly foreshortened and fibrotic. Although there is controversy over the true incidence of the short esophagus, we believe that this entity exists.

A variety of issues involving fundoplication construction can contribute to failed anti-reflux surgery (Figure 8.4). The easiest failure to diagnose and repair is the "missin' Nissen"—a fundoplication that is disrupted or completely undone. A "slipped" Nissen results when the body of the stomach intussuscepts through the fundoplication. This creates an hourglass defect with part of the stomach residing above the wrap and part below. Patients with a "slipped" fundoplication often experience severe reflux and regurgitation because the pouch of stomach above the wrap traps food and serves as a reservoir of acid-rich refluxate below an incompetent esophageal sphincter. Similarly, a wrap may be misplaced around the upper stomach rather than around the esophagus. This creates an hourglass defect in which the wrap is below the diaphragmatic hiatus, but the upper stomach and gastroesophageal junction are above the diaphragm. Another common error particularly in the laparoscopic era is use of the body or even antrum of the stomach to construct a Nissen fundoplication (Figure 8.5). This leads to a twisted, bulky wrap that fails to function properly. Lastly, a fundoplication that is too tight may result in dysphagia. Since the work of

Dunnington and DeMeester[8] established the efficacy of the floppy fundoplication, most surgeons construct 360° wraps over a 56–60 French dilator to avoid this problem. However, constructing a wrap over a large dilator without adequate fundic mobilization can still lead to tension. By routinely dividing the short gastric vessels and approximating the crura, Soper and Dunnegan[1] reported the failure rate of primary laparoscopic fundoplication decreased from 19% to 4%. Whereas others have demonstrated that division of the short gastric vessels does not improve the clinical outcome of laparoscopic fundoplication, the Nissen procedure performed in this study as the control was not the classic "floppy" fundoplication with full mobilization.[9] As such, we believe that the short gastric vessels should be divided with full mobi-

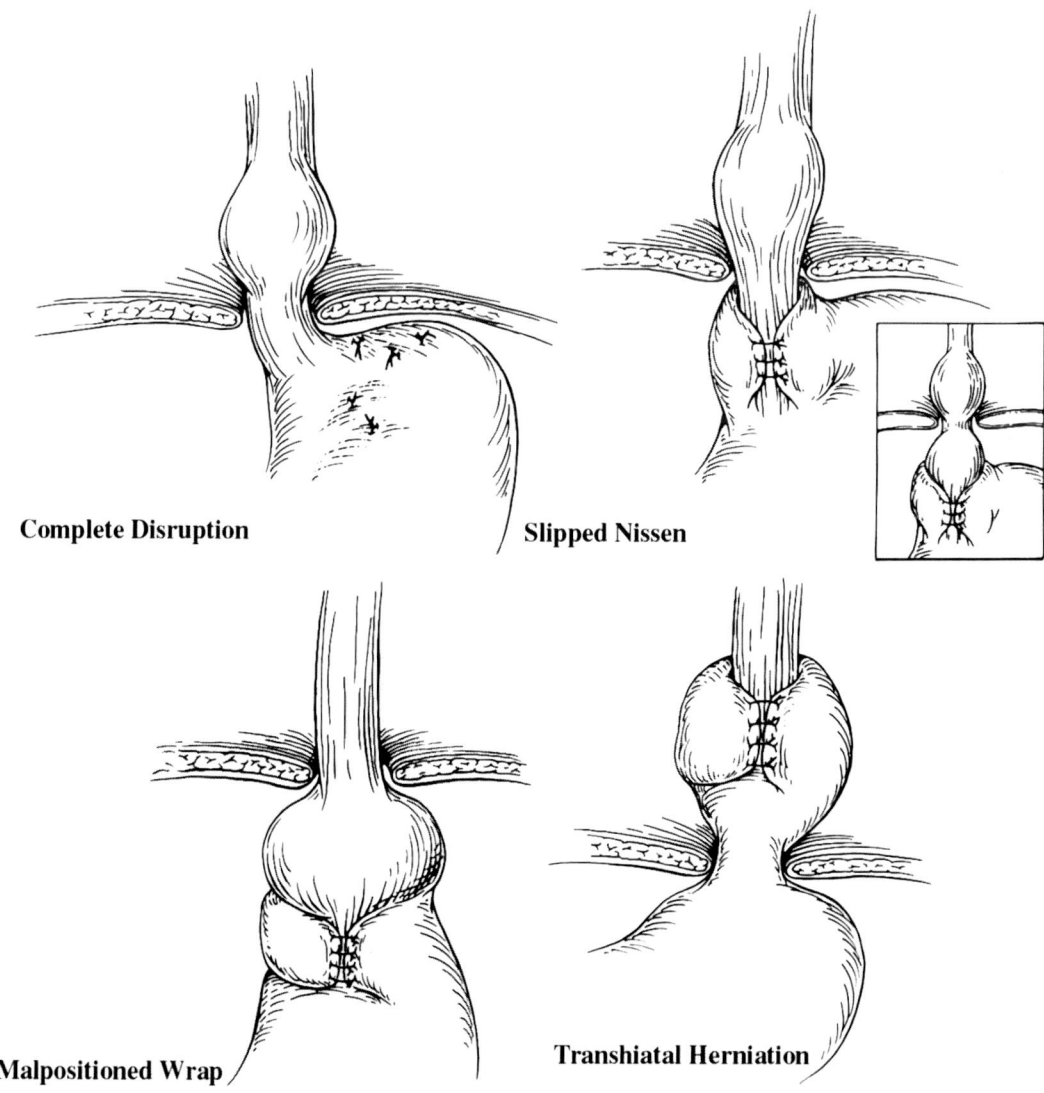

Complete Disruption

Slipped Nissen

Malpositioned Wrap

Transhiatal Herniation

Figure 8.4. Types of surgical failure of Nissen fundoplication. (Reprinted from Hinder RA. Gastroesophageal reflux disease. In: Bell RH Jr, Rikkers LF, Mulholland MW, eds. Digestive Tract Surgery: A Text and Atlas. Philadelphia: Lippincott-Raven Publishers; 1996:19, with permission.)

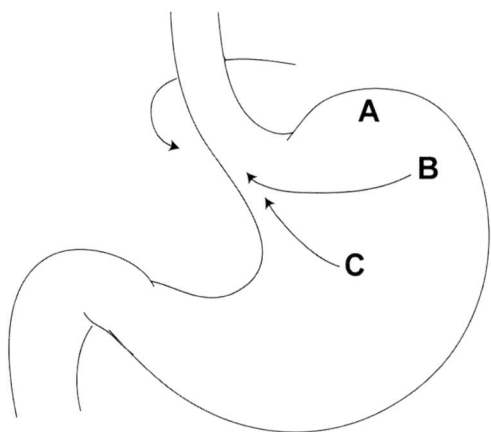

Figure 8.5. The body or antrum of the stomach can be mistakenly used to form the fundoplication. A proper fundoplication is constructed by wrapping "A" around the distal esophagus and bringing "B" anterior to the esophagus to join "A." By bringing "C" anteriorly to complete the wrap, a malformed fundoplication will be created.

lization of the fundus in order to create a wrap that lies comfortably around the esophagus.

There are a myriad of partial fundoplications in use today. The most common laparoscopic partial fundoplication is the posterior fundoplication described by Andre Toupet. Because few surgeons had experience with this repair in the open era, modern-day laparoscopic surgeons tend to make this fundoplication too short. In contrast to the Nissen fundoplication, longer is better for a Toupet procedure. The wrap should extend for at least 4 cm. Belsey fundoplication failures are usually attributed to inadequate esophageal mobilization or improper depth of suture placement when constructing the wrap.

The competency of the crural closure is critical in the performance of a successful fundoplication. The crural closure can either be too tight leading to dysphagia or too lax leading to transdiaphragmatic herniation of the wrap. In open operations, the crural closure should admit the tip of the surgeon's index finger snugly when a nasogastric tube lies in the esophagus. Obviously, this rule of thumb cannot be used for laparoscopic operations. We try to leave 1–1.5 cm of space between the anterior border of the esophagus and the anterior margin of the hiatus to approximate the degree of closure obtained in open operations. Although some use a bougie to calibrate the

hiatal closure[5] we find this method both inaccurate and dangerous. The quality of the crura and ability to obtain a well-approximated and tension-free closure are essential. Patients with large hiatal hernias at the time of their initial surgery are three times more likely to develop a recurrence.[1] Recent publications have demonstrated the feasibility and utility of judiciously placing prosthetic material to buttress the crural closure when the crural fibers are attenuated.[10,11]

Without a doubt, the best time to prevent recurrence is at the time of the original procedure. Anticipating potential pitfalls and problems at the esophageal, wrap and crural level during the initial procedure will prevent later complications. We recommend esophageal manometry for all patients before anti-reflux surgery and if weak peristalsis is present, a partial, rather than a total fundoplication, should be performed. The esophagus should be adequately mobilized such that 2–3 cm of tension-free intraabdominal esophagus can be obtained. If a foreshortened esophagus is discovered preoperatively or intraoperatively, an esophageal lengthening procedure should be performed. The establishment of a 2- to 4-cm length of intraabdominal esophagus is a fundamental principle of anti-reflux surgery. If tension is required to keep a fundoplication in the abdomen, transdiaphragmatic herniation will ultimately result. The crura should always be closed with a nonabsorbable suture, often reinforced with the use of pledgets.

Treatment Options

Appropriate treatment of failed anti-reflux surgery may range from reassurance to re-operative therapy. Revisional surgery can be recommended when the preoperative evaluation identifies a surgically correctable problem corresponding to the patient's symptoms. In general, operations that have failed for technical reasons can be corrected by a second operation. The most appropriate surgical approach will depend on the patient's previous operation and the results of the preoperative evaluation (see Chapter 11).

For patients with persistent dysphagia, esophageal dilation should be the first line of therapy. Often, multiple dilations can loosen a tight, but properly oriented wrap. However, if dysphagia is caused by a tight crural closure, dilation usually will not work and reoperation is often necessary. Similarly, if the wrap is malpositioned, conservative therapy is unlikely to provide benefit. Patients whose dysphagia fails to respond to 2 or 3 dilations should be suspected of having a poorly constructed wrap or an overly tight crural closure. Reoperation should be considered if symptoms persist for more than 3–4 months.

What Is the Best Surgical Approach to a Reoperation?

The most important factor a surgeon should consider in choosing the surgical approach for reoperation is the likelihood that he or she can perform a safe and technically proper reconstruction of the anti-reflux mechanism. Irrespective of the surgical approach and choice of operation, the surgeon must establish a 3- to 4-cm segment of intraabdominal esophagus, improve the lower esophageal sphincter resting pressure, and reestablish a valve mechanism at the gastroesophageal junction. Multiple studies have demonstrated the safety and efficacy of laparoscopic reoperations, but all these reports come from high-volume experienced centers.[5,12–16] Whereas some surgeons are extremely skilled in laparoscopic techniques, others are less facile. Laparoscopic reoperations are clearly more difficult than primary anti-reflux procedures and the potential for serious complications (e.g., unrecognized perforation of the stomach and esophagus, vagal nerve injury) should not be underestimated.

Patients whose initial anti-reflux surgery was performed via laparotomy are more difficult to approach laparoscopically than those whose primary procedure was laparoscopic. If the reoperation fails, patients may become esophageal cripples with irreparable motility disorders and face the prospect of esophageal replacement surgery. Hence, the stakes are extremely high in the reoperative setting.

In general, patients who have previously had open surgery should have open revisional surgery to avoid unnecessary risk and prolonged operative times. When reoperating on patients with longstanding reflux disease, it is essential that the surgeon have the capability to perform an esophageal lengthening procedure. Large iatrogenic paraesophageal hernias can be very difficult to reduce laparoscopically. Finally, in obese male patients, laparoscopic exposure of the scarred hiatus may be difficult and one should consider a transthoracic approach (Table 8.1). If a patient is deemed not to be a candidate for a laparoscopic reoperation, the choice of transabdominal versus transthoracic approach depends on the perceived need for esophageal mobilization/lengthening and body habitus. A thoracotomy provides the best opportunity to fully mobilize the esophagus up to the level of the aortic arch and overcomes difficulty exposing the hiatus in obese patients. However, if a transthoracic approach is chosen, the abdomen must be prepped and draped into the operative field. Difficult reoperations often require a combined thoracic and abdominal approach to dissect the hiatus and mobilize the fundus if it is heavily scarred from prior surgery. Although the peritoneal cavity can be accessed through a counter incision in the diaphragm, extending a

Table 8.1. Choosing a laparoscopic or open approach for redo fundoplication.

Factor	Laparoscopic Approach	Laparotomy	Thoracotomy
Prior repair via laparotomy	↓	→	→
Prior laparoscopic repair	↑	→	→
Large hiatal hernia	→*	↓	↑*
Obesity	→	↓	↑
Concern of short esophagus	→*	↓	↑*

↑ = good choice.
→ = no contraindication.
↓ = poor choice.
* Must have skills to perform lengthening procedure.

thoracotomy incision across the costal margin often provides the best exposure to deal with particularly difficult cases.

Choosing a Partial or a Total Fundoplication

The surgical literature is replete with articles debating the pros and cons of the Nissen fundoplication. Advocates of partial fundoplications such as the Toupet and Belsey fundoplication point out advantages of less dysphagia and preservation of the ability to vomit. Proponents of the Nissen fundoplication claim superior control of acid reflux as well as ease of performance of the procedure. In fact, there is little level 1 evidence to support the superiority of one procedure over another when performing a redo fundoplication. The choice of fundoplication should be tailored to the symptom or anatomic defect needing correction. Patients who had a good short-term result from a Nissen fundoplication should probably have a full wrap reconstructed. Those patients who had a partial fundoplication with poor control of acid reflux should be considered for conversion to a Nissen. If a clear technical error can be identified that caused a full fundoplication to fail, one should not hesitate to reconstruct the 360° fundoplication in a proper manner. However, it is logical to perform partial fundoplications on patients that have had a prior Nissen fundoplication and complain of persistent dysphagia or gas bloat syndrome. Patients who undergo reoperation to correct wrap herniation may benefit from a procedure that anchors the fundus to the hiatus such as a Hill repair, Belsey procedure, or Toupet procedure. When an esophageal lengthening procedure is performed, a partial fundoplication has theoretical advantages because the gastric tube that becomes the distal neoesophagus is aperistaltic.

Considerations for Esophageal Lengthening Procedures

It is essential that the gastroesophageal junction lie tension free in the abdomen before creating a fundic wrap. The length of tension-free intraabdominal esophagus should be measured after closing the crural defect. When the crura are closed from the caudal condensation of the crural fibers toward the anterior margin of the hiatus, the hiatal orifice is effectively displaced cephalad. This transposition of the hiatal orifice lengthens the intraabdominal segment of esophagus because the anterior portion of the hiatus is cephalad to the posterior portion of the hiatus. If the gastroesophageal junction lies at the level of the hiatal closure, one must do something to achieve an adequate intraabdominal segment of esophagus. The first step should be esophageal mobilization. This can be done transhiatally or transthoracically. If the segmental arteries to the esophagus are divided to the level of the aortic arch and the vagal branches to the hilum of the lungs are divided, one can generally gain 2 cm of esophageal length. If the intraabdominal esophageal segment is still inadequate, there are several methods for lengthening the intraabdominal segment (see Chapter 14).

The Collis gastroplasty is the most widely used technique to lengthen the esophagus. First described in conjunction with transthoracic hiatal hernia repairs, the Collis gastroplasty can also be performed with minimally invasive approaches. Although some have reported outstanding long-term results with the Collis gastroplasty,[17] the neoesophagus may contain acid-secreting mucosa causing concern that patients with Barrett's esophagus may continue to be exposed to acidic irritation. In the current era wherein most reoperations follow failed laparoscopic Nissen fundoplication, the proximal end of the Collis gastroplasty may become ischemic because the short gastric vessels have been previously divided. This may result in a stricture that is very difficult to treat by dilation.

In 1996, Swanstrom et al.[18] described a minimally invasive transthoracic Collis gastroplasty technique (see Chapter 13). For this approach, a 12-mm trocar is placed in the right anterior axillary line in the third or fourth intercostal space. A 35-mm tissue stapler is introduced into the right chest and passed along the posterior medial sulcus until it can be seen laparoscopically from the abdomen indenting the mediastinal pleura. The pleura is incised and the stapler is advanced parallel to the esophagus. A 46- to 48-French bougie is advanced into the stomach along the lesser curvature. While the fundus is retracted laterally, the stapler is advanced along the bougie, adjacent to the angle of His. The stapler is fired creating a 3-cm gastric tube. The crura are closed in standard manner and a fundoplication is performed (Figure 8.6).

A Collis gastroplasty can also be performed laparoscopically without violating the thoracic cavity (see Chapter 12). An esophageal bougie is advanced along the lesser curvature. A circular stapling device is used to create a "buttonhole" in the gastric fundus adjacent to the bougie. A 35-mm tissue stapler is passed into the "buttonhole" and advanced parallel to the bougie toward the angle of His. The linear stapler is then fired creating a neoesophagus[19] (Figure 8.7). The introduction of roticulating endoscopic staplers has greatly simplified laparoscopic esophageal lengthening procedures. Many surgeons now resect a wedge-shaped segment of the fundus to create a neoesophagus rather than using the buttonhole technique described above. Once the short gastric vessels have been divided and with a bougie in the esophagus, a linear stapler is fired across the

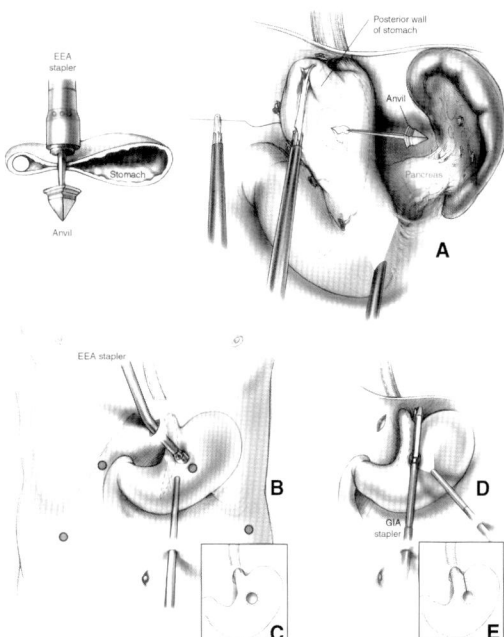

Figure 8.7. This laparoscopic method of addressing the foreshortened esophagus requires two types of staplers. The anvil of a circular stapler is brought through and through the body of the stomach, following a stitch on a straight needle (A). The stapler is fired, creating an aperture through the stomach (B). A linear cutting stapler is fired from this aperture to the gastroesophageal junction, completing the lengthening gastroplasty. (Reprinted from Horvath et al.,[22] with permission.)

fundus near the gastroesophageal junction, perpendicular to the esophagus. This then permits the surgeon to divide the fundus adjacent to the dilator and parallel to the esophagus creating the neoesophagus. A fundoplication is then performed.

Management of the Difficult Hiatus

Closing the crura in reoperative surgery can be challenging. The first and most important step in repairing hiatal defects is to avoid destroying the crural fibers while performing the initial dissection of the area. Spending the extra time to dissect this area carefully will be rewarded later in the operation when it becomes time to close the hiatus. On rare occasions, the crura will be very fibrotic creating esophageal obstruction at the hiatal level. This problem is easily remedied by dividing a portion of the

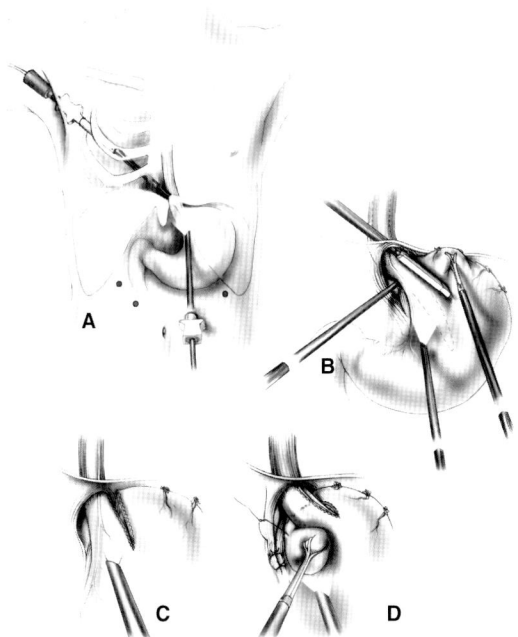

Figure 8.6. A minimally invasive transthoracic method of creating a Collis gastroplasty entails visualization of the hiatus from above. After the proximal stomach is mobilized, a linear stapler is brought through the thoracic port and fired alongside a bougie in the stomach (B). This creates a lengthening gastroplasty (C) that is used to form a fundoplication (D). (Reprinted from Horvath et al.,[22] with permission.)

crus. The most common problem, however, is dealing with a large hiatal defect. In most instances, primary closure can be accomplished. The stoutest crural fibers are the posterior fibers so sutures should be placed deeply to encompass them. In laparoscopic reoperations, the intraabdominal pressure should be lowered to 8 or 10 mm Hg in order to diminish the diaphragmatic stretch.

There are situations in which primary closure seems impossible. When this occurs, the options are to make a relaxing incision in the diaphragm and close this defect with prosthetic material or to place prosthetic material directly into the hiatus. Surgical dogma has been that placement of prosthetic material in the hiatus would lead to erosion of the foreign body into the esophagus. In the laparoscopic era, however, there are numerous reports claiming both the safety and benefit of using prosthetic material for difficult hiatal closures. Although there is relatively limited follow-up, the use of mesh at the esophageal hiatus has been associated with significantly reduced recurrence rates with minimal morbidity. Laparoscopic refundoplication with a circular polypropylene mesh was performed in 24 patients with intrathoracic herniation of the wrap. Although one patient had severe dysphagia requiring pneumatic dilation postoperatively, all patients had good to excellent functional outcome at 1 year follow-up.[11] Prosthetic material may be useful in reinforcing the crural closure, particularly if the hiatal disruption is large or if the tissue is less than robust. The use of polytetrafluoroethylene mesh in conjunction with a Nissen fundoplication was investigated in patients with a hiatal defect >8 cm. With at least 1 year follow-up, this prospective, randomized controlled study demonstrated that 8 of the 36 patients undergoing simple cruroplasty developed recurrences, whereas none of the 36 patients with polytetrafluoroethylene mesh recurred.[20] This benefit of prosthetic reinforcement has been observed in multiple other studies.[10,20,21] Although there has been concern regarding the possibility of erosion of the mesh into the stomach or esophagus, these fears have not materialized—at least in the short term. Most recently, biodegradable small intestinal submucosal patches have become available and appear to hold promise as an adjunct to closing large hiatal defects.

Technical Tips for Laparoscopic Reoperations

A five trocar technique described for primary laparoscopic fundoplication can be used for redo surgery (see Chapter 12). Adhesiolysis may be challenging and is best accomplished with cold scissors to avoid thermal or conductive injury to the esophagus and vagi. The liver is almost invariably stuck to the site of the previous fundoplication and needs to be freed as the first step of the procedure. As with primary surgery, the crura are identified and dissected. In general, the left crus is more easily identified. If the short gastric vessels have not been taken previously, they should be divided to facilitate identification of the left crus. The right crus can be more challenging and is best isolated by finding the caudate lobe and proceeding superiorly and to the left. The crura are dissected in a 360° manner such that a Penrose drain can be passed behind the esophagus (or stomach if there is a herniated fundoplication). Once the hiatus has been delineated clearly, attention is turned to the prior fundoplication. We routinely take down the previous fundoplication, try to restore normal anatomy, and then reconstruct the fundoplication again. The retained sutures are divided sharply and the fundus is peeled away from the stomach and esophagus circumferentially. Sharp dissection is continued in order to avoid inadvertent injury to the vagi. Special attention is required along the left lateral wall of the esophagus to ensure that the prior fundoplication is fully mobilized.

With the fundoplication taken down, an assessment of the intraabdominal esophageal length is made. When necessary additional esophageal length is obtained as previously described. The crura are reapproximated with nonabsorbable pledgetted sutures starting caudally and progressing cephalad toward the esophageal hiatus. Generous crural bites should be taken. If closing the hiatus is difficult, tension on the diaphragm can be reduced by lowering the intraabdominal insufflation pressure. If the crural closure remains under tension, mesh reinforcement should be considered. Attention is turned to the recreation of the fundoplication. A 56-French esophageal bougie is passed orally into the stomach. The fundus should easily pass posterior to the esophagus and its orientation should be confirmed by the "shoe shine" test. For a Nissen fundoplication, the wrap should not be under any tension. Nonabsorbable pledgetted sutures are used to approximate the fundus around the distal 2–3 cm of esophagus with each suture incorporating a generous purchase of stomach and esophagus. By anchoring fundoplication to the esophagus, migration is less likely. Further steps to prevent herniation of the fundoplication include fixation of the posterior portion of the wrap to the crural closure and performance of an anterior gastropexy or gastrostomy.

Conclusion

Patients who experience technical failures after anti-reflux surgery typically complain of dysphagia, heartburn, vomiting, or a combination of these symptoms. Understanding why the original procedure failed and establishing the physiologic basis of the patient's symptoms are critical elements in choosing management options. Evaluation typically includes a careful history and a complete physical examination, barium swallow, upper endoscopy, esophageal manometry, esophageal pH monitoring, and often an assessment of gastric emptying. Symptom recurrence in the absence of important anatomic abnormalities can often be managed medically. When a technical failure has occurred that results in symptoms that are difficult to control or an important anatomic abnormality, reoperation is necessary. Choosing the right approach to reoperation requires honest appraisal of the surgeon's experience and capabilities as well as tailoring the operative procedure to solve the patient's physiologic abnormality. Because the stakes are high in reoperative esophageal surgery, consideration should be given to referring such cases to surgeons or centers doing a high volume of anti-reflux surgery.

References

1. Soper NJ, Dunnegan D. Anatomic fundoplication failure after laparoscopic anti-reflux surgery. Ann Surg 1999; 229:669–677.
2. Galvani C, Fisichella PM, Gorodner MV, Perretta S, Patti MG. Symptoms are a poor indicator of reflux status after fundoplication for gastroesophageal reflux disease: role of esophageal functions tests. Arch Surg 2003;138: 514–519.
3. Perdikis G, Hinder RA, Lund RJ, Raiser F, Katada N. Laparoscopic Nissen fundoplication: where do we stand? Surg Laparosc Endosc 1997;7:17–21.
4. Carlson MA, Frantzides CT. Complications and results of primary minimally invasive anti-reflux procedures: a review of 10,735 reported cases. J Am Coll Surg 2001; 193:428–439.
5. Hinder RA, Klinger PJ, Perdikis G, Smith SL. Management of the failed anti-reflux operation. Surg Clin North Am 1997;77:1083–1098.
6. Hunter JG. Approach and management of patients with recurrent gastroesophageal reflux disease. J Gastrointest Surg 2001;5:451–457.
7. Stylopoulos, Bunker CJ, Rattner DW. Development of achalasia secondary to laparoscopic Nissen fundoplication. J Gastrointest Surg 2002;6:368–376.
8. Dunnington GL, DeMeester TR. Outcome effect of adherence to operative principles of Nissen fundoplication by multiple surgeons. The Department of Veterans Affairs Gastroesophageal Reflux Disease Study Group. Am J Surg 1993;166:654–657.
9. O'Boyle CJ, Watson DI, Jamieson GG, Myers JC, Game PA, Devitt PG. Division of short gastric vessels at laparoscopic Nissen fundoplication: a prospective double-blind randomized trial with 5 year follow up. Ann Surg 2002;235:165–170.
10. Carlson MA, Richards CG, Frantzides CT. Laparoscopic prosthetic reinforcement of hiatal herniorrhaphy. Dig Surg 1999;16:407–410.
11. Ganderath FA, Kamolz T, Schweiger UM, Pointer R. Laparoscopic refundoplication with prosthetic hiatal closure for recurrent hiatal hernia after primary failed anti-reflux surgery. Arch Surg 2003;138:902–907.
12. Bais JE, Horbach JMLM, Masclee AAM, Smout AJPM, Terpstra J, Gooszen HG. Surgical treatment for recurrent gastro-oesophageal reflux disease after failed anti-reflux surgery. Br J Surg 2000;87:243–249.
13. Floch NR, Hinder RA, Kingler PJ, et al. Is laparoscopic reoperation for failed anti-reflux surgery feasible? Arch Surg 1999;134:733–737.
14. Granderath FA, Kamolz T, Schweiger UM. Long-term follow-up after laparoscopic refundoplication for failed anti-reflux surgery: quality of life, symptomatic outcome and patient satisfaction. J Gastrointest Surg 2002;6: 812–818.
15. Pointer R, Bammer T, Then P, Kamolz T. Laparoscopic refundoplications after failed anti-reflux surgery. Am J Surg 1999;178:541–544.
16. Watson DI, Jamieson GG, Game PA, Williams RS, Devitt PG. Laparoscopic reoperation following failed anti-reflux surgery. Br J Surg 1999;86:98–101.
17. Luketich JD, Grondin SC, Pearson FG. Minimally invasive approaches to acquired shortening of the esophagus: laparoscopic Collis-Nissen gastroplasty. Semin Thorac Cardiovasc Surg 2000;12:173–178.
18. Swanstrom LL, Marcus DR, Galloway GQ. Laparoscopic Collis gastroplasty is the treatment of choice for the shortened esophagus. Am J Surg 1996;171:477–481.
19. Johnson AB, Oddsdottir M, Hunter JG. Laparoscopic Collis gastroplasty and Nissen fundoplication: a new technique for the management of esophageal foreshortening. Surg Endosc 1998;12:1055–1060.

20. Frantzides CT, Madan AK, Carlson MA, Stavropoulos GP. A prospective, randomized trial of laparoscopic polytetrafluoroethylene (PTFE) patch repair vs simple cruroplasty for large hiatal hernia. Arch Surg 2002;137: 649–653.

21. Basso N, De Leo A, Genco A, et al. 360 degrees laparoscopic fundoplication with tension-free hiatoplasty in the treatment of symptomatic gastroesophageal reflux disease. Surg Endosc 2000;14:164–169.

22. Horvath KD, Swanstrom LL, Jobe BA. The short esophagus: pathophysiology, incidence, presentation, and treatment in the era of laparoscopic anti-reflux surgery. Ann Surg 2000;232:630–640.

23. Hunter JG, Smith CD, Branum GD, et al. Laparoscopic fundoplication failures: patterns of failure and response to fundoplication revision. Ann Surg 1999;230:595–604.

9

Symptoms after Anti-Reflux Surgery: Everything is not always caused by Surgery

Kenneth R. DeVault

Anti-reflux surgery controls reflux symptoms in a majority of patients. Unfortunately, that control comes with a price in some patients with the development of new, postoperative symptoms. These symptoms vary widely and can include dysphagia, increased abdominal gas (gas bloat syndrome), and several other symptoms. All of these are very common if inquired for by questionnaire. For example, in a study of 60 patients with 1-year follow-up, some gastrointestinal symptom was present in 93% of patients, but only 19% said that they had symptom that disturbed their lifestyle.[1] There are many symptoms that may accompany both typical (heartburn and regurgitation) and atypical (pulmonary or ears, nose, and throat) presentations of reflux. These include dysphagia, epigastric pain, nausea, and vomiting.[2] If the primary symptoms are relieved by surgery, there is a chance that a preexisting less-appreciated symptom may now become primary and appear to be attributable to surgery when, in fact, it was really present all along. In addition to new symptoms, the persistence or return of the reflux symptoms that resulted in the surgery initially is an important issue. Whereas much attention is given to each of these recurrent gastroesophageal reflux disease (GERD)-attributed symptoms in other chapters in this book, our goal will be to explore symptoms occurring after surgery, but not related to the surgery itself.

Dysphagia

Dysphagia is a common symptom after anti-reflux surgery. Mild dysphagia has been reported in up to 40% of patients,[3] and more severe dysphagia, resulting in the need for esophageal dilation, in >10% of patients.[4] It has been suggested that the type of anti-reflux surgery may influence postoperative dysphagia. In a randomized, controlled trial of open versus laparoscopic fundoplication, dysphagia was more common after the laparoscopic approach.[5] In fact, the randomized study was closed early because of that dysphagia, although many surgeons do not believe that the laparoscopic approach predisposes to dysphagia. Another study compared outcomes in 185 laparotomy patients with 200 laparoscopy patients.[6] Recurrent heartburn and subjective dissatisfaction with the surgery were both more common in the laparoscopy group. Esophageal manometry has been used as a tool to "tailor" anti-reflux surgery to the patient's underlying motility. This "tailoring" of anti-reflux surgery, by performing a partial fundoplication in patients with poor motility, is currently loosing favor in some centers because of the finding of a lack of utility in several randomized trials.[7,8] However, the knowledge of preoperative motility in patients experiencing postoperative dysphagia is very helpful in both managing and prognosticating, because the knowledge of normal or near-normal preoperative motility may provide some comfort to patient and surgeon when dysphagia develops. An Australian study of 262 patients with 5-year follow-up suggested that a normal preoperative pH test and prior abdominal surgery were associated with an increased risk of dysphagia.[9] There are few other data in regard to the evaluation of other preoperative factors that might be predictive of postoperative dysphagia.

Patients with severe reflux disease will occasionally develop significant stricturing of their esophagus. These strictures were once considered a contraindication to surgery, but we have reported successful outcomes with an improvement in both dysphagia and the need for esophageal dilation after surgery.[10] If a stricture is present before surgery, it should be dilated and the patient placed on proton pump inhibitor (PPI) therapy to ensure healing of the stricture before surgery. If a stricture is missed in the preoperative evaluation, dysphagia caused by that stricture postoperatively could erroneously be attributed to the surgery.

Dysphagia is common in GERD patients before anti-reflux surgery, even in those without demonstrable strictures. This is a finding that must be considered when discussing postoperative dysphagia. For example, in patients with chronic GERD, up to 14% may be expected to complain of dysphagia.[2] Interestingly, some of that dysphagia may improve with surgical control of the patient's reflux and is likely related to reflux-induced dysmotility or symptom.[11] To truly attribute dysphagia to surgery, it should not be present before and be documented to only develop after surgery. Dysphagia was about equally common before and after surgery in a 312-patient trial with prospective pre- and postoperative symptom assessment.[12] In that trial, dysphagia for liquids improved in 88 patients (28%) and deteriorated in 20 (6%) and dysphagia for solids improved in 53 (17%) and deteriorated in 96 (31%) after operation. Despite this new postoperative symptom of dysphagia, most patients were still satisfied with their surgery and would do it again if given the choice. Many other studies that attribute dysphagia to surgery are biased against surgery by recall bias in that questionnaires about dysphagia ask the patient to compare their current symptoms to those before surgery and only rarely has dysphagia been assessed prospectively. Patients with severe reflux, particularly when they are older, have decreased esophageal motility that may at times also contribute to postoperative dysphagia.[13]

Dysphagia, like many other symptoms, is subjective. A patient may complain of dysphagia and yet their evaluation yields no objective evidence of bolus transport or motility abnormalities. If the fundoplication is causing dysphagia, this is often best demonstrated with a barium examination, especially if a solid bolus is documented to "hang up" at the esophagogastric junction. In our experience, the majority of patients with postoperative dysphagia respond to esophageal dilation and, if they do not, they usually have anatomical evidence of problems related to their surgery.[4] These patients with "abnormal wraps" tend to have persistent dysphagia despite dilation and often require revision of their surgery.

Gas Bloat and Upper Abdominal Discomfort

A bloated, uncomfortable feeling in the upper abdomen is common after reflux surgery. This has been described as "gas bloat" by many authors. Belching is normally initiated by distention of the proximal stomach, which leads to transient lower esophageal sphincter (LES) relaxation.[14] This is followed by either an episode of secondary peristalsis pushing the air back into the stomach or a relaxation of the upper esophageal sphincter and venting of the gas (a belch). Fundoplication alters the physiology of the proximal stomach by both tightening the LES and by partially obliterating the fundus. In addition, the fundus of the stomach normally receptively relaxes and has classically been thought to be a storage location for liquids after a meal.[15] Using a barostat, accommodation of the proximal stomach to a liquid meal has been shown to be lessened (higher pressures produced with same volume of meal) after fundoplication.[16] The wrap of the fundus increases basal LES pressure, decreases transient LES relaxations, and partially obliterates the fundus. These physiologic changes not only prevent reflux of liquid material from the stomach to the esophagus, but also prevent the normal venting of gas. Therefore, symptoms such as gas bloat seem to be a predictable result of surgery.

Lundell et al.[17] reported that 76% of their patients complained of early satiety, 56% of postprandial pain, and 80% of one or more new upper gastrointestinal symptoms 1 year after surgery. When asked, 20–57% of patients will report that they cannot belch after anti-reflux surgery.[18,19] Patients are about twice as likely to indicate that they cannot belch after, compared with before surgery.[12] In a large trial randomizing patients to either open anti-reflux surgery or omeprazole therapy, bloating was much more common in the surgery group.[20] Patients' symptoms and our ability to document physiologic differences to explain those symptoms often differ. A small study compared symptoms to physiology in fundoplication patients and controls.[21] They found that transient LES relaxations did not occur with gastric distention in the fundoplication patients and that when fundoplication patients felt the need to belch, there was no common cavity between the stomach and esophagus. They also found that patients with a fundoplication frequently reported the desire to belch and hypothesized that this was related to retained air in the esophagus rather than air being vented after a transient LES relaxation (the physiology in patients without a fundoplication). Their findings also suggest that almost no fundoplication patients can truly belch (pass air from the stomach to the esophagus via a common cavity) whether or not the patient believes that they can belch. In addition, surgery may change the way the body handles meals (particularly the liquid portion) because of the partial loss of the reservoir function of the fundus. This is a mechanical effect and may also be related to changes in vagus nerve function in some patients.[22] Interestingly, postoperative changes in gastric compliance have been suggested to be associated with the development of a sensation of fullness reported by some patients.[23]

Documented delayed gastric emptying is another potential cause of bloating that has been reported in several patients after anti-reflux surgery,[24] although there have been no systematic studies of the incidence of this problem. Gastric emptying disturbances have been reported in up to 40% of patients with GERD,[25] although the exact prevalence of clinically significant disorders is unknown. An early report suggested that most patients with symptomatic delayed gastric emptying after surgery actually had the problem before surgery.[26] Some centers routinely check for gastric emptying abnormalities before surgery, although normalization of delayed gastric emptying has also been reported after anti-reflux surgery.[27] Some authors have suggested that changes in emptying, whether delay or acceleration, can cause symptoms in some patients.[28] Others advocate a pyloroplasty in anti-reflux surgery patients with significantly delayed gastric emptying.[29,30] We only test gastric emptying before surgery in patients with symptoms suggestive of gastroparesis (nausea, vomiting, or weight loss).[31] This approach leaves us at a disadvantage if the patient develops delayed gastric emptying postoperatively in that we then are unable to determine if the problem was present before, or a result of, the surgery.

It has been suggested that many GERD patients swallow air as a response to esophageal reflux.[32] If this is true, then the surgery may be bound to produce symptoms. Also, some GERD patients tend to both overeat and eat very quickly, two factors that increase air swallowing. In fact, whereas inability to belch increased in patients after surgery, the symptom of bloating was less common and fullness or early satiety were equally common after surgery.[12] Using means and medians to report changes in symptoms can be misleading; a better approach is to look at symptoms in individual patients before and after surgery. For example, Anvari and Allen[33] found that patients with gas bloat symptoms before surgery were very common (73%) and likely to improve, but those without bloating before surgery often developed symptoms, resulting in about the same percentage of patients with symptoms after surgery. Another study attempted to correlate preoperative testing to postoperative gas bloat.[34] The researchers found that among patients without bloating before surgery, those who refluxed during the day were more likely to develop postoperative symptoms and those who refluxed predominantly at night did not. In addition, patients who were bloated before surgery tended to improve, not worsen. They hypothesized that the daytime refluxers were more likely to be air swallowers. Other investigators have also observed that patients with predominantly upright reflux tend to not do as well and have more postoperative symptoms than those with nighttime reflux.[35] There is considerable overlap between the symptoms of dyspepsia and those of reflux.[36] Because dyspepsia patients have been suggested to have both changes in gastric accommodation and altered visceral perception,[37] patients with an overlap between GERD and dyspepsia may be predisposed to demonstrate or unmask postoperative symptoms similar to gas bloat.

Flatulence, Diarrhea, and Irritable Bowel Syndrome

Problems related to flatulence, diarrhea, and irritable bowel syndrome (IBS) are very common among adult patients with or without GERD.[38] It is therefore to be expected that many patients will have these symptoms both before and after anti-reflux surgery. In a study from our institution, diarrhea was present in 14% of patients before surgery and 29% after. Other symptoms included bloating (3% preoperative, 19% postoperative), constipation (15 and 18%, respectively), and abdominal pain (2 and 8%, respectively) (Figure 9.1).[39] Flatulence has been reported in 12–88% of patients after anti-reflux surgery.[40,41] It has been suggested that this flatulence is attributable to the patient's inability to belch and subsequent passage of more gas into and then through the gastrointestinal tract.[42] Most of these studies are retrospective and at risk for recall bias, because many only surveyed patients after surgery and asked them to recall how they were before the surgery. In general, the suggested causes for increased flatulence after

anti-reflux surgery are the same as those listed for gas bloat. This is a very common symptom in the general population and care must be taken not to inappropriately attribute it to the effect of surgery.

If diarrhea develops after fundoplication, it tends to be low volume and occur after meals, but can be explosive at times. Postfundoplication diarrhea has been attributed to dumping syndrome, vagus nerve injury with subsequent bacteria overgrowth, and to exacerbation of underlying IBS. The loss of the fundus accelerates gastric emptying in some patients, which may result in overloading the small intestine's ability to handle the bolus. Classical dumping syndrome has been reported after anti-reflux surgery, particularly in infants and children.[43] A small series found evidence of dumping (by glucose tolerance test or gastric emptying study) in 15 of 50 (30%) infants after anti-reflux surgery.[44] In addition to classical dumping, rapid gastric emptying may result in diarrhea attributed to overloading the small bowel with poorly digested, high osmotic material. Impairment in vagus nerve function can cause diarrhea by changing the body's ability to clear bacteria and maintain bile acid homeostasis because of alterations in small bowel motility.[45,46] Attributing diarrhea to a specific etiology can be quite difficult. For example, our center reported a case of a patient with severe diarrhea believed to be the result of vagus nerve injury (documented by an abnormal pancreatic polypeptide response to a sham meal).[47] In a subsequent, larger study in which the test was performed before and after surgery, there was very little correlation between the results of the pancreatic polypeptide test and postoperative diarrhea[48] (Figure 9.2).

There is considerable overlap between GERD (particularly nonerosive disease) and IBS.[49] Nonulcer dyspepsia also overlaps with heartburn and it is possible that some patients may have been operated on for reflux when their preoperative symptom was actually more attributable to nonulcer dyspepsia.[50] This diagnostic confusion has been exacerbated by the tendency to use response to PPI therapy as a diagnostic test for GERD. This approach actually has poor sensitivity[51] and we believe that pathologic reflux should be documented before considering surgery in any patient. Therefore, a positive "PPI test" should not be considered sufficient

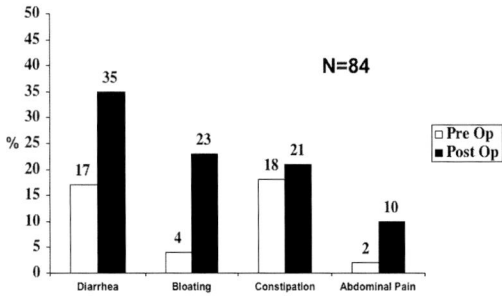

Figure 9.1. Prevalence (%) of bowel symptoms before and after anti-reflux surgery in 84 patients. (Adapted from Klaus et al.[39])

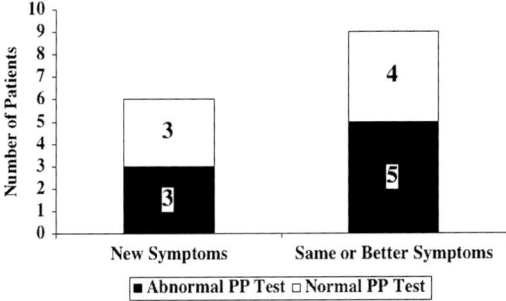

Figure 9.2. Lack of association between abnormal vagus nerve function as measured by the meal-stimulated pancreatic polypeptide (PP) test and development of new lower gastrointestinal symptoms. In this study, 6 of 15 patients developed new lower gastrointestinal symptoms after anti-reflux surgery and the PP test was only abnormal in half of those 6. In contrast, 9 patients either had no new symptoms or an improvement in their symptoms, yet 5 of those 9 also had an abnormal PP test of vagus function. (Adapted from DeVault et al.[48])

documentation of GERD before surgery. In addition, patients have been documented to "migrate" from one functional symptom (heartburn for example) to others (IBS). This was highlighted by a recent retrospective study of 155 patients finding that a coexisting diagnosis of a nonreflux functional bowel disorder (usually IBS or dyspepsia) more than doubled the risk of a loosely defined "poor outcome" after anti-reflux surgery.[52] When one is confronted with a patient with postoperative bowel symptoms, determining whether their symptom complex was really present before surgery is difficult and perhaps impossible. Ideally, the same physician should evaluate the patient before and after the surgery, but this is often not practical in our health care system.

Recurrent Heartburn

Much interest and research has recently focused on the durability of anti-reflux surgery. For example, a large randomized trial of medical versus surgical therapy initially reported superiority for the surgical approach.[53] A follow-up of these patients >10 years later found that 92% of the patients who were initially randomized to surgery to still be on medication and 62% of patients who were operated on to be back on reflux medications (about half PPI and half histamine-2-receptor antagonist)[54] (Figure 9.3).

Univariate analysis of several factors suggested that previous abdominal surgery, female gender, lower socioeconomic status, and a normal preoperative pH study were predictive of persistent, postoperative heartburn.[9]

Does the fact that the patient is back on PPI prove that their surgery has failed? In a small study from our institution with 5-year follow-up, continuous PPI use was actually fairly rare (14%) and perhaps more importantly, many of these patients did not have classic heartburn or regurgitation and appeared to be on PPI for more vague abdominal and chest symptoms.[55] The actual prevalence of postoperative GERD symptoms in that study was regurgitation in 6.4% and heartburn in 5.8%. In a later preliminary report of a different cohort of patients, we found a greater percentage of patients back on medications at 2 years (39%), although interestingly 84% of the patients were happy with their outcome and this satisfaction was not worse in those who were back on medications.[56] Others have also suggested that many patients who are restarted on reflux medications after surgery actually do not have either typical reflux symptoms or demonstrable acid reflux on testing.[57] A recent study has also suggested that obese patients with a body mass index of >30 have an increased risk of surgical failure[58] (Figure 9.4), although we continue to perform surgery on selected obese patients. Proton pump inhibitor therapy is certainly effective in controlling acid reflux and is becoming less expensive, therefore it remains reasonable to offer an empiric trial in the patient with recurrent symptoms after surgery. However, before considering anything

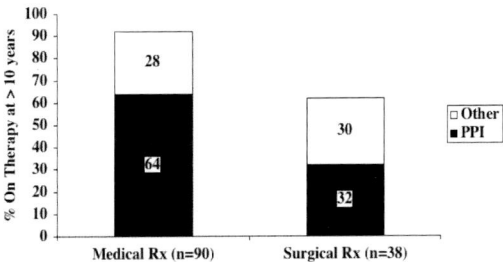

Figure 9.3. Use of acid suppressant medications >10 years after randomization to either medical or surgical therapy for reflux. Reflux medications were being used in 92% of patients originally randomized to medical therapy and 62% of patients who underwent fundoplication. About half the medications in each group were PPIs. (Adapted from Spechler et al.[54])

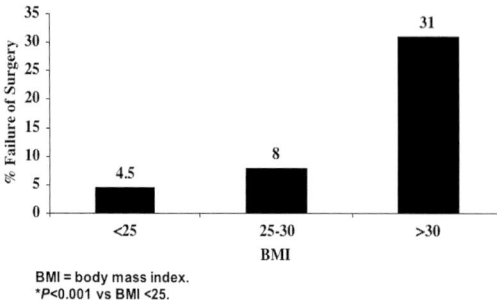

Figure 9.4. Risk of failure of surgery correlates with body mass index. (Adapted from Perez et al.[58])

more aggressive and perhaps before trying progressively higher doses of PPI, it is important to document that the patients actually have recurrent reflux. Ambulatory pH testing has been the standard for that documentation and the recent development of more comfortable "tubeless" equipment will make that testing more patient friendly.[59]

Recurrent "Atypical" Symptoms

This is a particularly common and important problem. Whereas well-documented heartburn and regurgitation tend to respond to medicine or surgery in 85–95% of patients, pulmonary and atypical symptoms are less likely to respond to either type of therapy[60] (Figure 9.5). It seems that a smaller amount of acid reflux is required to produce these symptoms than is needed to produce typical symptoms and routine esophagitis. This suggests that failure to control symptoms could be the result of incomplete control of small amounts of acid reflux. An alternative explanation is that many of these symptoms were never caused by reflux, even before the surgery.

Asthma and GERD often coexist, although it is not always easy to determine if the two are truly related.[61] However, medical and surgical therapy both have been demonstrated to improve or control both esophageal and pulmonary symptoms in many asthma patients.[62,63] Objective evidence of improvement using pulmonary function testing has been more difficult to document. Because causality is so difficult to prove, recurrent asthma after anti-reflux surgery

should not be blamed on failure of surgery unless pathologic acid reflux can be documented using ambulatory esophageal testing. Proving that reflux is causing cough is even more difficult because so many other common problems can cause cough such as postnasal drip, common medications, and occult asthma.[64] When patients who have GERD and a cough that does not respond to medical therapy for reflux undergo surgery, it is our experience that the cough often returns. In addition, despite the return of that symptom, we are able to document outstanding acid control with ambulatory testing. Laryngeal symptoms are also problematic and a large portion of that problem surrounds our imprecise ability to definitively determine the etiology of both laryngeal symptoms and laryngoscopic findings. Most patients with symptoms or signs suggestive of laryngopharyngeal reflux (LPR) will have normal esophageal endoscopy and often fairly modest overall esophageal acid exposure on pH testing.[65] Interesting, preliminary reports have shed more doubt on LPR. The first study performed pH monitoring of the hypopharynx, proximal and distal esophagus in patients with presumed reflux-related, endoscopic laryngeal findings.[66] An abnormal study was noted in only 15% of hypopharyngeal probes, 29% of distal probes, and 9% of proximal probes indicating that most patients with symptoms and signs of LPR do not have documented abnormal acid exposure. This was followed by a

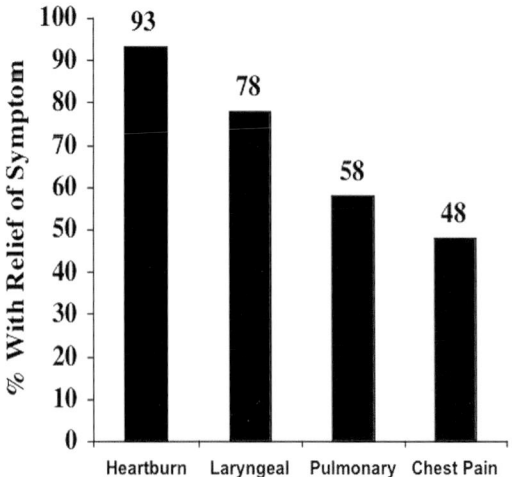

Figure 9.5. Response of atypical symptoms to laparoscopic anti-reflux surgery is less likely than the response of typical symptoms such as heartburn. (Adapted from So et al.[60])

randomized, placebo-controlled trial of esomeprazole 40mg twice daily in the same patients finding a 42% response rate on esomeprazole and a 46% response rate on placebo.[67] If these findings are true, then it is certainly not surprising that these supraesophageal symptoms either do not respond to surgery or recur after surgery.

Noncardiac chest pain (NCCP) is often attributed to GERD. This is supported by both physiologic studies using ambulatory pH testing[68] and by a few appropriately designed trials.[69,70] Limited data from surgical series suggest that this symptom does not respond well to anti-reflux surgery.[60] Patients with NCCP have clearly been demonstrated to have increased sensitivity to both acid perfusion and distention of the esophagus.[71] It is plausible that manipulation of the esophagogastric junction is likely to produce new symptoms in these patients who may have abnormal visceral sensitivity. We hesitate to offer surgery to chest pain patients even if they have demonstrable reflux attributed to these issues.

Summary

New or recurrent symptoms are common after fundoplication whether performed through an open or laparoscopic approach. Obtaining a careful, complete, and accurate gastrointestinal history before surgery will frequently reveal symptoms that may persist after surgery and if not ascertained preoperatively can be errantly attributed to the surgery. In addition, new symptoms such as diarrhea are very common with a high incidence in the general population and are not always caused by the surgery itself. However, if the symptom is physiologically plausible and definitely appeared after surgery, then it may well be related to the surgery. Certain patient groups, such as those with NCCP and coexistent IBS, may be predisposed to the development or new recognition of pre-existing symptoms after surgery, although additional study is needed to accurately characterize that predisposition. The first approach to recurrent reflux symptoms after surgery is to ensure that the patient actually has recurrent reflux. This can be accomplished with a therapeutic trial, but ambulatory pH testing provides stronger evidence. An appropriate and detailed evaluation of these patients is especially important if additional surgery is being considered, because the results of "redo" fundoplication are certainly inferior to those expected with a first fundoplication.

References

1. Beldi G, Glattli A. Long-term gastrointestinal symptoms after laparoscopic Nissen fundoplication. Surg Larparosc Endosc Percutan Tech 2002;12:316–319.
2. Locke GR III, Talley MJ, Fett SL, et al. Prevalence and clinical spectrum of gastroesophageal reflux: a population-based study in Olmsted County, Minnesota. Gastroenterology 1997;112:1448–1456.
3. Watson DI, Jamieson GG, Pike GK, Davies N, Richardson M, Devitt PG. Prospective randomized, double-blind trial between laparoscopic Nissen fundoplication and anterior partial fundoplication. Br J Surg 1999;86:123–130.
4. Malhi-Chowla N, Gorecki P, Bammer T, et al. Dilation after fundoplication: timing, frequency, indications and success. Gastrointest Endosc 2002;55:219–223.
5. Bias JE, Bartelsman JFWM, Bonjer HJ, et al. Laparoscopic or conventional Nissen fundoplication for gastro-oesophageal reflux disease: randomized clinical trial. The Netherlands Anti-reflux Surgery Study Group. Lancet 202;355:170–174.
6. Sandbu R, Khamis H, Gustavsson S, Haglund U. Long-term results of anti-reflux surgery indicate the need for a randomized clinical trial. Br J Surg 2002;89:225–230.
7. Oleynikov D, Eubanks TR, Oelschlager BK, Pellegrini CA. Total fundoplication is the operation of choice for patients with gastroesophageal reflux and defective peristalsis. Surg Endosc 2002;16:909–913.
8. Fernando HC, Luketich JD, Christie NA, Ikramuddikng S, Schauer PR. Outcomes of laparoscopic Toupet compared to laparoscopic Nissen fundoplication. Surg Endosc 2002;16:905–908.
9. O'Boyle CJ, Watson DI, DeBeaux AC, Jamieson GG. Preoperative prediction of long-term outcome following laparoscopic fundoplication. ANZ J Surg 2002;72:471–475.
10. Klingler PJ, Cina RA, DeVault KR, et al. Laparoscopic anti-reflux surgery for the treatment of esophageal strictures refractory to medical therapy. Am J Gastroenterol 1999;94:632–636.
11. Wetscher GJ, Glaser K, Gadenstaetter M, et al. The effect of medical therapy and anti-reflux surgery on dysphagia in patients with gastroesophageal reflux disease without esophageal stricture. Am J Surg 1999;177:189–192.
12. de Beaux AC, Watson DI, O'Boyle C, Jamieson GC. Role of fundoplication in patient symptomatology after laparoscopic anti-reflux surgery. Br J Surg 2001;88:1117–1121.
13. Achem AC, Achem SR, Stark ME, DeVault KR. Failure of esophageal peristalsis in older patients: association with esophageal acid exposure. Am J Gastroenterol 2003;98:35–39.

14. Wyman JB, Dent J, Heddle R, et al. Control of belching by the lower oesophageal sphincter. Gut 1990;31:639–646.

15. Kelly KA. Gastric emptying of liquids and solids: roles of proximal and distal stomach. Am J Physiol 1980;239: G71–76.

16. Wijnhoven BPL, Salet GAM, Roelofs JMM, et al. Function of the proximal stomach after Nissen fundoplication. Br J Surg 1998;85:267–271.

17. Lundell LR, Meyers JC, Jamieson GG. Delayed gastric emptying and its relationship to symptoms of "gas float" after anti-reflux surgery. Eur J Surg 1994;160:161–166.

18. DeMeester TR, Johnson LF. Evaluation of the Nissen anti-reflux procedure by esophageal manometry and twenty four hour pH monitoring. Am J Surg 1975;129: 94–100.

19. Ellis FH Jr, Crozier RE. Reflux control by fundoplication: a clinical and manometric assessment of the Nissen operation. Ann Thorac Surg 1984;38:387–392.

20. Lundell L, Dalenvack J, Hattlevakk J, et al. Continued (5-year) followup of a randomized clinical study comparing anti-reflux surgery and omeprazole in gastroesophageal reflux disease. J Am Coll Surg 2001; 192:172–179.

21. Tew S, Ackroyd R, Jamieson GG, Holloway RH. Belching and bloating: facts and fantasy after anti-reflux surgery. Br J Surg 200;87:477–481.

22. Engel JJ, Spellberg MA. Complications of vagotomy. Am J Gastroenterol 1978;70:55–60.

23. Vu MK, Ringers J, Arndt JW, Lamers CB, Masclee AA. Prospective study of the effect of laparoscopic hemifundoplication on motor and sensory function of the proximal stomach. Br J Surg 2000;87:338–343.

24. Stein NJ, Feussner H, Siewert JR. Failure of anti-reflux surgery. Causes and management strategies. Am J Surg 1996;171:36–40.

25. McCallum RW, Berkowitz DM, Lerner E. Gastric emptying in patients with gastroesophageal reflux. Gastroenterology 1981;80:285–291.

26. Lundell LR, Meyer JC, Jamieson GG. Delayed gastric emptying and its relationship to symptoms of "gas bloat" after anti-reflux surgery. Eur J Surg 1994;160: 161–166.

27. Bias JE, Samson M, Boudesteijn EAJ, et al. Impact of delayed gastric emptying on the outcome of anti-reflux surgery. Ann Surg 2001;234:139–146.

28. Hinder RA, Stein HJ, Bremner CG, et al. Relationship of a satisfactory outcome to normalization of delayed gastric emptying after Nissen fundoplication. Ann Surg 1989;210:458–464.

29. Farrell TM, Richardson WS, Halkar R, et al. Nissen fundoplication improves gastric motility in patients with delayed gastric emptying. Surg Endsoc 2001;15: 271–274.

30. Patti MG, Arcerito M, Pellegrini CA, et al. Minimally invasive surgery for gastroesophageal reflux disease. Am J Surg 1995;170:614–617.

31. DeVault KR. Gas bloat syndrome: a pre- or postoperative dysmotility syndrome. Am J Gastroenterol 1995;90:1536–1537.

32. Hinder RA, Klingler PJ, Perdikis G, et al. Management of the failed anti-reflux operation. Surg Clin North Am 1997;77:1083–1098.

33. Anvari M, Allen C. Postprandial bloating after laparoscopic Nissen fundoplication. Can J Surg 2001;44: 440–444.

34. Papasavas PK, Keenan RJ, Yeaney WW, et al. Prediction of postoperative gas bloating after laparoscopic anti-reflux procedures based on 24-h pH acid reflux pattern. Surg Endosc 2002;17:381–385.

35. Winslow ER, Frisella MM, Soper NH, Clouse RE, Klingensmith ME. Patients with upright reflux have less favorable postoperative outcomes after laparoscopic anti-reflux surgery than those with supine reflux. J Gastrointest Surg 2002;6:819–829.

36. Talley NJ, Boyce P, Jones M. Identification of distinct upper and lower gastrointestinal symptom groupings in an urban population. Gut 1998;42:690–695.

37. Tack J, Piessevaux H, Coulie B, et al. Role of impaired gastric accommodation to a meal in functional dyspepsia. Gastroenterology 1998;115:1346–1352.

38. Talley NJ, Dennis EH, Schettler-Duncan VA, et al. Overlapping upper and lower gastrointestinal symptoms in irritable bowel syndrome patients with constipation or diarrhea. Am J Gastroenterol 2003;98:2454–2459.

39. Klaus A, Hinder RA, DeVault KR, Achem SR. Bowel dysfunction after laparoscopic anti-reflux surgery: incidence, severity and clinical course. Am J Med 2003; 114:6–9.

40. Kivilutoto T, Siren J, Farkkila M, et al. Laparoscopic Nissen fundoplication: a prospective analysis of 200 consecutive patients. Surg Larparosc Endosc 1998;8: 429–434.

41. Swanstrom L, Wayne R. Spectrum of gastrointestinal symptoms after laparoscopic fundoplication. Am J Surg 1994;167:538–541.

42. Negre JB. Post-fundoplication symptoms. Do they restrict the success of Nissen fundoplication? Ann Surg 1983;198:698–700.

43. Meyer S, Deckelbaum RJ, Lax E, Schiller M. Infant dumping syndrome after gastroesophageal reflux surgery. J Pediatr 1981;99:235–237.

44. Samuk I, Afriat R, Horne F, et al. Dumping syndrome following Nissen fundoplication, diagnosis and treatment J Pediatr Gastroenterol Nutr 1996;23:235–240.

45. Blake G, Kennedy TL, McKelvey ST. Bile acids and postvagotomy diarrhea. Br J Surg 1983;70:177–179.

46. Condon JR, Robinson V, Suleman MI, Fan VS, McKeown MD. The cause and treatment of postvagotomy diarrhoea. Br J Surg 1975;62:309–312.

47. Ukleja A, Woodward TA, Achem SR. Vagus nerve injury with severe diarrhea after laparoscopic anti-reflux surgery. Dig Dis Sci 2002;47:1590–1593.

48. DeVault KR, Wentling GK, Achem SR, Hinder RA. Evaluation of vagus nerve integrity before and after anti-reflux surgery. Gastroenterology 2004;126: A772–773.

49. Pimentel M, Rossi F, Chow EJ, et al. Increased prevalence of irritable bowel syndrome in patients with gastroesophageal reflux. J Clin Gastroenterol 2002;34:221–224.

50. Talley NJ, Dennis EH, Schettler-Duncan VA, et al. Overlapping upper and lower gastrointestinal symptoms in irritable bowel syndrome patients with constipation or diarrhea. Am J Gastroenterol 2003;98:2454–2459.

51. Numans ME, Lau J, de Witt NJ, Bonis PA. Short-term treatment with proton-pump inhibitors as a test for gastroesophageal reflux disease. A meta-analysis of

diagnostic test characteristics. Ann Intern Med 2004; 140:518–527.

52. Axelrod DA, Divi V, Ajluni MM, Eckhauser FE, Colletti LM. Influence of functional bowel disease on outcome of surgical anti-reflux procedures. J Gastrointest Surg 2002;6:632–637.

53. Spechler SJ. Comparison of medical and surgical therapy for complicated gastroesophageal reflux disease in veterans. N Engl J Med 1992;326:786–792.

54. Spechler SJ, Lee E, Ahnen D, et al. Long-term outcome of medical and surgical therapies for gastroesophageal reflux disease. Follow-up of a randomized controlled trial. JAMA 2001;285:2331–2338.

55. Bammer T, Hinder RA, Klaus A, Klingler PJ. Five- to eight-year outcome of the first laparoscopic Nissen fundoplications. J Gastrointest Surg 2001;5:42–48.

56. Bammer T, Achem SR, DeVault KR, et al. Use of acid suppressive medications after laparoscopic anti-reflux surgery: prevalence, clinical indications and causes. Gastroenterology 2000;118:A478.

57. Lord RV, Kaminski A, Oberg S, et al. Absence of gastroesophageal reflux disease in a majority of patients taking acid suppression medications after Nissen fundoplication. J Gastrointest Surg 2002;6:3–10.

58. Perez AR, Moncure AC, Rattner DW. Obesity adversely affects the outcome of anti-reflux operations. Surg Endosc 2001;15:986–989.

59. Ward EM, DeVault KR, Bouras EP, et al. Successful esophageal pH monitoring with a catheter-free system. Aliment Pharmacol Ther 2004;19(4):449–454.

60. So JBY, Zeitels SM, Rattner DW. Outcomes of atypical symptoms attributed to gastroesophageal reflux treated by laparoscopic fundoplication. Surgery 1998;124:28–32.

61. DeVault KR. Overview of therapy for the extraesophageal manifestations of GERD. Am J Gastroenterol 2000;95:S39–44.

62. Field SK, Sutherland LR. Does medical anti-reflux therapy improve asthma in asthmatics with gastroesophageal reflux? A critical review of the literature. Chest 1998;114:275–283.

63. Field SK, Gelfand GA, McFadden SD. The effects of anti-reflux surgery on asthmatics with gastroesophageal reflux. Chest 1999;116:766–774.

64. Irwin RS, Curley FJ, French CL. Chronic cough. The spectrum and frequency of causes, key components of the diagnostic evaluation, and outcome of specific therapy. Am Rev Respir Dis 1990;141:640–647.

65. Koufman JA. Laryngopharyngeal reflux testing. Ear Nose Throat J 2002;82(suppl 2)S14–18.

66. Richter J, Vaezi M, Stasney CR, et al. Baseline pH measurements for patients with suspected signs and symptoms of reflux laryngitis. Gastroenterology 2004; 126:A536–537.

67. Vaezi M, Richter J, Stasney CR, et al. A randomized, double blind, placebo-controlled study of acid suppression for the treatment of suspected laryngopharyngeal reflux. Gastroenterology 2004;126:A22.

68. Peters L, Maas L, Petty D, et al. Spontaneous noncardiac chest pain. Evaluation by 24-hour ambulatory esophageal motility and pH monitoring. Gastroenterology 1988;94:878–886.

69. Achem SR, Kolts BE, MacMath T, et al. Effects of omeprazole versus placebo in treatment of noncardiac chest pain and gastroesophageal reflux. Dig Dis Sci 1997;42: 2138–2145.

70. Fass R, Fennerty MB, Ofman JJ, et al. The clinical and economic value of a short course of omeprazole in patients with noncardiac chest pain. Gastroenterology 1998;115:42–49.

71. Richter JE, Barish CF, Castell DO. Abnormal sensory perception in patients with esophageal chest pain. Gastroenterology 1986;91: 845–852.

10

The Medical and Endoscopic Management of Failed Surgical Anti-Reflux Procedures

M. Brian Fennerty and John G. Hunter

Surgical anti-reflux procedures, both open and laparoscopic, when performed by an experienced surgeon have been shown to be extremely effective in eliminating the major symptoms (heartburn and regurgitation) associated with gastroesophageal reflux disease (GERD) as well as heal erosive esophagitis and prevent stricture. The results of surgical anti-reflux surgery have also demonstrated durability in maintaining symptomatic and endoscopic remission in most of the patients who have an initial response. However, not all patients exhibit an initial or permanent satisfactory outcome from surgery, and surgical failure is even more prevalent when surgery is performed outside community and academic anti-reflux surgery centers of excellence. Thus, both the anti-reflux surgeon and his/her gastroenterology colleague likely will see an increasing number of their own or other physicians' patients that either failed to obtain initial symptom relief after anti-reflux surgery or whose symptoms have returned after an initial symptomatic improvement following their operation. This chapter will discuss the medical and endoscopic management of these patients and leave the surgical management of such patients for Drs. Kieran and Curet to discuss in Chapter 11 of this book.

Magnitude of the Problem

When a well-trained, competent surgeon performs anti-reflux surgery in a patient presenting with heartburn and regurgitation, 80–95% of patients obtain satisfactory relief of their reflux symptoms once recovered from the operation and eating normally again.[1–14] Unfortunately, this degree of success cannot be matched outside of surgical centers of excellence and some data indicate that failure rates at 1 year as high as 50–60% may occur in less-experienced surgical centers.[15,16] Furthermore, even in the best of hands, some patients will symptomatically relapse over time, with approximately 15–25% or more of patients reexperiencing symptoms of GERD five or more years after surgery despite initial success being achieved.[17,18] Given the hundreds of thousands of anti-reflux procedures performed in the last few years and the continued rapid increase in the number of these procedures being performed,[14,19,20] and with most of these being performed outside of highly skilled surgical centers, the problem of persisting or recurrent reflux symptoms after surgery is indeed a common one that will continue to grow and challenge the team caring for patients with GERD for the foreseeable future.[21–27]

Documentation of Recurrent Reflux after Surgical Anti-Reflux Therapy

The first step in deciding how best to manage a patient with persistent or recurrent GERD symptoms after anti-reflux surgery is to ensure that the symptoms are actually reflux related.

Patients are notoriously unreliable in understanding or describing what the term heartburn refers to and a word description such as "a substernal burning sensation rising towards the neck" is a much more objective and reliable term to define reflux-related heartburn than the word "heartburn" itself.[28] Thus, the first step one should take when a patient says they have heartburn after anti-reflux surgery is to ask them to carefully describe their symptom(s). Furthermore, the ability of physicians to adequately predict recurrent GERD in the postoperative state based on symptoms alone is also questionable.[22] In patients who underwent anti-reflux surgery for the symptoms of heartburn and regurgitation and where preoperatively objective evidence had linked these specific symptoms to pathological reflux (esophagitis on endoscopy or esophageal pH monitoring documenting pathological intraesophageal acid exposure, especially when the symptoms of GERD correlated with reflux events) persistence or return of these symptoms after anti-reflux surgery is likely to be associated with persistent or recurrent reflux. However, in patients who underwent anti-reflux surgery for atypical symptoms of GERD (nausea, dyspepsia, cough, hoarseness, etc.), persistence or return of these symptoms after surgery does not necessarily predict a return of reflux. Furthermore, the new onset of symptoms such as dyspepsia and upper abdominal pain after anti-reflux surgery in no way can be taken as firm evidence that reflux is still occurring or has recurred regardless of what the preoperative physiological assessment determined regarding GERD. As a matter of fact, there are few data regarding the effect anti-reflux surgery has on upper gastrointestinal symptom characteristics and it is possible that surgery alters the way a patient perceives or communicates symptoms related to a persistence or return of reflux, accounting for some of the difficulty in evaluating patient symptoms after anti-reflux surgery.[22] Thus, in all of these clinical situations, when reflux is thought to be present in the postoperative state, it is necessary to objectively link persistent or recurrent symptoms to reflux events through a thorough and careful diagnostic evaluation. Only when this link is established unequivocally can one then reliably recommend a therapeutic option to a patient aimed at managing their postoperative GERD-related symptoms.

Once one is convinced that the postoperative symptom(s) may be related to persistent or recurrent GERD, the second step is to objectively evaluate the upper gastrointestinal tract anatomically and physiologically, before suggesting one of the therapeutic alternatives. Although the preoperative diagnostic evaluation for anti-reflux therapy has evolved over time, and not all agree that a comprehensive preoperative esophageal physiological evaluation is necessary in all cases, the preoperative presence of some or all of the following tests can prove to be enormously useful in making postoperative management decisions in these patients: endoscopy, barium swallow, esophageal manometry, ambulatory esophageal pH testing, and/or gastric emptying study.[11,29] Although not all of these tests can be considered mandatory, some or all of these tests when performed preoperatively are very helpful in determining whether the recurrent symptoms are attributable to GERD (by comparing pre- and postoperative test results) and whether the preoperative physiology has been altered postoperatively to possibly account for the apparent failure of the procedure or a cause of any atypical symptoms.[30]

This diagnostic approach for what are thought to be persistent or recurrent GERD symptoms by definition requires the presence of preoperative anatomic and physiological information in order to compare postoperative findings, and therefore in our opinion, a complete and comprehensive preoperative evaluation is not only helpful in planning the original antireflux surgery and predicting outcome as it was previously used, but now is also helpful in accurately evaluating what is thought to be postoperative symptoms of GERD. Thus, it is our firm opinion that these tests, or some of them (endoscopy, pH monitoring, and esophageal manometry at a minimum), should always be performed preoperatively if at all possible.

The most important, and we believe mandatory, postoperative anatomic assessment in the patient thought to have persistent or recurrent reflux is a careful and complete endoscopic inspection of the surgical wrap to determine if anatomic disruption and/or migration have occurred or whether other pathology may account for the postoperative symptoms that otherwise may be wrongly attributed to GERD (see Chapter 9).

The most important physiological test to assess whether postoperative symptoms are related to reflux is ambulatory pH monitoring and possible impedance testing if this latter test becomes widely available. If persistent pathological acid reflux is documented by ambulatory esophageal pH monitoring along with other physiological [an esophageal manometry documenting an ineffective lower esophageal sphincter (LES) barrier] and/or anatomic (a disrupted or migrated wrap demonstrated endoscopically) evidence of an ineffective surgical procedure, then the decision must be made between another surgical anti-reflux procedure (see Chapter 11), an endoscopic anti-reflux procedure, or institution of pharmacological therapy for GERD (see Chapter 3). The final treatment decision will obviously depend on several factors including patient (their personal choices, or their specific physiology and anatomy) and physician (his or her surgical skills with a repeat anti-reflux procedure, availability of endoscopic anti-reflux expertise, etc.) factors and should be made only after a frank and realistic discussion of all of these available therapeutic options with the patient.

Endoscopic Assessment of a Prior Surgical Anti-Reflux Procedure

Whereas in the past the postoperative assessment of a surgical anti-reflux repair was often made by using esophageal manometry to measure the LES length and pressure as an indicator of the competence of the postoperative valve, this has largely been supplanted by direct endoscopic assessment of the surgical repair. Much has since been written regarding the normal and disrupted endoscopic appearance of the various surgical anti-reflux procedures.[21,31-33] However, many endoscopists continue to be unaware of the appearance of a normal, much less disrupted, anti-reflux surgery valve appearance or the technique of endoscopic inspection or information that is needed by the treating physician in order to determine whether the wrap is functionally competent or has been compromised. It has been taught that

the squamocolumnar junction usually approximates the proximal border of the lower esophageal sphincter and as such its location should be just above or within the surgical anti-reflux repair. When the location of the squamocolumnar junction is proximal to the wrap, this usually indicates a slipped or inappropriately placed repair. Additionally, the presence of esophagitis should be considered ample evidence of an incompetent repair and the return or persistence of reflux. Furthermore, on an endoscopic retroflexed view, it is expected that the wrap should appear to have a telescoping effect with the folds tightly adherent to the endoscope (Figures 10.1–10.5). Unfortunately, these various endoscopic findings are often subjectively appraised and not evaluated in a uniform or systematic way by the endoscopist attempting to assess the competency of a surgical anti-reflux repair.

Recently, a method to systematically endoscopically appraise the appearance and function of the various surgical anti-reflux procedures has been described and physicians that deal with these patients need to be aware of this classification scheme in order to accurately appraise the integrity of the surgical repair and effectively communicate their findings to others caring for the patient[31] (Table 10.1). In this proposed scheme, Jobe and colleagues[31] have char

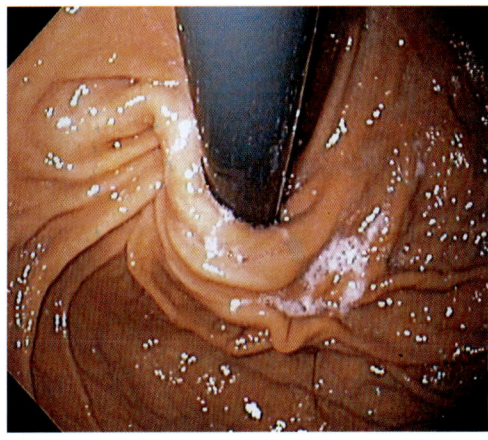

Figure 10.1. Retroflexed endoscopic view of the normal postoperative appearance of a "Nissen" fundoplication. Note the thin lip, adequate length, tight adherence around the scope, and intraabdominal location.

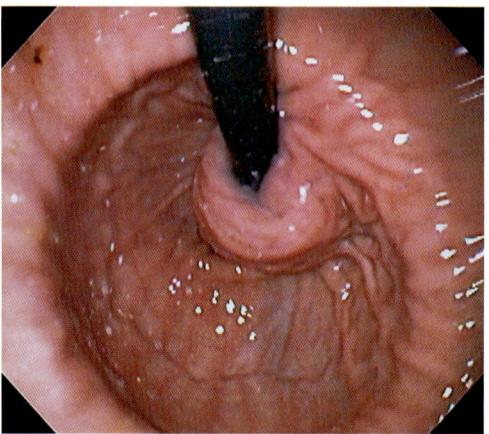

Figure 10.2. Retroflexed endoscopic view of the appearance of a "slipped" Nissen fundoplication with the wrap and fundus herniated across the diaphragm. Note the thicker than normal lip.

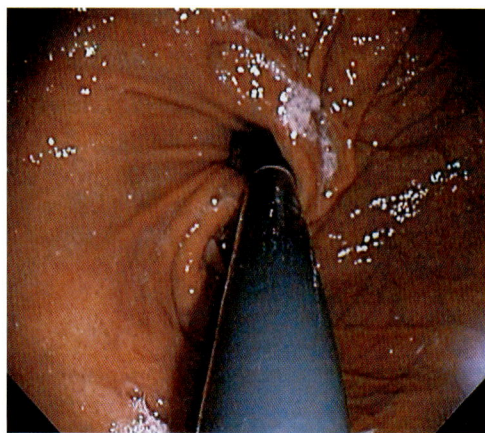

A

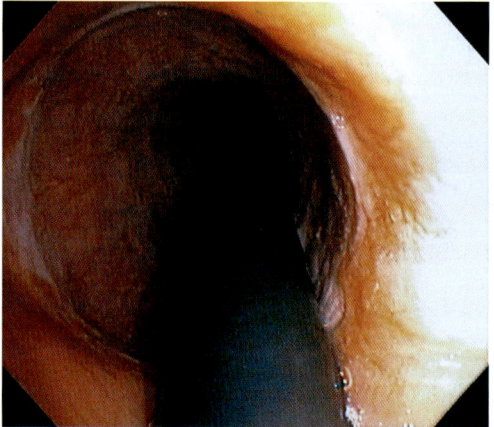

B

Figure 10.3. Retroflexed endoscopic view of a disrupted surgical anti-reflux repair with (A) valve laxity such that the retroflexed endoscope can be withdrawn (B) into the lower esophageal sphincter (LES) visualizing the squamocolumnar junction.

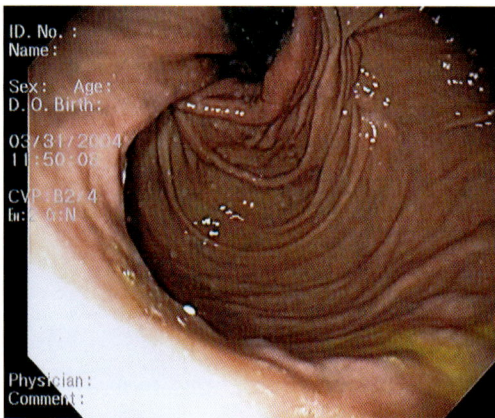

Figure 10.4. Retroflexed endoscopic view of a disrupted anti-reflux surgical repair with valve laxity, short intraabdominal length, etc.

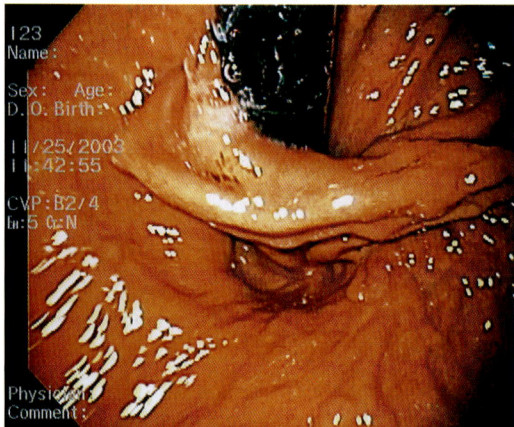

Figure 10.5. Retroflexed endoscopic view of a disrupted anti-reflux surgical repair with valve laxity, short intraabdominal length, and periesophageal hernia.

acterized the normal "valve" appearance of the Nissen, Collis-Nissen, Toupet, Dor, and Hill anti-reflux surgical procedures and have suggested a common medical terminology that should be used to describe the appearance of the postsurgical repair. In this classification scheme, they used 10 criteria by which to judge the valve appearance and used this information to determine the competence of the surgical repair. Endoscopic valve criteria included the lip (thin vs broad), body (length in centimeters), anterior (absent, shallow, or deep) and posterior (absent, shallow, or deep) grooves, lesser curve appearance (narrow or wide), adherence to the scope on retroflexion (loose, moderate, or tight), effect of respiration (laxity at any time during respiration), valve "type" (flat or nipple), intraabdominal location being present as the normal finding, repair position 3 cm proximal to the gastroesophageal junction, and the unique appearance characteristics specific to each surgical repair. For instance, in the commonly performed Nissen procedure, they determined a normal postoperative valve should have a thin lip, 3- to 4-cm body, shallow anterior and deep posterior groove, narrow lesser curve, tight adherence to the scope at baseline and during respiration, nipple-type valve appearance, intraabdominal position, typical repair position, and a body appearing like a "stacked coil." Each of the various anti-reflux surgical procedures has its own unique endoscopic features that need to be appreciated in order to judge competency of the specific surgical repair with this endoscopic method. In the case in which the repair appears to be intact using these endoscopic criteria, then serious consideration of alternative explanations for the patient's recurrent or persistent symptoms needs to undertaken. At a minimum, further physiological testing is now mandatory to prove reflux as a cause of the symptom(s). Hopefully, this carefully constructed endoscopic 10-item valve evaluation scheme can be demonstrated to be a reliable indicator of valve competency in prospective studies. Regardless, at this time, we believe that the above-described endoscopic evaluation of the valve remains the best initial test when evaluating a patient with suspected recurrent reflux after anti-reflux surgery before recommending further anti-reflux therapy of any sort.

Ambulatory Esophageal pH Monitoring in Patients with Prior Anti-Reflux Procedures

One of the great fallacies in managing patients with GERD is that pharmacological, endoscopic, or surgical anti-reflux therapy normalizes intraesophageal acid exposure in most patients. The reality is that many GERD patients, even those with complete resolution of heartburn and healing of esophagitis, often have improved but persistent pathological intraesophageal acid exposure, despite apparent adequate pharmacological, endoscopic, or surgical therapy. Thus, pathological intraesophageal acid exposure after anti-reflux surgery in of itself is not necessarily indicative of a failed surgical procedure. A postoperative esophageal pH assessment is difficult to reconcile with postoperative symptoms if the preoperative pH values are not known and unless a symptom correlation is performed between reflux events and symptoms with the follow-up study. Unfortunately, this later symptom assessment during interpretation of pH monitoring is not routinely performed by all that read these tests, but in the case of suspected postoperative GERD, a symptom correlation should be part of the routine assessment of these tracings. Clearly, unimproved or worsening intraesophageal acid exposure from preoperative to postoperative studies is likely to suggest an incompetent repair as does a good correlation between symptoms and reflux events.[21] In cases in which there has been a decrease or normalization of esophageal acid exposure between studies and no or little correlation with symptoms, then it is unlikely that reflux related to a defective surgical repair is responsible for the patient's postoperative symptoms. Whether a dual probe assessing proximal as well as the more usual distal esophageal acid exposure or a 48-hour study with the Bravo system (Medtronics, Minneapolis, MN) increases the sensitivity of this physiological test in the postoperative state is unknown. Our personal bias is that patients are more tolerant of the tubeless Bravo probe and more likely to maintain normal diet and activity while being studied and therefore more likely to demonstrate pathological reflux if present. However, not all centers performing anti-reflux surgery evaluations have access to a Bravo system nor has it been shown to improve diagnostic outcome in this specific clinical situation.

Other Tests of Gastrointestinal Physiology and Function

Esophageal manometry has been used in the past to assess the length of the LES, its pressure, and intraabdominal location as a surrogate of valve competency after surgical treatment of GERD. There are no data demonstrating that this is a reliable means of assessing postsurgical valve competence, but nonetheless the procedure has been widely adopted and implemented into clinical practice.[21] Our experience suggests that the normal range in length and pressure of the LES after otherwise effective anti-reflux surgery is so great that unless the pressure is minimal (<8 mm Hg) or the length is extremely short, competency of the valve in the postoperative state is nearly impossible to determine by this test alone. However, manometry can be complementary to other tests of valve function (e.g., endoscopy, pH monitoring) or diagnostic when other unusual diseases that can mimic GERD in the postoperative state are present (e.g., achalasia).

The barium swallow has also been used in the past to detect recurrent hiatus hernia or marked displacement of wrap location after anti-reflux surgery.[21] However, this test is only sensitive to gross disruption of the surgical repair, and likely adds little to the preferred method for assessing valve anatomy after anti-reflux surgery, a careful and descriptive endoscopic examination (Table 10.1).

Endoscopic and Pharmacological Therapy after Failed Anti-Reflux Surgery

Once it has been objectively determined through the above diagnostic testing strategy that the symptoms the patient has are related to continued or recurrent reflux, the next decision one needs to make is how best to manage the patient's GERD. Options include repeat anti-reflux surgery in centers with skill and experience in this type of surgery, endoscopic anti-reflux procedures, or pharmacological anti-reflux therapy. The choice will depend in part on the patient's preference as well as their unique physiology and anatomy as well as the availability of surgical or endoscopic skill in performing these types of procedures. There are no comparative trials in the medical literature evaluating these different management strategies versus each other. Furthermore, although there are numerous case series demonstrating success in treating failed anti-reflux surgery with reoperation,[34–56] there is no literature regarding efficacy of anti-reflux endoscopic procedures (despite personal and anecdotal reports of success) and surprisingly little written regarding the utility of standard anti-reflux drug therapy (although most of us have a firm clinical impression that these drugs perform similarly in the postoperative patient to the efficacy demonstrated in unoperated individuals with GERD).

Endoscopic Anti-Reflux Procedures in General

Endoscopic anti-reflux procedures have been in development for a number of decades and available for clinical use in the United States for approximately 5 years. They can be thought of largely to consist of three categories of interventions: 1) injection of substances into the deep muscle layer of the cardia meant to either bolster the esophagogastric junction and thereby increase LES pressure or stiffen the cardia thereby preventing distension of the cardia and subsequent transient LES relaxations (tLESRs) that allow reflux events to occur; 2) plication of the cardia and gastro-esophageal junction, using either a submucosal suture or a full-thickness suture or pin plication, thereby increasing the LES yield pressure and perhaps stiffening the cardia as well (see above); and 3) application of radiofrequency energy to the deep muscle layer of the gastroesophageal junction and cardia resulting in either a "neurolysis" and loss of sensation to refluxate or creating other effects on LES physiology in a way that decreases reflux events or duration of acid exposure. The theoretical basis for all of these endoscopic approaches is similar to those of surgery (improve valve function through anatomic and or physiological remodeling of the LES), but none of the current endoscopic anti-reflux techniques impact anatomically or physiologically the LES valve mechanism to the degree that can be achieved with surgery.[57–64] Additionally, the exact mechanism of effect leading to improved GERD symptoms with any of these techniques is incompletely understood. However, all of these endoscopic anti-reflux techniques appear to decrease tLESRs and thus are presumed to work in part by decreasing cardia distension. However, none of the devices normalizes tLESRs, thus another mechanism(s) must also be effected in order to explain their efficacy in managing GERD symptoms. Neurolysis in the case of radio frequency ablation (RFA), increased yield pressure with plication, etc., are but some of the many additional mechanisms that have been postulated to explain the efficacy of these procedures. Furthermore, it is plausible that the physiological effects that these endoscopic procedures have in the postoperative stomach may be very different and unique conferring an adjunctive effect to surgery that could be greater than expected based on what is known regarding these devices. Surprisingly, normalization of intraesophageal pH exposure occurs in 50% or less of patients undergoing endoscopic anti-reflux procedures and although there is some correlation between normalization of intraesophageal pH and clinical response, this is not a direct relationship.[65–69] The effect of these devices on LES length and pressure has been variable but in general the devices have very little effect on esophageal manometry. Nonetheless, each of the above approaches seems to be effective in treating GERD.[57–69] The magnitude of this treatment effect is still under evaluation as sham trials comparing each device to a "placebo sham" are just now being reported or performed.[65]

Food and Drug Administration Status of Endoscopic Anti-Reflux Procedures

Four endoscopic anti-reflux devices have been cleared or approved for use in the United States: the Stretta procedure (Curon Medical, Sunnyvale, CA), the EndoCinch device (Bard, Billerica, MA), Plicator (NDO Surgical, Mansfield, MA), and Enteryx (Boston Scientific, MA). Many other plicator and injection endoscopic anti-reflux devices are currently in development and are expected to be marketed over the next few years. Most have been cleared through a 510k mechanism and only Enteryx has been approved through the pre-market approval (PMA) process that involves a public hearing and a data presentation to an independent Food and Drug Administration (FDA) Advisory Panel. None of the devices have been specifically "labeled" for use in patients failing or recurring after anti-reflux surgery although there are no warnings or precautions against using these devices in this clinical situation that we are aware of.

Reimbursement Status of Endoscopic Anti-Reflux Procedures

A CPT Level I code for one of the endoscopic anti-reflux devices (Stretta) is forthcoming and goes into effect in 2005. Until now, most of these devices either did not have a CPT code or were assigned lower Level III codes (EndoCinch) making reimbursement for these procedures a problem in many locations. This is especially problematic given that the cost of the devices is approximately $2000 and when the endoscopic procedure and physician payment is also included, the entire cost of the procedure can be as much as $3000–4000. If the procedure is not covered by insurance, many patients are understandably reluctant to pay this much out of pocket when other medical and surgical anti-reflux therapies are covered by their insurer.

Short- and Long-term Outcomes of Endoscopic Anti-Reflux Procedures

All four of the FDA cleared and approved devices either have completed sham trials (Stretta, EndoCinch, Enteryx-European) or have them underway (Plicator, Enteryx-United States) and in general the success rates with these devices in these studies is 60–70%.[57,58,60,65–69] Previous uncontrolled studies of endoscopic anti-reflux devices indicated clinical response rates of 90% or more, but these earlier studies' results are not nearly as reliable as the data we are deriving from the sham-controlled studies because uncontrolled trials tend to overestimate treatment effect. Furthermore, the endpoint of many of these early trials was less than optimal because the primary endpoint for success was often a decrease, not elimination of proton pump inhibitor (PPI) use. It must also be appreciated that both the preliminary studies and the newer sham-controlled trials only enrolled patients with GERD that were responsive to PPIs and having no more than mild to moderate reflux disease determined endoscopically (generally hiatus hernias <2–3 cm and nonerosive reflux disease or at most Los Angeles grade A or B erosive esophagitis). Response rates in those with more severe disease (larger hiatal hernias, or those with more severe esophagitis) or atypical symptoms (dyspepsia, cough, asthma, etc.) have not been adequately studied but likely will be less than observed in the pivotal trials that only included patients with more mild or moderate forms of GERD. However, partial improvement in reflux physiology with a prior anti-reflux surgical procedure may make patients previously thought to have anatomy not applicable for endoscopic anti-reflux therapy, now possible candidates for those procedures. Although there are no controlled trial data regarding success of these procedures in GERD patients with atypical symptoms or in those with an incomplete response to antisecretory drugs, anecdotal experience and uncontrolled observational studies suggest some success in this situation as well.

However, again it is unlikely that success rates >50% will be demonstrated in these types of patients.

Use of Endoscopic Anti-Reflux Procedures in This Clinical Situation

There are only anecdotal reports of use of endoscopic anti-reflux procedures as an adjunct to therapy in patients who have failed anti-reflux surgery. Although it is intuitive that some or all of these devices could augment the effect of an ineffective anti-reflux surgical procedure based on their anatomic and physiological effects at the LES, there are still no reliable data documenting efficacy in this specific situation. Nonetheless, we are aware of at least three of the endoscopic devices being used to augment a less than optimal anti-reflux surgical outcome with at least verbal reports of success in some cases. Hopefully, we will see more reliable data from clinical trials become available in the near future regarding the use of these devices as augmentation of either an initial suboptimal surgical outcome or later with relapse of symptoms. Until then, one needs to make sure that the patient and referring physician are aware that we do not know what the magnitude of treatment success, if any, is with endoscopic anti-reflux procedures used in the postoperative state and that patients being treated with these devices may fail this therapy as well (Figure 10.6).

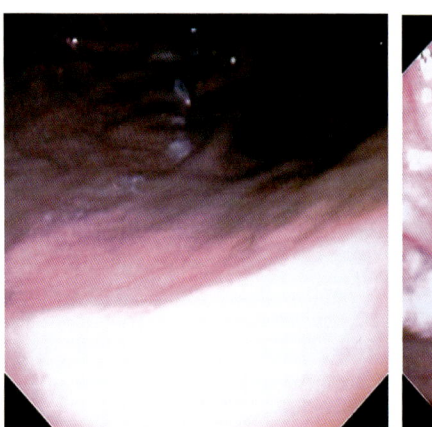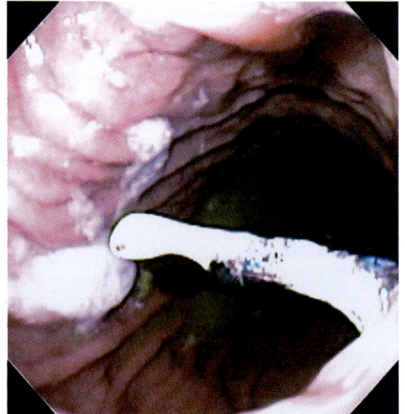

Figure 10.6. Retroflexed endoscopic view of an anti-reflux surgical repair that (A) has had an attempt at bolstering with EndoCinch endoscopic plication. (B) Close-up antegrade view demonstrating plication disruption.

One other consideration regarding endoscopic anti-reflux therapy versus other management approaches after failed surgery includes the issue of cost of therapy. In this era of health care, the issue of cost-effectiveness of a therapy will always remain a critical question. Payers not only are demanding efficacy be proven before paying for new therapies, they often require proof that new therapies are as, or more, cost-effective than currently used therapies. All of the endoscopic anti-reflux devices have high initial cost, related in part to the need for endoscopy to apply or direct therapy, but also related to the device itself and/or its associated equipment costs (radiofrequency generators, etc.) as well. If repeat applications of these techniques are required to maintain remission or co-therapy with drugs are still needed once these devices have been applied (e.g., they downgrade the severity of GERD but do not eliminate symptoms), these costs will have to be taken into consideration as well, along with indirect costs (lost work time, etc.). However, given the enormous upfront cost of repeat laparoscopic anti-reflux surgery, if efficacy and durability with these endoscopic techniques similar to surgery can be demonstrated, it is intuitive that these devices would then be cost-effective alternatives to repeat surgery. Whether cost-effectiveness of endoscopic anti-reflux devices can be demonstrated versus medical therapy for treatment of failed anti-reflux surgery will be more difficult to prove.[70–73]

The availability of over-the-counter and generic histamine-2-receptor antagonists (H2RAs) and PPIs, make the comparable cost-effectiveness of these endoscopic techniques less likely to be achievable. However, if one-time applications of endoscopic anti-reflux procedures results in substantial efficacy and prove to be durable in the postoperative patient, it is at least likely that these therapies would be competitive from a cost standpoint, even with the availability of inexpensive generic pharmacological therapies. Formal cost studies will be required to definitively answer these important clinical questions.

We believe that endoscopic therapies for GERD are promising technologies that likely will find clinical application in at least a subset of patients with persistent or recurrent GERD after anti-reflux surgery. But integration of these new endoscopic GERD therapies into clinical practice will require more information from carefully performed and analyzed trials. Issues that still need to be addressed include the efficacy of these devices compared with repeat surgery or PPI therapy and which, if any, endoscopic technique works best in this clinical situation. Once efficacy has been established, durability of response also needs to be clearly determined. Intensive postmarketing surveillance, device registries, and long-term clinical follow-up studies should be able to document durability. The impact of the learning curve for endoscopic anti-reflux procedures on outcomes including efficacy and safety should also be studied.

Despite these seemingly large hurdles that still have to be surmounted, we are confident that one, if not more, of these technologies will prove to be an effective, durable, safe, and cost-effective treatment option(s) for patients with recurrent or persistent GERD after a surgical anti-reflux procedure.

Pharmacological Therapy for Failed Anti-Reflux Surgery

Pharmacological therapy of GERD with antisecretory agents dates back to the mid-1970s when H2RAs first became available.[28,74] These agents demonstrated healing and symptom relief in approximately 50% of patients treated. In the 1980s–1990s, use of prokinetic compounds (cisapride) was also being used primarily or adjunctively to treat GERD symptoms, with efficacy similar to that demonstrated with H2RAs.[75] In 1989, the first PPI, omeprazole, was introduced and recently a second-generation PPI (esomeprazole) has become available. Substantial data from well-designed clinical trials with these drugs demonstrated healing and symptom response rates of 75–95%.[76] We now have at our disposal substantial short- and long-term PPI efficacy data demonstrating that 80–95% of patients with GERD treated with these agents obtain symptom relief and can be maintained in clinical remission.[77]

Interestingly, in studies in which pharmacological therapy is directly compared with surgical therapy for GERD, surgical therapy usually performs as well or better.[17,18,78,79] Some have noted that many of these trials were in the era before PPI use; however, there are also data comparing PPI therapy to open fundoplication that also demonstrate equal if not superior efficacy obtained with surgical therapy.[17] Nonetheless, we believe that both well-performed anti-reflux surgery and PPI therapy are effective primary therapies for GERD and although repeat anti-reflux surgery for failure has been well documented as an effective management option but PPI therapy has not, it is likely that PPIs are similarly effective as repeat surgery in treating postoperative GERD.

Use in This Clinical Situation

Why choose medical therapy over a repeat operation or an endoscopic therapy for recurrent GERD symptoms after surgery? The most obvious reason would be that the patient chose to be placed back on pharmacological therapy rather than undergo a second operation or have an invasive endoscopic anti-reflux procedure. This is not an evidence-based decision but one based solely on patient preference (perhaps with some understanding of the outcomes of the other various treatment options). Another reason for this choice would be that pharmacological therapy was superior in outcomes versus a repeat anti-reflux surgical or endoscopic procedure.

However, there have been no comparative studies of these differing management approaches nor are we aware of any trials comparing these therapeutic approaches being planned. However, there are limited data suggesting that pharmacological therapy remains effective (as it would be expected to be) after anti-reflux surgical failure. In a study of children who had postsurgical failure and a return of GERD, both symptoms and complications could be effectively managed with PPI therapy and none of the 18 children presenting with recurrent GERD symptoms or findings "required" a second operation.[80] In the Veterans Affairs Cooperative randomized trial comparing medical and surgical therapy, patients originally treated surgically and now on medical therapy expressed similar satisfaction with their outcome as those still in surgically induced remission.[18] These findings would imply that pharmacological therapy after failed surgery remains effective. Indeed, most clinicians have found similarly. We have never encountered a patient successfully treated with PPIs before

surgery whose typical GERD symptoms that recurred after surgery could not be effectively retreated by reinstitution of PPI therapy. The same success with PPIs cannot be assumed for new or atypical symptoms. A third reason to choose drugs over endoscopic or repeat surgical anti-reflux therapy may be one of cost-effectiveness. It has long been debated as to whether the long-term costs of therapy for GERD are greater with pharmacological versus surgical therapy and more recently endoscopic therapy has entered this debate.[70-73] Part of the difficulty in determining which management approach is more cost-effective has to do with the difficulties in relying on models of economic outcomes given the near absence of directly measured costs from randomized controlled trials comparing these various strategies. Myrvold et al.[72] as part of a previously reported randomized controlled trial, measured the direct costs of PPI therapy versus surgical therapy in a number of European countries participating in the study. Costs for surgical therapy were higher in Sweden, Denmark, and Norway but not Finland. Although both therapies were equally effective in controlling GERD symptoms, it was stated that PPI therapy was more cost-effective. What was ignored in the study was the fact that surgery demonstrated statistically significant reductions in heartburn scores although "treatment failure" was not different between arms.

Thus, without reporting confidence intervals for the treatment effect to allow insight into potential sample size limitations of a study, it may be that one strategy is not really economically dominant over another and therefore cost alone should not be a basis for a decision regarding choice of therapy for GERD. Additionally, given there are no comparative cost data for any therapy after failed anti-reflux surgery, this issue of cost in making a decision regarding therapy after failed anti-reflux surgery becomes a moot point in helping one select therapy in this clinical situation.

Thus, it really comes down to patient preference based in part on local availability of endoscopic or surgical anti-reflux therapy expertise that will determine the treatment decision. The only downside to this clinical approach is that in a patient who chooses surgical anti-reflux therapy because of the inconvenience, intolerance, or cost of continuous PPI therapy, may be back to where they started from without resolution of their problem. Thus, offering them PPI therapy to manage their recurrent GERD symptoms after anti-reflux surgery may not be an option they wish to consider.

Conclusions

Failure after surgical anti-reflux therapy is an increasingly common clinical condition that we will continue to encounter for years to come. Once it has been determined that the patient's postoperative symptoms are likely representative of GERD and a careful diagnostic strategy has confirmed a disrupted surgical repair and objectively confirmed pathological reflux as a cause of the patient's symptoms, then three therapeutic options can be considered: a repeat surgical procedure, reinstitution of pharmacological therapy (usually a PPI), or an attempt at adjunctive therapy via an endoscopic anti-reflux procedure. There are no clinical trial data with the latter two options, although there is substantial experience with the successful use of pharmacological therapy in this clinical situation. Intuitively, an endoscopic anti-reflux procedure may be effective because of its ability to possibly augment a less than optimal surgical repair. Although there is anecdotal evidence supporting this approach, its cost and invasiveness mandates that more substantial information documenting its effectiveness as a salvage therapy be available before it can be recommended for widespread use in this situation. Ultimately, the choice of therapy resides with the patient's wishes and it is our role to make sure that the choices that are available are objectively discussed along with the specific issues of their individual anatomy and physiology in order to assist them in making their decision.

References

1. Menon VS, Manson JM, Baxter JN. Laparoscopic fundoplication: learning curve and patient satisfaction. Ann R Coll Surg Engl 2003;85(1):10–13.
2. Novitsky YW, Zawacki JK, Irwin RS, French CT, Hussey VM, Callery MP. Chronic cough due to gastroesophageal reflux disease: efficacy of anti-reflux surgery. Surg Endosc 2002;16(4):567–571.
3. Khoursheed MA, Al-Asfoor M, Al-Shamali M, et al. Effectiveness of laparoscopic fundoplication for gastro-oesophageal reflux. Ann R Coll Surg Engl 2001;83(4): 229–234.
4. Althar RA. Laparoscopic anti-reflux surgery in the community hospital setting: evaluation of 100 consecutive patients. JSLS 1999;3(2):107–112.
5. Kimber C, Kiely EM, Spitz L. The failure rate of surgery for gastro-oesophageal reflux. J Pediatr Surg 1998;33(1): 64–66.
6. Rantanen TK, Halme TV, Luostarinen ME. The long term results of open anti-reflux surgery in a community-based health care center. Am J Gastroenterol 1999;94: 1777–1781.
7. So JB, Zeitels SM, Rattner DW. Outcomes of atypical symptoms attributed to gastroesophageal reflux treated by laparoscopic fundoplication. Surgery 1998;124:28–32.
8. Hinder RA, Filipi CJ, Wetscher G, et al. Laparoscopic Nissen fundoplication is an effective treatment for gastroesophageal reflux disease. Ann Surg 1994;46:527–531.
9. DeMeester TR, Bonavina L, Albertucci M. Nissen fundoplication for gastroesophageal reflux disease. Evaluation of primary repair in 100 consecutive patients. Ann Surg 1986;204:9–20.
10. Peters JH, Heimbucher J, Incarbone R, et al. Clinical and physiologic comparison of laparoscopic and open Nissen fundoplication. J Am Coll Surg 1995;180: 385–393.
11. Hunter JG, Trus TL, Branum GD, et al. A physiologic approach to laparoscopic fundoplication for gastroesophageal reflux disease. Ann Surg 1996;223:673–685.
12. Bremner RM, DeMeester TR, Crookes PF, et al. The effects of symptoms and nonspecific motility abnormalities on outcomes of surgical therapy for gastroesophageal reflux disease. J Thorac Cardiovasc Surg 1994;107:1244–1249.
13. Champion JK. Thorascopic Belsey fundoplication with 5-year outcomes. Surg Endosc 2003;17:1212–1215.
14. Flum D, Koepsell T, Heagerty P, Pelligrini C. The nationwide frequency of major adverse events in anti-reflux surgery and the role of surgeon experience 1992–1997. J Am Coll Surg 2002;195:611–618.
15. Vakil N, Shaw M, Kirby R. Clinical effectiveness of laparoscopic fundoplication in a US community. Am J Med 2003;114:1–5.
16. Khaitan L, Ray W, Holzman M, Smalley W. Healthcare utilization following medical and surgical therapy for GERD: a population-based study, 1996–2000. Gastroenterology 2000;122:A-67.
17. Lundell L, Mietten P, Myrvold H, et al. Continued (5 year) follow-up of a randomized clinical study comparing anti-reflux surgery and omeprazole in gastro-oesophageal reflux disease. J Am Coll Surg 2001;192: 172–179.
18. Spechler SJ, Lee E, Ahnen D, et al. Long-term outcome of medical and surgical therapies for gastroesophageal reflux disease: follow-up of a randomized controlled trial. JAMA 2001;285:2331–2338.
19. Finlayson SR, Birkmeyer JD, Laycock WS. Trends in surgery for gastroesophageal reflux disease: the effect of laparoscopic surgery on utilization. Surgery 2003; 133(2):147–153.
20. Urbach D, Ungar W, Rabeneck L. Whither surgery in the treatment of gastroesophageal reflux disease? CMAJ 2004;170:219–221.
21. Spechler SJ. The management of patients who have "failed" anti-reflux surgery. Am J Gastroenterol 2004; 99(3):552–561.

22. Galvani C, Fisichella PM, Gorodner MV, Perretta S, Patti MG. Symptoms are a poor indicator of reflux status after fundoplication for gastroesophageal reflux disease: role of esophageal functions tests. Arch Surg 2003; 138(5):514–518.

23. Langer JC. The failed fundoplication. Semin Pediatr Surg 2003;12(2):110–117.

24. Stein HJ, Feussner H, Siewert JR. Failure of anti-reflux surgery: causes and management strategies. Am J Surg 1996;171(1):36–39; discussion 39–40.

25. Waring JP. Management of postfundoplication complications. Semin Gastrointest Dis 1999;10:121–129.

26. Hinder RA, Klingler PJ, Perdikis G, Smith SL. Management of failed anti-reflux operation. Surg Clin North Am 1997;77:1083–1098.

27. Low D. Management of the problem patient after anti-reflux surgery. Gastroenterol Clin North Am 1994; 23:371–389.

28. Fennerty MB, Castell D, Fendrick AM, et al. The diagnosis and treatment of gastroesophageal reflux disease in a managed care environment: suggested disease management guidelines. Arch Intern Med 1994; 156:477–484.

29. Waring JP, Hunter JG, Oddsdottir M, et al. The preoperative evaluation of patients considered for laparoscopic anti-reflux surgery. Am J Gastroenterol 1995;90:35–38.

30. Mathew G, Watson DI, Myers JC, et al. Oesophageal motility before and after laparoscopic Nissen fundoplication. Br J Surg 1997;84:1465–1469.

31. Jobe BA, Kahrilas PJ, Vernon AH. Endoscopic appraisal of the gastroesophageal valve after anti-reflux surgery. Am J Gastroenterol 2004:233–243.

32. Oberg S, Peters JH, DeMeester TR, et al. Endoscopic grading of the gastroesophageal valve in patients with symptoms of gastroesophageal reflux disease (GERD). Surg Endosc 1999;13:1184–1188.

33. Johnson DA, Younes Z, Hogan WJ. Endoscopic assessment of hiatal hernia repair. Gastrointest Endosc 2000; 52:650–659.

34. Granderath FA, Kamolz T, Schweiger UM, Pointner R. Laparoscopic refundoplication with prosthetic hiatal closure for recurrent hiatal hernia after primary failed anti-reflux surgery. Arch Surg 2003;138(8):902–907.

35. Granderath FA, Kamolz T, Schweiger UM, Pointner R. Failed anti-reflux surgery: quality of life and surgical outcome after laparoscopic refundoplication. Int J Colorectal Dis 2003;18(3):248–253.

36. Johnsson E, Lundell L. Repeat anti-reflux surgery: effectiveness of a Toupet partial posterior fundoplication. Eur J Surg 2002;168(8–9):441–445.

37. Granderath FA, Kamolz T, Schweiger UM, Pointner R. Long-term follow-up after laparoscopic refundoplication for failed anti-reflux surgery: quality of life, symptomatic outcome, and patient satisfaction. J Gastrointest Surg 2002;6(6):812–818.

38. Braghetto I, Csendes A, Burdiles P, Botero F, Korn O. Results of surgical treatment for recurrent postoperative gastroesophageal reflux. Dis Esophagus 2002;15(4): 315–322.

39. Velanovich V, Ben Menachem T. Laparoscopic Nissen fundoplication after failed endoscopic gastroplication. J Laparoendosc Adv Surg Tech A 2002;12(5):305–308.

40. Kamolz T, Granderath FA, Bammer T, Pasiut M, Pointner R. Failed anti-reflux surgery: surgical outcome of laparoscopic refundoplication in the elderly. Hepato-gastroenterology 2002;49(45):865–868.

41. Watson AJ, Krukowski ZH. Revisional surgery after failed laparoscopic anterior fundoplication. Surg Endosc 2002;16(3):392–394.

42. Granderath FA, Kamolz T, Schweiger UM, et al. Is laparoscopic refundoplication feasible in patients with failed primary open anti-reflux surgery? Surg Endosc 2002; 16(3):381–385.

43. Legare JF, Henteleff HJ, Casson AG. Results of Collis gastroplasty and selective fundoplication, using a left thoracoabdominal approach, for failed anti-reflux surgery. Eur J Cardiothorac Surg 2002;21(3):534–540.

44. Serafini FM, Bloomston M, Zervos E, et al. Laparoscopic revision of failed anti-reflux operations. J Surg Res 2001;95(1):13–18.

45. Szwerc MF, Wiechmann RJ, Maley RH, Santucci TS, Macherey RS, Landreneau RJ. Reoperative laparoscopic anti-reflux surgery. Surgery 1999;126(4):723–728; discussion 728–729.

46. Floch NR, Hinder RA, Klingler PJ, et al. Is laparoscopic reoperation for failed anti-reflux surgery feasible? Arch Surg 1999;134(7):733–737.

47. Curet MJ, Josloff RK, Schoeb O, Zucker KA. Laparoscopic reoperation for failed anti-reflux procedures. Arch Surg 1999;134(5):559–563.

48. Watson DI, Jamieson GG, Game PA, Williams RS, Devitt PG. Laparoscopic reoperation following failed anti-reflux surgery. Br J Surg 1999;86(1):98–101.

49. Pointner R, Bammer T, Then P, Kamolz T. Laparoscopic refundoplications after failed anti-reflux surgery. Am J Surg 1999;178(6):541–544.

50. Bonavina L, Chella B, Segalin A, Incarbone R, Peracchia A. Surgical therapy in patients with failed anti-reflux repairs. Hepatogastroenterology 1998;45(23): 1344–1347.

51. Frantzides CT, Carlson MA. Laparoscopic redo Nissen fundoplication. J Laparoendosc Adv Surg Tech A 1997; 7(4):235–239.

52. Dalla Vecchia LK, Grosfeld JL, West KW, Rescorla FJ, Scherer LR III, Engum SA. Reoperation after Nissen fundoplication in children with gastroesophageal reflux: experience with 130 patients. Ann Surg 1997; 226(3):315–321; discussion 321–323.

53. O'Reilly MJ, Mullins S, Reddick EJ. Laparoscopic management of failed anti-reflux surgery. Surg Laparosc Endosc 1997;7(2):90–93.

54. Deschamps C, Trastek VF, Allen MS, Pairolero PC, Johnson JO, Larson DR. Long-term results after reoperation for failed anti-reflux procedures. J Thorac Cardiovasc Surg 1997;113(3):545–550; discussion 550–551.

55. Lim JK, Moisidis E, Munro WS, Falk GL. Re-operation for failed anti-reflux surgery. Aust N Z J Surg 1996; 66(11):731–733.

56. Ellis FH Jr, Gibb SP, Heatley GJ. Reoperation after failed anti-reflux surgery. Review of 101 cases. Eur J Cardiothorac Surg 1996;10(4):225–231; discussion 231–232.

57. Edmundowicz SA. Injection therapy of the lower esophageal sphincter for the treatment of GERD. Gastrointest Endosc 2004;59(4):545–552.

58. Kahrilas PJ. Radiofrequency therapy of the lower esophageal sphincter for treatment of GERD. Gastrointest Endosc 2003;57:723–731.

59. Swain P, Park PO, Mills T. Bard EndoCinch: the device, the technique, and pre-clinical studies. Gastrointest Endosc Clin N Am 2003;13:75–88.

60. Fennerty MB. Endoscopic suturing for treatment of GERD. Gastrointest Endosc 2003;57:390–395.

61. O'Connor KW, Lehman GA. Endoscopic placement of collagen at the lower esophageal sphincter to inhibit gastroesophageal reflux: a pilot study of 10 medically intractable patients. Gastrointest Endosc 1988;34:106–112.

62. Ferretis C, Benakis P, Dimapoulos C, et al. Endoscopic implantation of Plexiglas (PMMA) microspheres for the treatment of GERD. Gastrointest Endosc 2001;53: 423–426.

63. Fockens P. Gatekeeper reflux repair system: technique, pre-clinical and clinical experience. Gastrointest Endosc 2003;13:179–189.

64. Deviere J, Pastorelli A, Louis H, et al. Endoscopic implantation of a biopolymer in the lower esophageal sphincter for gastroesophageal reflux: a pilot study. Gastrointest Endosc 2002;55(3):335–341.

65. Corley DA, Katz P, Wo J, et al. Temperature controlled radiofrequency energy delivery to the gastroesophageal junction for the treatment of GERD (the Stretta procedure): a randomized, double-blind, sham controlled, multi-center clinical trial. Gastroenterology 2003;125:668–676.

66. Filipi CJ, Lehman GA, Rothstein RI, et al. Transoral, flexible endoscopic suturing for treatment of GERD: a multicenter trial. Gastrointest Endosc 200;53:416–422.

67. Mahmood Z, McMahon B, Weir D, et al. Endocinch therapy for gastro-oesophageal reflux disease: a one year prospective follow-up. Gut 2003;52:34–39.

68. Mahmood Z, Byrne PJ, McCullough J, et al. A comparison of Bard endocinch transesophageal endoscopic plication (BTEP) with laparoscopic Nissen fundoplication (LNF) for the treatment of gastroesophageal reflux disease. Gastrointest Endosc 2002;55:90.

69. Johnson DA, Ganz R, Aisenberg J, et al. Endoscopic, deep mural implantation of Enteryx for the treatment of GERD: 6 month follow-up of a multicenter trial. Am J Gastroenterol 2003;98:250–258.

70. Swanstrom LL. Motion—laparoscopic Nissen fundoplication is more cost effective than oral PPI administration: arguments for the motion. Can J Gastroenterol 2002;16(9):621–623.

71. Sonnenberg A. Motion—laparoscopic Nissen fundoplication is more cost effective than oral PPI administration: arguments against the motion. Can J Gastroenterol 2002;16(9):627–631.

72. Myrvold HE, Lundell L, Miettinen P, et al. The cost of long term therapy for gastro-oesophageal reflux disease: a randomised trial comparing omeprazole and open anti-reflux surgery. Gut 2001;49:488–494.

73. Viljakka M, Nevalainen J, Isolauri J. Lifetime costs of surgical versus medical treatment of severe gastro-oesophageal reflux disease in Finland. Scand J Gastroenterol 1997;32:766–772.

74. Fennerty MB. Medical treatment of gastroesophageal reflux disease in the managed care environment. Semin Gastrointest Dis 1997;8:90–99.

75. Robinson M. Prokinetic therapy for gastroesophageal reflux disease. Am Fam Physician 1995;52(3):957–966.

76. Chiba N, De Gara CJ, Wilkinson JM, Hunt RH. Speed of healing and symptom relief in grades II to IV gastroesophageal reflux disease: a meta-analysis. Gastroenterology 1997;112:1798–1810.

77. Klinkenberg-Knol EC, Festen HP, Jansen JB, et al. Long-term treatment with omeprazole for refractory reflux oesophagitis: efficacy and safety. Ann Intern Med 1994; 121:161–167.

78. Walker SJ, Baxter ST, Morris DI, et al. Review article: controversy in therapy of gastro-esophageal reflux disease—long-term proton pump inhibitor or laparoscopic anti-reflux surgery. Aliment Pharmacol Ther 1997;11:249–260.

79. Spechler SJ. The Department of Veteran's Affairs Gastroesophageal Reflux Disease Study Group; comparison of medical and surgical therapy for complicated gastroesophageal reflux disease in veterans. N Engl J Med 1992;326:786–792.

80. Pashankar D, Blair GK, Israel DM. Omeprazole maintenance therapy for gastroesophageal reflux disease after failure of fundoplication. J Pediatr Gastroenterol Nutr 2001;32(2):145–149.

11

Reoperation for Failed Anti-Reflux Surgery

Jennefer A. Kieran and Myriam J. Curet

Recurrent gastroesophageal (GE) reflux symptoms after fundoplication have been reported in 6–20% of open fundoplications and in 6–17% of laparoscopic fundoplications.[1–6] The most common symptoms are recurrent reflux (30–60%) and dysphagia (10–20%). The majority of these patients can be treated medically with only 4–6% requiring reoperation.[4,6] Only patients with persistent, severe, refractory symptoms should be considered for reoperation. Recurrence and technical failures are discussed in detail in Chapter 8. In those patients chosen for reoperative surgery, it is imperative that one determines the cause of failure of the original operation to ensure that patients receive the appropriate treatment. The best results for fundoplication occur with primary operation with success rates reported to be 90–95%. When recurrences require reoperation, the success of the operation declines precipitously with the number of subsequent surgeries. Success rates for reoperations are 85% for patients who have had one previous operation, 66% who have had two previous operations, and only 42% for patients with three or more previous operations.[2,6–9] Choosing the correct operation for the individual patient during the original surgery will decrease the risk of recurrent disease and the need for reoperation.[10]

Preoperative Evaluation

The preoperative evaluation of patients being considered for reoperation should include pH studies, manometry, upper gastrointestinal (GI) series, endoscopy, and gastric emptying studies if symptoms indicate. This evaluation has been discussed in detail in previous chapters, but is essential to mention here because the results dictate the operative strategy. The upper GI series can demonstrate anatomic reasons for failure including paraesophageal hernia, wrap herniation into the chest, stricture, a wrap that is too tight, or a short esophagus. Similarly, endoscopy can identify a disrupted wrap, a recurrent hiatal hernia, poor gastric motility, or esophagitis. Manometry can confirm that a wrap is too tight, poor esophageal motility, undiagnosed achalasia, or an incompetent lower esophageal sphincter. Finally, pH studies can identify recurrent reflux without other evidence of anatomic abnormalities.

The goal of this chapter is to identify the appropriate operation for the individual patient with failed prior anti-reflux surgery and describe the different operative techniques used for such patients. Reoperative choices include: an open laparotomy, laparoscopy, or a thoracic approach; partial or total fundoplication; gastric bypass; pyloroplasty; gastropexy; antrectomy and vagotomy; Roux-en-Y biliary diversion; and esophageal resection.[5,11] Some of these techniques are addressed in other Chapters 2, 5, 11–14. This chapter will focus on laparoscopic, open, and transthoracic approaches with partial or total fundoplication.

Operative Techniques

Reoperative surgery is inherently more difficult than the original procedure. For this reason, a preoperative cardiopulmonary evaluation is necessary to ensure optimal physiologic status before surgery.

Regardless of the method used to gain access in the reoperative fundoplication, the surgical principles remain the same. These include meticulous technique with adhesiolysis, adequate esophageal mobilization, crural closure, appropriate fundoplication, and anchoring of the wrap within the abdomen.[6,12] Many authors believe that the original wrap needs to be completely undone as part of the reoperative strategy. The only potential exception to this might be a patient who, on preoperative studies and intraoperative examination, clearly has an intact and properly performed wrap that had herniated into the mediastinum. All patients undergo an appropriate preoperative evaluation as previously described. Deep venous thrombosis (DVT) prophylaxis with sequential compression devices and preoperative subcutaneous heparin are instituted. Preoperative prophylactic antibiotics are given and a Foley catheter is placed.

Open Laparotomy for Reoperative Fundoplication

The most common approach for reoperative anti-reflux surgery is revision fundoplication via laparotomy, or the so-called open technique. Once in the operating room, the patient is placed in the supine position. The abdomen is prepped and draped in a sterile fashion. An upper midline incision is performed and extensive adhesiolysis may be necessary. Use of meticulous technique is important to minimize gastrotomies, enterotomies, or esophagotomies. If created, they are repaired primarily and, if at all possible, are subsequently contained within the wrap. A lighted bougie or endoscope can aid in the identification of the hiatal structures. The first step is to dissect the liver off the anterior surface of the stomach and wrap. Identification of either the right or left crus as an initial step is very helpful in confirming the location of dissection and in helping to identify the wrap. Dissection of both crura should continue until the wrap is completely dissected free. Retroe-

sophageal dissection is then performed with care taken not to injure the aorta. A Penrose drain can be placed around the esophagus to aid in mobilization.

The cause of technical failure is then assessed. Possible causes include wrap migration or herniation, wrap failure with either a too loose or too tight wrap, paraesophageal hernia formation, and slipped fundoplication onto the stomach body (see Chapter 8). The wrap is taken down completely and both vagal nerves are identified and spared. If the short gastric vessels had not previously been divided, this is performed before wrap formation. It may be necessary to dissect the fundus off the spleen if the short gastric vessels have already been divided. If a paraesophageal hernia is the cause of failure, the hernia sac is excised.

Before creating the fundoplication, it is imperative that the GE junction is well within the abdomen. At least 5 cm of esophagus above the GE junction is mobilized. After releasing tension on the stomach, the GE junction must remain below the diaphragm without retracting into the mediastinum. If this is not possible with esophageal mobilization, an esophageal lengthening procedure such as the Collis gastroplasty is performed.[2,11] Additionally, as Hunter et al.[15] detail, a Collis gastroplasty may be indicated in patients who appear to have adequate esophageal length, but have herniated their wrap more than once. A Collis gastroplasty is performed by placing a GIA stapler at the angle of His and creating a longitudinal staple line that effectively recreates the GE junction further distally on the stomach (Figure 11.1). The wrap is then performed at the new GE junction while ensuring adequate intraabdominal length.

Regardless of the cause of failure, the hiatus is closed posteriorly with nonabsorbable sutures in all patients. The revision fundoplication is performed over a 56- to 60-French bougie to ensure a "floppy" wrap. Partial or total fundoplication is selected based on preoperative manometric studies. Patients with poor esophageal motility are considered for a partial or Toupet fundoplication in order to decrease the risk of postoperative dysphagia. If esophageal motility is adequate, the preferred operation is the Nissen fundoplication. In patients with paraesophageal hernias, surgeons may prefer a Toupet wrap because that will better anchor the GE junction in the

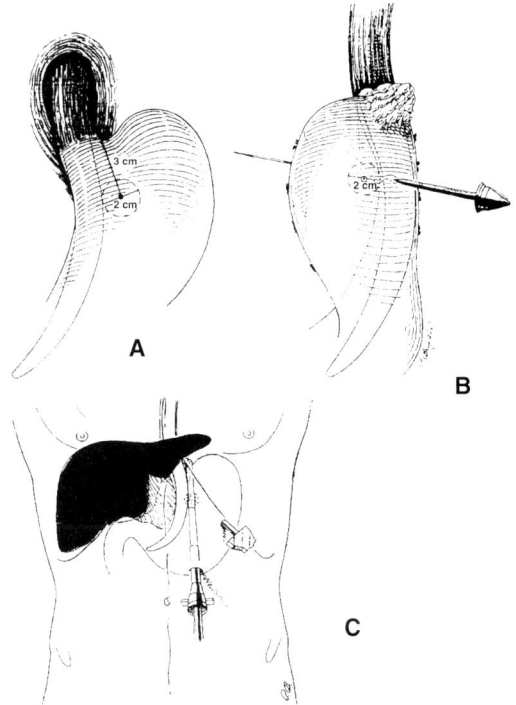

Figure 11.1. Collis gastroplasty. A, An area for the initial gastrotomy is selected that is adjacent to the indwelling bougie and 3 cm from the esophagogastric junction. B, A through-and-through gastrotomy is performed with an EEA stapler. C, A linear cutting stapler is positioned through the gastrotomy and is fired parallel to the lesser curve of the stomach to complete the gastroplasty. (Zucker KA. Surgical Laparoscopy. 2nd ed. Baltimore: Lippincott Williams & Wilkins; 2000:462.)

sary is seeing the spleen pulled medially when the fundus is brought posteriorly to create the fundoplication. Once the fundus is adequately mobilized, it is passed posteriorly to the GE junction again. A 56- to 60-French bougie is passed down the esophagus and positioned across the GE junction. The anterior portion of the wrap is secured to the esophagus and the posterior portion of the wrap with two sutures approximately 1 cm apart, followed by a fundofundal suture at the level of the GE junction. Pledgets can be used to reinforce the sutures (Figure 11.3). There should be no tension on the wrap. This is assessed by passing an instrument between the wrap and the esophagus to see how much tension there is. The bougie is then removed. Given the difficult dissection that is typically experienced during reoperative surgery, intraoperative endoscopy with leak test should be performed at the conclusion of the operation. The leak test is performed by submerging the wrap under saline, insufflating at the GE junction with the endoscope, and observing for bubbles. If bubbles are seen, the enterotomy is sutured closed, and the leak test is repeated.

abdomen and may decrease the risk of recurrent herniation.

For a total fundoplication, the fundus is passed posteriorly around the esophagus. Performance of the "shoe-shine" maneuver, in which the fundus is grasped on either side of the esophagus and moved back and forth, ensures the appropriate amount of fundus is passed posteriorly and the wrap is in the correct orientation (Figure 11.2). The portion of the fundus now on the right of the GE junction is released. If the fundus retracts under the esophagus back to the left of the GE junction, there is excessive tension on the wrap and further attempts to mobilize the fundus need to be undertaken. Another sign that further mobilization is neces-

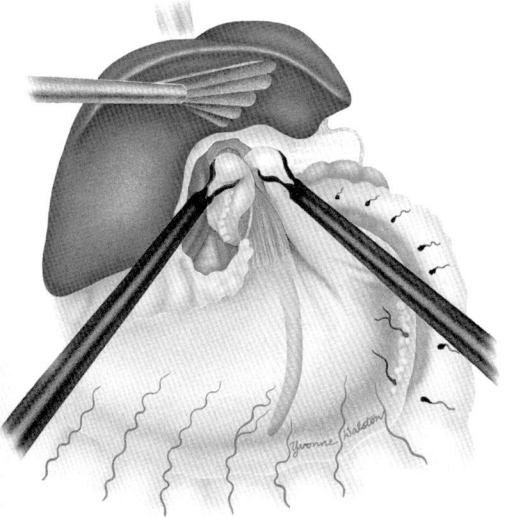

Figure 11.2. Performing a "shoe-shine" maneuver before suturing a Nissen fundoplication. (Reproduced with permission from Phillips EH, Rosenthal J, eds. Operative Strategies in Laparoscopic Surgery. New York: Springer-Verlag; 1995:121.)

A partial posterior, or Toupet, fundoplication is indicated for patients who have inadequate esophageal motility. Patients with dysphagia from a fundoplication that is too tight may also benefit from a partial fundoplication if it is not possible to create a total fundoplication that is floppy secondary to scarring or ischemia. Although some authors recommend liberal use of a Toupet fundoplication, there are higher failure rates with a Toupet compared with a Nissen fundoplication.[16,17] The Toupet is performed by wrapping the fundus posteriorly and securing the fundus to the esophagus and crura bilaterally. Two sutures are placed from the fundus to the crus on the right, and four fundus to esophagus sutures are placed, two on each side. Sutures along the esophagus are placed 1 cm apart to create a 2-cm fundoplication (Figure 11.4).

If the patient had signs of vagal denervation preoperatively manifested by prolonged gastric emptying, then pyloric dilation, pyloroplasty, or pyloromyotomy should be performed to alleviate the symptoms of delayed gastric emptying. Rieger et al.[18] caution against pyloroplasty because complication rates are significantly higher in these patients.

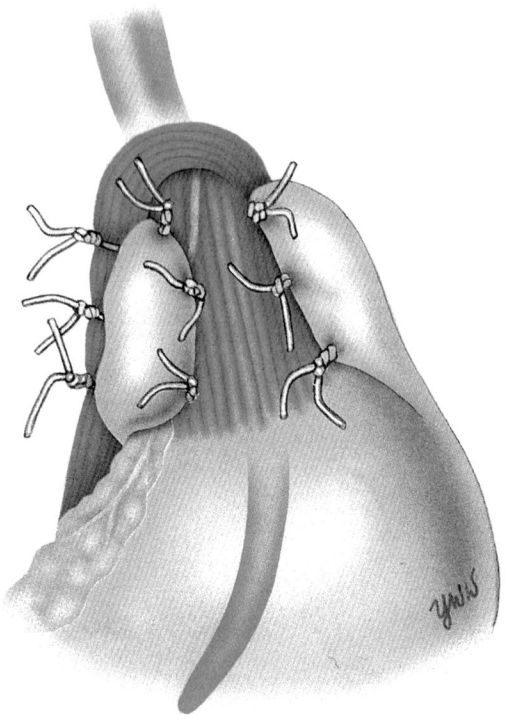

Figure 11.4. Completed Toupet fundoplication. (Zucker KA. Surgical Laparoscopy. 2nd ed. Baltimore: Lippincott Williams & Wilkins; 2000:406.)

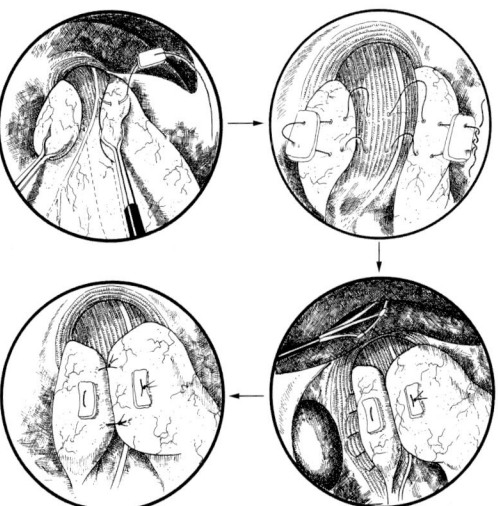

Figure 11.3. Use of Teflon pledgets to reinforce a fundoplication. (Reproduced with permission from Phillips EH, Rosenthal J, eds. Operative Strategies in Laparoscopic Surgery. New York: Springer-Verlag; 1995:121.)

Siewert et al.[5,11] summarized the morbidity and mortality data reported for open redo fundoplications. The authors identified a wide range of morbidity reported, ranging from 20 to 40% and a mortality rate of 2%. Good to excellent results were reported in 80–85% of selected patients undergoing reoperation for failed anti-reflux surgery. They reemphasized what Little et al.[8] reported: that multiple operations significantly and adversely affect the success rate to the point that, after three operations, one should consider esophageal resection.

Laparoscopic Revision of Fundoplication

Operative access for technical failures of fundoplications was originally described using an open abdominal technique or a thoracic approach. In the past 10 years, there have been multiple retrospective reviews of personal expe-

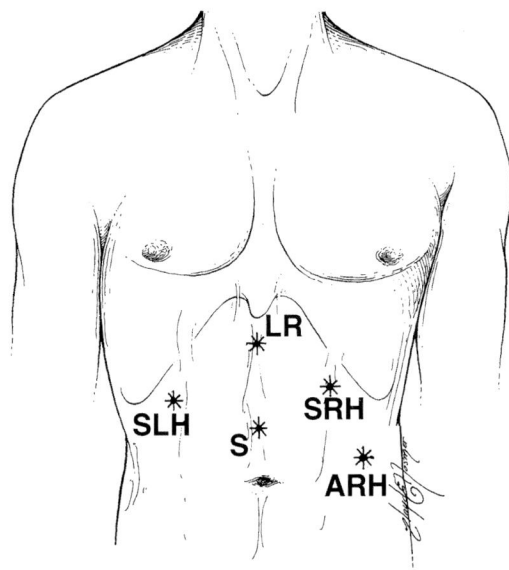

Figure 11.5. Port placement for laparoscopic reoperative fundoplication surgery. LR, liver retractor; S, telescope; SLH, surgeon's left hand; SRH, surgeon's right hand; ARH, assistant's right hand. (Reproduced with permission from Dallemagne B, Weerts JM, Jehaes C, et al. Laparoscopic Nissen fundoplication: preliminary report. Surg Laparosc Endosc 1991;1(3):138–143.)

riences with laparoscopic reoperative fundoplication. The overall conclusion to date is that laparoscopic reoperation is safe and effective if performed by an experienced laparoscopic surgeon. In addition, most reports indicate that laparoscopic reoperative fundoplication is associated with fewer complications, shorter length of stay, and better patient satisfaction.

Laparoscopic refundoplication is performed with a five-trocar technique similar to the initial fundoplication procedure (Figure 11.5). Initial access to the abdomen is obtained either with an open technique with insertion of a Hasson trocar or placement of a Veress needle away from the original operative site, e.g., the left subcostal region. Adhesiolysis is then performed as necessary to insert the subsequent ports. Initially, it may be necessary to place ports in nontraditional locations to aid in lysis of adhesions. The operating ports are then inserted once the abdominal wall is cleared of adhesions.

The type of device used for hemostasis is surgeon dependent. Ultrasonic shears can minimize heat conduction to surrounding tissue and reduce the risk of inadvertent enterotomies.

If cautery is used, one must clearly visualize adhesions and ensure that no conduction to surrounding tissue occurs. Some surgeons prefer sharp dissection with use of cautery only when hemorrhage occurs. Regardless of the hemostatic technique chosen, meticulous adhesiolysis is imperative to prevent gastrotomy or esophagotomy. If created, these are repaired primarily and the operation can continue laparoscopically if deemed safe. If possible, the repair is included in the new wrap to protect it.

Once operative trocars are placed, adhesions from the left lobe of the liver to the fundoplication are taken down. The liver retractor may need to be adjusted periodically to aid in the dissection. Once the liver is retracted, both crura are identified. To enable the identification and dissection of the esophagus, an endoscope or lighted bougie can be placed at the GE junction. After the crura are identified, the wrap is encircled with a Penrose drain to aid in retraction. Both vagal nerves are identified and spared if possible. The wrap is taken down either by removing the previous fundic sutures, or by stapling the fundo-fundic connection with the EndoGIA stapler. The anterior vagus is usually identified in the wrap. If the posterior vagus was included in the wrap previously, it is much easier to identify and spare. The short gastric vessels are divided with the ultrasonic shears if this was not previously performed. If the short gastric vessels were previously divided, the fundic adhesions to the spleen are carefully lysed.

A crural closure is performed in all patients (Figure 11.6). This is done with nonabsorbable suture and may be buttressed with pledgets or mesh. The data of Granderath et al.[19–21] on the routine use of polypropylene mesh in crural closure for both primary and recurrent fundoplication reveal that recurrent herniation is significantly lower in the mesh group (Figure 11.7). They reported 24 patients who underwent revisional fundoplication.[19] All patients had hiatal disruption and all had been previously closed primarily. There were no intraoperative complications and only one patient had severe postoperative dysphagia that responded to dilation. A barium swallow test was performed at 1 year in 19 of the 24 patients, which revealed no hiatal recurrence. The remaining 5 patients were asymptomatic. They support the use of mesh in all patients undergoing fundoplication. This is

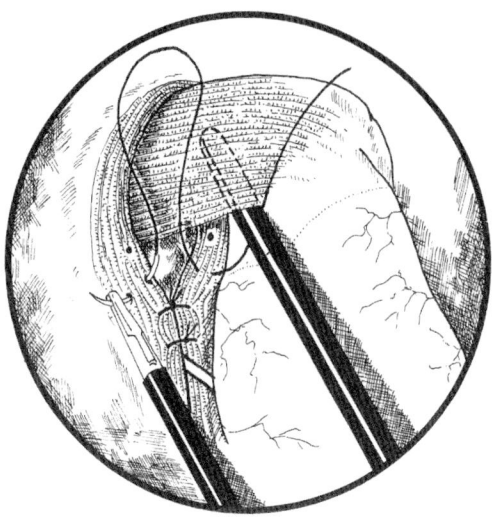

Figure 11.6. Closure of the hiatus with crural sutures. Phillips EH, Rosenthal RJ. Operative Strategies in Laparoscopic Surgery. Springer-Verlag 1995, 119.

also supported by Frantzides and Carlson[22] in a prospective, randomized trial of 72 patients who had either suture cruroplasty or polytetrafluoroethylene mesh repair. This study determined that the frequency of recurrent hiatal hernia was significantly higher in the primary repair group (22%) versus the mesh group (0%). Carlson et al.[23] had similar results in 31 patients who were randomized to simple suture closure versus mesh closure. Whereas some authors report mesh erosion into the esophagus, Granderath et al.[19] state that mesh erosion is a very rare complication.

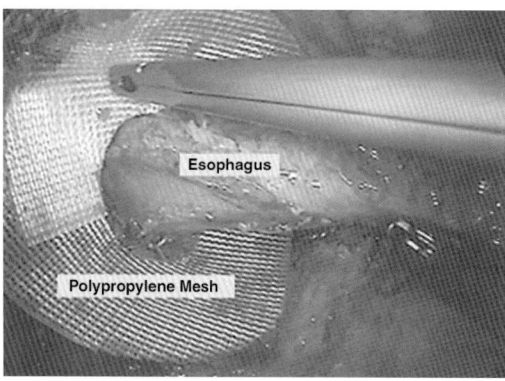

Esophagus

Polypropylene Mesh

Figure 11.7. Mesh closure of the hiatus. (Reproduced with permission from Granderath et al.,[18] Copyright ©2003, American Medical Association. All rights reserved.)

Once the crura are reapproximated posteriorly, the endoscope is removed and a 56- to 60-French bougie dilator is placed. A Nissen fundoplication or Toupet fundoplication is then performed based on the preoperative manometry as previously described. Some authors secure the Nissen fundoplication to the crura with collar sutures. There are no studies currently that evaluate recurrence based on securing the wrap to the crura. In contrast to the Nissen, the Toupet fundoplication is routinely secured to both crura. Finally, upper endoscopy is performed to evaluate the new wrap for leak. The liver retractor and all ports are removed under direct vision and the ports >5 mm are closed at the fascial level.

Most authors agree that laparoscopy is a safe and effective tool in reoperative surgery when performed by an experienced laparoscopist. Hunter et al.[2,15] begin laparoscopically in all patients who underwent previous laparoscopic fundoplication and usually approach patients who have undergone previous open surgery either with a laparotomy or thoracotomy. Other authors attempt laparoscopy in all patients, but have a low threshold to convert to open laparotomy if adhesions preclude laparoscopic completion.[15,6,24,25] Overall conversion rates vary from 9 to 60%. In the studies presented, recurrent symptoms were evaluated preoperatively as previously described. Among the technical causes of failure that were identified for the initial operation, crural failure with hiatal herniation of the wrap was the number one cause of recurrent symptoms,[1,15,24–26] followed by wrap failure, slipped Nissen, and a wrap that was too tight.[27–29]

When choosing the appropriate reoperation, one must consider the preoperative workup, which should clearly document the cause of the failure. Most authors agree that a tailored approach to each patient based on the cause of the recurrent symptoms is essential, rather than attempting the same operation in everyone.[25] As is summarized in Table 11.1, most studies are small retrospective reviews of single surgeons' personal experience. However, in combining these data, of 505 total patients, 385 were completed laparoscopically for an overall conversion rate of 23.8%. The majority underwent Nissen fundoplication (56%), followed by Toupet partial fundoplication (17%), then miscellaneous operative procedures including

Table 11.1. Results of laparoscopic reoperation after failed fundoplication.

Authors	Patients (n)	Operative Time (min)	Conversion Rate (%)	Morbidity (%)	Length of Stay (days)	Follow-up (months)	Success Rate (%)
Awad et al.[1]	37	240	13.5	—	4	26.5	65
Curet et al.[6]	27	250	3.7	65.3	3.7	22	96
DePaula et al.[30]	19	210	5.2	15.8 intraop 15.8 postop	3.1	13	84.3
Dutta[31]	28	55.4	7.1	0	3	25.1	96.2
Floch et al.[32]	46	210	19.6	40.5	2.3	17.2	89
Granderath et al.[33]	51	L-80 O-245	0	11		12	96
Heniford et al.[25]	45	L 234 O 261	17.8	12.7	4.6	21.3	92.5
Horgan et al.[34]	31	307	9.7	32.3	4.1	25	87
Hunter et al.[15]	75	199	13.3	5	2.6	—	87
Kamolz et al.[35]	11	L 80 O 200	9.0	—	11	26	91
Khaitan et al.[36]	16	—	56.3	—	5.3	32.6	75
O'Reilly et al.[37]	8	—	25	50	2.2	12–42	100
Pointner et al.[38]	30	L 135 O 315	6.7	25	8	29	93
Serafini et al.[39]	28	L-184 O-216	10.7	16.2 intraop 37.8 postop	5	20	89
Soper and Dunnegan[26]	8		25.0	—			
Szwerc et al.[40]	15	135	0	—	2.3	3	87
Watson and Krukowski[41]	11	141	9.0	20	3	29	91
Watson et al.[42]	27	L-80 O-105	22.2	0	3	12	92.5
Yau[43]	28	73.4	32.1	—	4	24	

L = previous laparoscopic operation.
O = previous open operation.

Collis gastroplasty and anterior fundoplication (12%) with 15% not reported. Operative times were significantly longer in the patients who had undergone previous open surgery than those who had undergone previous laparoscopic surgery. Average length of stay for all studies except the Austrian group (government-mandated longer length of stay) was 4.4 days, which is shorter than reported in most open reoperative literature. Mean follow-up was 21.6 months with an average success rate of 90%. Success rates in most studies were based on patient satisfaction and not on scientific data. The relatively short average follow-up in most studies, although definitely a shortcoming, was not considered a problem because most recurrences occur in the first year. Complication rates were not consistently reported but ranged from 10 to 65% (Table 11.1). Previous open surgery was associated with a significantly higher complication rate than previous laparoscopic surgery. Common complications included

pneumothorax, enterotomy, postoperative leak, dysphagia, and gas bloating. There were no operative mortalities reported in any of these studies. From these data, we conclude that laparoscopic refundoplication, especially in patients with previous laparoscopic repair, is associated with minimal morbidity, no mortality, a decreased length of hospital stay, and improved patient satisfaction compared with both open and thoracic reoperative surgery. Most authors agree that in the hands of an experienced laparoscopic surgeon, reoperative laparoscopy for failed fundoplication is safe and effective.

Comparison of Open Versus Laparoscopic Refundoplication

Hunter et al.[15] reviewed 100 patients undergoing reoperative fundoplication. Seventy-five of these operations were initiated laparoscopically, with 6 being converted to open (8%). Patients were offered laparoscopic revision only if they had undergone a single previous laparoscopic fundoplication initially. As the authors gained experience, they offered a laparoscopic approach to previous laparotomy patients. Their operative times were reported as 210 minutes, 203 minutes, and 183 minutes for the first, second, and last 25 patients in the laparoscopic group. The median operative time for open laparotomy was 211 minutes. The length of stay was significantly shorter in the laparoscopic group (2.6 days vs 7.5 days). Complication rates were also lower in the laparoscopic group (5% vs 9%). The only mortality was a patient who underwent laparotomy who succumbed to pneumonia postoperatively. Although this was not a randomized, controlled trial comparing open versus laparoscopy, it is the most comprehensive study to date comparing the two types of experiences.

Laparoscopic Gastric Bypass for Recurrent Reflux

Several studies mention the use of gastric bypass as an alternative and superior technique for morbidly obese patients who present with primary GE reflux disease.[44,45] Perez et al.[46] identified a higher rate of recurrent reflux in obese patients undergoing laparoscopic Nissen fundoplication compared with their normal-weight cohorts. Applying this theory to patients with recurrent symptoms, Heniford et al.[25] described using the Roux-en-Y gastric bypass in obese patients with recurrent reflux symptoms after failed anti-reflux surgery. Patients should meet the National Institutes of Health 1991 Consensus criteria of a body mass index (BMI) >40 or >35 when associated with significant comorbidities. They must have also tried and failed multiple diets. If the recurrent reflux patient meets these criteria, a gastric bypass should be offered rather than simply revising the previous fundoplication.

Laparoscopic gastric bypass is performed with the patient in a split-legged position. Preoperative DVT prophylaxis and antibiotics are given and a Foley catheter is placed. Five ports are placed as seen in Figure 11.8. The original wrap is taken down completely. Once this is

accomplished, a 15- to 30-cc pouch is created based on the lesser gastric curve. This can be performed with an EEA anvil, by visualization, or by using a 36-French orogastric tube. Next, the jejunum is divided approximately 20–30 cm from the ligament of Trietz. A 75- to 150-cm Roux limb is measured and a jejunojejunostomy is created with the EndoGIA stapler. Some surgeons base the Roux limb lengths on preoperative BMI with BMI >50 necessitating a 150-cm Roux limb and a BMI <50 receiving a 100-cm Roux limb. Other surgeons use the same Roux limb length in every case. The Roux limb is passed antecolic or retrocolic. If an antecolic route is used, the omentum must be divided to ensure a tension-free anastomosis. If the limb is positioned retrocolic, the mesenteric defect is closed with running, nonabsorbable suture to prevent internal herniation through the mesocolic window.

The gastrojejunostomy can be created using the circular stapler, the linear stapler, or a hand-sewn technique. The final anatomy is detailed in Figure 11.9. An intraoperative leak test is performed with either air or methylene blue dye. Because leaks are more prevalent in reoperative surgery, placement of a drain is recommended.

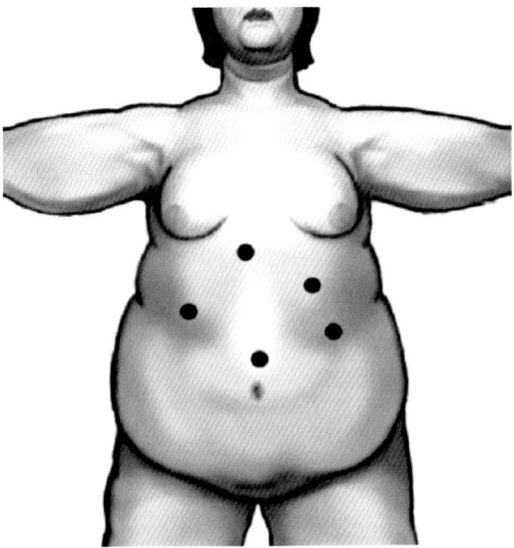

Figure 11.8. Port placement for Roux-en-Y gastric bypass for patients with morbid obesity and recurrent gastroesophageal reflux disease. Courtesy of Ethicon Endo-Surgery, Inc., a Johnson & Johnson company. All rights reserved.

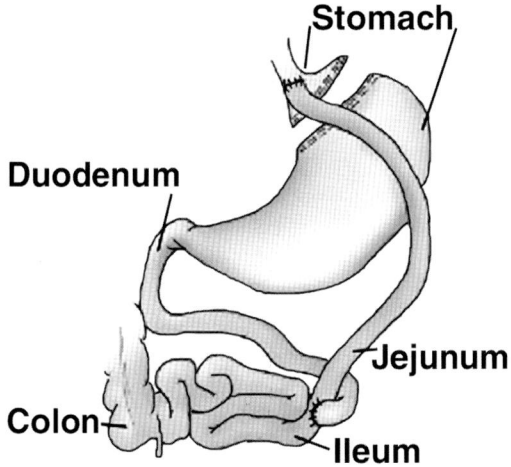

Figure 11.9. Roux-en-Y gastric bypass for patients with morbid obesity and gastroesophageal reflux disease. Courtesy of Ethicon Endo-Surgery, Inc., a Johnson & Johnson company. All rights reserved.

The report by Heniford et al.[29] of 55 patients undergoing reoperative anti-reflux surgery included two patients who met the National Institutes of Health criteria for morbid obesity and subsequently underwent gastric bypass. They both reported good resolution of symptoms. As of 2004 there were no other published reports describing gastric bypass for revisional anti-reflux surgery.

Thoracotomy

Several approaches to a failed fundoplication can be applied through a thoracotomy including a redo Nissen fundoplication and a Belsey Mark IV. Many authors believe that if the original operation was performed transabdominally, a transthoracic approach should be utilized in reoperations. Others believe that only thoracic surgeons should perform thoracic surgery and general surgeons will feel more comfortable, and will have better results, with a laparotomy even in redo operations. Currently, transthoracic Belsey Mark IV can be useful in patients who have had multiple abdominal procedures, and may be considered as an alternative to transabdominal approaches for surgeons who are well trained in thoracic procedures.[13,47,48] Deschamps et al.[48] reported their experience with 185 patients who had recurrent reflux after

previous fundoplication. They performed a thoracotomy in 133 of these patients and a Belsey Mark IV in 47 (25%). Their median follow-up was 31 months (range, 3–283 months). Complications occurred in (25%) of patients. Mean length of stay was 9 days (range, 5–58 days). Excellent or good results were reported in only 60.2%. Migliore et al.[49] found that 12.5% of patients undergoing thoracotomy reported poor results. They advise patients that laparoscopy provides better cosmetic results, has comparable results to open surgery, has less incisional pain, and offers a quicker return to normal life. The authors believe the indications for thoracotomy should be limited to reoperative fundoplication in patients that have concurrent esophageal pathology or extensive intraabdominal adhesions. Many thoracic surgeons have adopted laparoscopic fundoplication into their repertoire with good to excellent results.[50]

Operative technique. The patient should have cardiac and pulmonary clearance before surgery. Once in the operating room, DVT prophylaxis and perioperative antibiotics are given. A thoracic epidural is placed for postoperative pain management. The patient is intubated with a double lumen tube to allow left lung collapse during the procedure. The patient is then placed in the semilateral position to allow for a thoracoabdominal incision, if needed. A left thoracotomy is performed in the 7th or 8th intercostal space and the left lung is excluded. The pulmonary ligament is divided and the esophagus is mobilized to the level of the aortic arch. The esophagus is encircled with a Penrose drain above the level of the inferior pulmonary vein. The middle esophageal artery is divided. The vagus nerves are identified and spared. The hiatal adhesions are lysed and the hernia sac, if present, is excised. Both crura are clearly defined and the previous fundoplication is taken down. The esophagogastric junction is identified and if it cannot be positioned intraabdominally without tension, a Collis gastroplasty is performed with a GIA stapler. Nonabsorbable crural stitches are placed but are not tied. A 56- to 60-French bougie is placed and either a Nissen (360°) or Belsey Mark IV (270°) wrap is performed based on preoperative manometric studies. The crural stitches are tied after the wrap has been completed. Pledgets or mesh can be used to buttress the crural closure. Pleural drainage tubes are placed and the thoracotomy is closed.[49,51]

Postoperative Management

Regardless of the operative approach, postoperatively, the patient is kept NPO overnight and an upper GI study is performed the next morning to evaluate the anatomy and to assess for leak. Once cleared, the patient is started on a clear liquid diet and advanced to full liquids. Over the next couple of weeks, they are advanced to pureed and soft food. Early dysphagia is common after anti-reflux surgery and can be managed conservatively with dietary modifications. Patients should avoid meat and bread initially. Most patients are discharged within 1 week, depending on the operative approach. As previously stated, laparoscopic technique allows for shorter hospital stays. One of the early postoperative factors that should be meticulously controlled whether in primary or reoperative anti-reflux surgery is retching.[1,15] Soper and Dunnegan[26] found that one-third of patients with early retching developed anatomic defects that required future intervention.[30] The use of perioperative ondansetron can aid tremendously in controlling retching within the first week of surgery.

Summary

Several technical points are important regardless of the method of access used for reoperative fundoplication. Meticulous adhesiolysis is essential in preventing inadvertent gastrotomies, esophagotomies, or enterotomies. If a perforation is identified, it is best to repair it primarily. If a laparoscopic approach is being used, laparoscopic repair of an enterotomy is acceptable unless visualization is poor or the repair appears inadequate. The fundoplication is used to buttress the gastrotomy. Adequate esophageal mobilization is essential to ensure the GE junction remains in the abdomen. A floppy wrap should be created by taking down the short gastric vessels, if not previously performed. It may be necessary to dissect the fundus off the spleen if the short gastric vessels have been previously divided. The crura are always closed with nonabsorbable suture. If they do not reapproximate easily, one may consider the use of mesh. It is imperative to identify the cause of failure and tailor the revision to the patient. Finally, laparoscopic reoperative surgery for previous failed anti-reflux procedures is technically feasible with minimal morbidity and mortality and excellent to good results. Reported conversion rates, even in the hands of laparoscopic specialists, are about 17%.[1,13,14,20,24,25,29,30,33,39–45] This approach should be used only by experienced laparoscopic surgeons, because reoperative laparoscopic surgery is significantly more difficult with higher conversion rates and higher morbidity than primary laparoscopic fundoplication.

References

1. Awad ZT, Anderson PI, Sato K, Roth TA, Gerhardt J, Filipi CJ. Laparoscopic reoperative anti-reflux surgery. Surg Endosc 2001;15:1401–1407.
2. Hunter JG. Approach and management of patients with recurrent gastroesophageal reflux disease. J Gastrointest Surg 2001;5(5):451–457.
3. Hinder RA, Klingler PJ, Perdikis G, Smith SL. Management of the failed anti-reflux operation. Surg Clin North Am 1997;77(5):1083–1098.
4. Jamieson GG. The results of anti-reflux and re-operative anti-reflux surgery. Gullet 1993;3:41–45.
5. Siewert JR, Isolauri J, Feussner H. Reoperation following failed fundoplication. World J Surg 1989;13(6):791–796; discussion 796–797.
6. Curet MJ, Josloff RK, Schoeb O, Zucker KA. Laparoscopic reoperation for failed anti-reflux procedures. Arch Surg 1999;134:559–563.
7. Johnsson E, Lundell L. Repeat anti-reflux surgery; effectiveness of a Toupet partial posterior fundoplication. Eur J Surg 2002;168(8–9):441–445.
8. Little AG, Ferguson MK, Skinner DB. Reoperation for failed anti-reflux operations. J Thorac Cardiovasc Surg 1986;91:511–517.
9. Luostarinen ME, Isolauri JO, Koskinen MO, Laitinen JO, Matikainen MJ, Lindholm TS. Refundoplication for recurrent gastroesophageal reflux. World J Surg 1993; 17(5):587–593; discussion 594.
10. Alexiou C, Beggs D, Salama FD, Beggs L, Knowles KR. A tailored surgical approach for gastro-oesophageal reflux disease: the Nottingham experience. Eur J Cardiothorac Surg 2000;17:389–395.
11. Siewert JR, Stein HJ, Feussner H. Reoperations after failed anti-reflux procedures. Ann Chir Gynaecol 1995; 84(2):122–128. Review.
12. Finley RJ. Reoperative anti-reflux surgery. Chest Surg Clin N Am 2001;11(3):583–587, vii.
13. Skinner DB. Surgical management after failed anti-reflux operations. World J Surg 1992;16(2):359–363.
14. Braghetto I, Csendes A, Burdiles P, Botero F, Kom O. Results of surgical treatment for recurrent postoperative gastroesophageal reflux. Dis Esoph 2002;15(4):315–322.

15. Hunter JG, Smith CD, Branum GD, Waring JP, Trus TL, Cornwell M, Galloway K. Laparoscopic fundoplication failures: patterns of failure and response to fundoplication revision. Ann Surg 1999;230(4):595–604; discussion 604–606.

16. Farrell TM, Archer SB, Galloway KD, Branum GD, Smith CD, Hunter JG. Heartburn is more likely to recur after Toupet fundoplication than Nissen fundoplication. Am Surg 2000;66:229–236.

17. Fernando HC, Luketich JD, Christie NA, Ikramuddin S, Schauer PR. Outcomes of laparoscopic Toupet compared to laparoscopic Nissen fundoplication. Surg Endosc 2002;16(6):905–908.

18. Rieger NA, Jamieson GG, Britten-Jones R, Tew S. Reoperation after failed anti-reflux surgery. Br J Surg 1994; 81(8):1159–1161.

19. Granderath FA, Kamolz T, Schweiger UM, Pointner R. Laparoscopic refundoplication with prosthetic hiatal closure for recurrent hiatal hernia after primary failed anti-reflux surgery. Arch Surg 2003;138(8):902–907.

20. Granderath FA, Schweiger UM, Kamolz T, Pasiut M, Haas CF, Pointner R. Laparoscopic anti-reflux surgery with routine mesh-hiatoplasty in the treatment of gastroesophageal reflux disease. J Gastrointest Surg 2002;6(3):347–353.

21. Kamolz T, Granderath FA, Bammer T, Pasiut M, Pointner R. Dysphagia and quality of life after laparoscopic Nissen fundoplication in patients with and without prosthetic reinforcement of the hiatal crura. Surg Endosc 2002;16(4):572–577. Epub 2002 Jan 09.

22. Frantzides CT, Carlson MA. Prosthetic reinforcement of posterior cruroplasty during laparoscopic hiatal herniorrhaphy. Surg Endosc 1997;11:769–771.

23. Carlson MA, Richards CG, Frantzides CT. Laparoscopic prosthetic reinforcement of hiatal herniorrhaphy. Dig Surg 1999;16.407–410.

24. Granderath FA, Kamolz T, Schweiger UM, Pasiut M, Haas CF, Wykypiel H, Pointner R. Is laparoscopic refundoplication feasible in patients with failed primary open anti-reflux surgery? Surg Endosc 2002;16(3):381–385.

25. Heniford BT, Matthews BD, Kercher KW, Pollinger H, Sing RF. Surgical experience in fifty-five consecutive reoperative fundoplications. Am Surg 2002;68(11):949–954; discussion 954.

26. Soper NJ, Dunnegan D. Anatomic fundoplication failure after laparoscopic anti-reflux surgery. Ann Surg 1999; 229(5):669–676; discussion 676–677.

27. Dallemagne B, Weerts JM, Jehaes C, Markiewicz S. Causes of failures of laparoscopic anti-reflux operations. Surg Endosc 1996;10:305–310.

28. Frantzides CT, Carlson MA. Laparoscopic redo Nissen fundoplication. J Laparoendosc Adv Surg Tech A 1997; 7(4):235–239.

29. Granderath FA, Kamolz T, Schweiger UM, Pasiut M, Haas CF, Wykypiel H, Pointner R. Long-term results of laparoscopic anti-reflux surgery: Surgical outcome and analysis of failure after 500 laparoscopic anti-reflux procedures. Surg Endosc 2002;16:753–757.

30. DePaula AL, Hashiba K, Bafutto M, Machado CA. Laparoscopic reoperations after failed and complicated anti-reflux operations. Surg Endosc 1995;9:681–686.

31. Dutta S, Bamehriz F, Boghossian T, Pottruff CG, Anvari M. Outcome of laparoscopic redo fundoplication. Surg Endosc 2004;18:440–443.

32. Floch NR, Hinder RA, Klingler PJ, Branton SA, Seelig MH, Bammer T, Filipi CJ. Is laparoscopic reoperation for failed anti-reflux surgery feasible? Arch Surg 1999; 134(7):733–737.

33. Granderath FA, Kamolz T, Schweiger UM, Pointner R. Failed anti-reflux surgery: Quality of life and surgical outcome after laparoscopic refundoplication. Int J Colorectal Dis 2003;18(3):248–253.

34. Horgan S, Pohl D, Bogetti D, Eubanks T, Pellegrini C. Failed anti-reflux surgery: what have we learned from reoperations? Arch Surg 1999;134(8):809–817.

35. Kamolz T, Granderath FA, Bammer T, Pasiut M, Pointner R. Failed anti-reflux surgery: surgical outcome of laparoscopic refundoplication in the elderly. Hepatogastroenterology 2002;49(45):865–868.

36. Khaitan L, Bhatt P, Richards W, Houston H, Sharp K, Holzman M. Comparison of patient satisfaction after redo and primary fundoplications. Surg Endosc 2003.

37. O'Reilly MJ, Mullins S, Reddick EJ. Laparoscopic management of failed anti-reflux surgery. Surg Laparosc Endosc 1997;7(2):90–93.

38. Pointner R, Bammer T, Then P, Kamolz T. Laparoscopic refundoplications after failed anti-reflux surgery. Am J Surg 1999;178(6):541–544.

39. Serafini FM, Bloomston M, Zervos E, Muench J, Albrink MH, Murr M, Rosemurgy AS. Laparoscopic revision of failed anti-reflux operations. J Surg Res 2001;95(1):13–18.

40. Szwerc MF, Wiechmann RJ, Maley RH, Santucci TS, Macherey RS, Landreneau RJ. Reoperative laparoscopic anti-reflux surgery. Surgery 1999;126(4):723–728; discussion 728–729.

41. Watson AJM, Krukowski ZH. Revisional surgery after failed laparoscopic anterior fundoplication. Surg Endosc 2002;16:392–394.

42. Watson DI, Jamieson GG, Game PA, Williams RS, Devitt PG. Laparoscopic reoperation following failed anti-reflux surgery. Br J Surg 1999;86(1):98–101.

43. Yau P, Watson DI, Devitt PG, Game PA, Jamieson GG. Early reoperation following laparoscopic anti-reflux surgery. Am J Surg 2000;179(3):172–176.

44. Patterson EJ, Davis DG, Khajanchee Y, Swanstrom LL. Comparison of objective outcomes following laparoscopic Nissen fundoplication vs laparoscopic gastric bypass in the morbidly obese with heartburn. Surg Endosc 2003;17:1561–1565.

45. Smith SC, Edwards CB, Goodman GN. Symptomatic and clinical improvement in morbidly obese patients with gastroesophageal reflux disease following Roux-en-Y gastric bypass. Obes Surg 1997;7:479–484.

46. Perez AR, Moncure AC, Rattner DW. Obesity adversely affects the outcome of anti-reflux operations. Surg Endosc 2001;15(9):986–989. Epub 2001 Jun 12.

47. Bais JE, Horbach TL, Masclee AA, Smout AJ, Terpstra JL, Gooszen HG. Surgical treatment for recurrent gastro-oesophageal reflux disease after failed anti-reflux surgery. Br J Surg 2000;87:243–249.

48. Deschamps C, Trastek VF, Allen MS, Pairolero PC, Johnson JO, Larson DR. Long-term results after reoperation for failed anti-reflux procedures. J Thorac Cardiovasc Surg 1997;113:545–550.

49. Migliore M, Arcerito M, Vagliasindi A, Puleo R, Basile F, Deodato G. The place of Belsey Mark IV fundoplication in the era of laparoscopic surgery. Eur J Cardiothorac Surg 2003;24(4):625–630.

50. Naunheim KS, Landreneau RJ, Andrus CH, Ferson PF, Zachary PE, Keenan RJ. Laparoscopic fundoplication: a natural extension for the thoracic surgeon. Ann Thorac Surg 1996;61(4):1062–1065.

51. Legare JF, Henteleff HJ, Casson AG. Results of Collis gastroplasty and selective fundoplication, using a left thoracoabdominal approach, for failed anti-reflux surgery. Eur J Cardiothorac Surg 2002;21(3): 534–540.

12

Management of Alkaline Reflux

Jose M. Clavero, Philippe Topart, and Claude Deschamps

Gastroesophageal reflux disease (GERD) is the most common disorder of the upper gastrointestinal tract and can lead to complications such as esophagitis, stricture, ulcerations, and Barrett's esophagus. About one-quarter of patients develop complications despite adequate medical treatment. A mechanically defective lower esophageal sphincter (LES), inefficient esophageal clearance, and abnormalities that decrease gastric emptying or increase intragastric pressure have been described as the main causes for increased exposure of the esophageal mucosa to refluxed gastric juices.[1] Duodenogastroesophageal reflux (DGER) is the regurgitation of duodenal contents into the stomach and esophagus.[2] It is a condition intimately associated with GERD, but can also occur after previous surgical procedures such as pyloroplasty and partial or total gastrectomy.

Pathogenesis

The composition of the refluxed juice has an important role in the genesis of mucosal damage and the progression from pure GERD to complications in the more severe forms of the disease (esophagitis, stricture, and Barrett's esophagus). Acid and pepsin have been recognized for a long time as the main agents involved in the mucosal damage of esophageal mucosa.[2] Over recent years, several studies have demonstrated that biliary and pancreatic secretions are as noxious to the esophageal mucosa

as acid-peptic secretions and that biliopancreatic secretions potentiate the damage produced to the esophageal mucosa by acid-gastric reflux.[3–9] Others have shown that conjugated bile salts remain soluble at low pH and cause esophageal mucosal damage in the presence of acid.[6,10,11] Trypsin is also believed to have a role in damaging esophageal mucosa, particularly in postgastrectomy patients.[9,12–14]

In patients with GERD, esophagitis, strictures, and Barrett's esophagus are more prevalent when there is an increased exposure to either acid or alkaline secretions.[15,16] These complications are more frequent in patients with combined acid and alkaline secretions than in patients with acid reflux only. In a study by Stein et al.,[17] 86% of patients with acid and alkaline reflux had esophagitis, stricture, or Barrett's esophagus compared with 51% of patients with only acid reflux. Simultaneous esophageal exposure to acid and duodenal reflux was found to be the most common pattern in a study by Vaezi and Richter,[18] occurring in 76% of patients with symptomatic GERD. Other studies have shown that combined acid and alkaline reflux correlates with an increase in complications.[13,18–21]

The greater number of complications related to this mixed refluxate has been attributed to the detergent effect of bile acids in an acidic environment. At low pH values, the ionized forms of conjugated bile acids that enter through the lipophilic membrane of mucosal epithelium predominate and accumulate in the intracellular space. The high intracellular concentration of bile salts can cause dissolution of cell membranes and tight junctions. The damage is likely to be accentuated by the noxious effect of acid and pepsin on membrane cells.[2,6,10,22]

Reflux of duodenal content into the stomach is most often asymptomatic.[23] Duodenogastric reflux has been shown to occur most often at night and after meals. A dysfunctional LES usually has an important role in patients with DGER, a factor that is critical in the surgical treatment of this problem.[2,13]

Stein et al.[17] used gastric and esophageal probes and documented duodenogastric reflux in 21% of patients with foregut symptoms without GERD and in 29% of GERD patients, but in none of the normal volunteers. Esophageal exposure to alkaline content was significantly higher in patients with GERD and duodenogastric reflux. Therefore, it seems that duodenogastric reflux is rare in normal people but increases in incidence in patients with acid reflux.[24]

Pure biliary-pancreatic esophagitis is almost exclusively iatrogenic, and is seen mainly in patients with defective LES with an achlorhydric stomach because of previous vagotomy and pyloroplasty, gastroenterostomy, or antrectomy with Billroth I or II reconstruction. Other patients at risk are those with a prior total gastrectomy, and those with an esophagogastrectomy with loss of sphincter, parietal cell mass, and vagus nerves.[20,23,25] Stein et al.[17] reported that 30 of 58 patients with duodenogastric reflux had previous foregut surgery.

Primary duodenogastric reflux is rare and might represent a global foregut motility disorder with gastric emptying problems and bile vomiting as its key features.[20] Manometric studies by Mason and DeMeester[23] in bile-vomiting patients demonstrated a dynamically defective LES that exhibited normal pressures when fasting. With gastric distension and accumulation of duodenogastric refluxate, gastric motility was inhibited by several intestinal hormones, including cholecystokinin, neurotensin, and peptide YY, which could increase alkaline esophageal reflux.[23]

The role of pure DGER in the absence of concomitant acid reflux in the damage of the esophageal mucosa is unclear. In 13 partial gastrectomy patients with reflux symptoms studied by Sears et al.,[26] 77% had DGER diagnosed by the Bilitec® probe but endoscopic esophagitis was present only in those with concomitant acid reflux. Vaezi and Richter[27] found that in partial gastrectomy patients, 24% of the upper gastrointestinal symptoms were caused by DGER without acid reflux. These results suggest that DGER could cause symptoms but in the absence of acid reflux does not produce esophagitis.

Diagnosis

Symptoms suggestive of alkaline reflux are epigastric pain, nausea, vomiting, and loss of appetite. Esophagitis caused by alkaline reflux should also be suspected in patients with obvious endoscopic esophagitis and normal 24-hour pH monitoring. The diagnosis of alkaline reflux can be made by endoscopy, 99Tc HIDA biliary scan, detection of bile acids by gastric aspiration, 24-hour pH monitoring, and bilirubin concentration measurement.[1,12,13,17,28-48] The available tests for the diagnosis of DGER are summarized in Table 12.1.

Endoscopy

The presence of bile in the stomach or esophagus is not accurate in the diagnosis of DGER. Stein et al.[29] found a sensitivity of 37%, a specificity of 70%, and positive predictive value of only 55%.

Scintigraphy

Duodenogastroesophageal reflux can also be documented by observing excessive presence of radioactivity in the esophagus after 99Tc HIDA biliary scan.[36,37] However, it is at best a semiquantitative and expensive test and is less physiologic and accurate than the more recent methods for the diagnosis of DGER. Also, several technical problems can interfere with the accuracy of the study.[30,38]

Aspiration Studies

Aspiration techniques that allow detection of duodenal contents using enzymatic or chromatographic measurements have been used for the diagnosis of DGER. In some early gastric aspiration studies, the concentration of fasting gastric bile salts was not found to be particu-

Table 12.1. Available tests for the diagnosis of duodenogastroesophageal reflux (DGER).

Method	Advantages	Disadvantages
Endoscopy	Easily available; allows mucosal biopsies	Poor sensitivity and specificity
Aspiration studies	Lower cost than endoscopy	Require enzymatic or chromatographic measurements; results difficult to interpret
Scintigraphy	Noninvasive	Semiquantitative; more expensive; radiation exposure; less physiologic; technically difficult
24-hour pH monitoring	Widespread use; familiar test to most centers; ambulatory prolonged monitoring in more physiologic conditions	pH > 4 is not a reliable indicator of DGER; concomitant use of gastric probe can increase its sensibility and specificity
24-hour bilirubin spectrophotometric measurement	Ambulatory prolonged monitoring in more physiologic conditions; can be use concomitantly with 24-hour pH monitoring	Not in widespread use; requires diet modification; bilirubin detection is underestimated in acidic environment in about 30%; fair to poor correlation with bile salts, pancreatic enzymes, and lysolecithin concentrations

larly helpful.[39,40] More recent studies, however, have shown that fasting gastric bile acid concentrations are increased in patients with GERD, being highest in patients with Barrett's esophagus.[28,33,34] The main limitation of these studies is that they assume that gastric bile acids are an indicator of esophageal exposure to these agents. Esophageal aspiration studies have also been performed to evaluate more precisely the role of duodenal content in the genesis of damage to the esophageal mucosa, but results have been conflicting because of various technical problems.[12,13,31,32,40,41]

Stein and coworkers[13] used a device that allows ambulatory aspiration of esophageal content in normal volunteers and patients with GERD and correlated the results with 24-hour pH monitoring. They found that the total bile acid concentration was higher in patients with GERD compared with controls. The total bile acids concentration showed a significant correlation with the time that the pH was >7. Patients with Barrett's esophagus or strictures had markedly increased bile acid concentration in the refluxed gastric juice and this correlated with the time pH was >7.[13]

Twenty-four-hour pH Monitoring

The interpretation of the 24-hour gastric pH monitoring for determining gastroduodenal reflux is more complex than its use for acid reflux diagnosis because of the interaction between mucous and acid secretions, ingested food, saliva, and duodenal, pancreatic, and biliary secretions.[42] The score proposed by Fuchs et al.[43] allows the quantification of duodenogastric reflux and gastric acid secretion and could be helpful in the assessment of DGER and gastric emptying disorders. The scoring had a sensitivity of 90% and a specificity of 100%. Alkaline reflux is confirmed by measurement of the time during which the esophageal pH is >7, but several considerations must be taken into account. Electrodes made of glass instead of antimony should be used, and extreme caution is exerted with the calibration method. The patient's diet should be restricted to food at a pH < 7, the patient should be examined for dental caries that can raise the salivary pH, and strictures should be dilated to prevent pooling of saliva.[13,17,37,43,44] The placement of a second probe in the stomach may be helpful in differentiating acid reflux, mixed, and alkaline reflux.[1] Mattioli et al.[24] used simultaneous esophageal, fundus, and antrum probes to demonstrate that 18% of patients with abnormal alkaline reflux could be considered normal based solely on standard 24-hour pH monitoring.[24] However, some authors have found a poor correlation between DGER and measured length of time of esophageal pH < 7, possibly because of increased saliva production or bicarbonate production by esophageal mucosal glands.[28,45,46]

Bilirubin Monitoring

Recently, a system designed to allow ambulatory monitoring of DGER has been developed (Bilitec®; Medtronic, Shoreview, MN). The system uses bilirubin as a marker of duodenal reflux and can be used concomitantly with 24-hour pH monitoring.[34] Continuous spectrophotometric measurement of luminal bilirubin concentration is made with a portable optoelectronic data logger and a fiberoptic probe passed transnasally and positioned in the foregut. The Teflon probe head has a 2-mm open groove across which two wavelengths of light are emitted and material is sampled. The light-emitting diodes have wavelengths of 470 and 565 nm, allowing the measurement of bilirubin and a reference signal. The photodiode system converts the light in an electrical signal through filtration and amplification, and a difference of the absorbance between the two wavelengths is calculated. This value is directly proportional to the bilirubin concentration. The system samples luminal concentration of bilirubin every 8 seconds. The continuously recorded data are downloaded into a computer and analyzed. A threshold of 0.14 absorbance units has been demonstrated by various authors as having a good correlation with the measurements of increased bile acid concentrations in gastric aspirates, and are considered diagnostic of DGER. Values <0.14 can be caused by the effect of suspended gastric particles or mucus. Other authors have used a threshold of 0.2 based on their studies in healthy volunteers. An increased esophageal exposure to bilirubin is identified when the percentage exposure time to bilirubin exceeds the 95 percentile level of the values obtained in normal subjects.[28,33–35,47,48]

It has been suggested that the amount of DGER determined by the Bilitec® probe can be underestimated when it is associated with acid reflux. Despite the high precision of this probe, the bilirubin measurement does not necessarily correlate with the amount of bile salts, pancreatic enzymes, and lysolecithin present in the esophageal refluxate.[47,49] It should also be noted that there is no standardization of the recommended diet while using the Bilitec®. Theoretically, a solid diet could interfere with the bilirubin measurement and the food could plug the tip of the probe. Therefore, most authors recommend a liquid diet. Some beverages such as coffee, tea, and cola should also be excluded because they have an absorbance close to that of bilirubin.[28,33,34,35] However, a liquid diet is less physiologic and could potentially interfere with the results of the 24-hour pH measurements obtained simultaneously with the continuous bilirubin determination. Even with these limitations, the spectrophotometric detection of bilirubin is the best method currently available for the diagnosis and measurement of DGER.

Treatment

Long-term medical treatment for true DGER (prokinetics, proton pump inhibitors, erythromycin, etc.) is notably ineffective and the condition usually requires surgical treatment. Topart and Vandenbroucke[20] have described the techniques thoroughly.

Bile Diversion Operations

Operations are designed to divert the duodenal content away from the stomach and, hence, from the esophagus. The total duodenal diversion (TDD) as based on the principles of Cesar Roux is the first and still the most popular operation used when the reflux occurs after gastric resection. Other operations that were subsequently developed include the Tanner 19 Roux-en-Y operation, the Braun enteroenterostomy, and the Henley anisoperistaltic jejunal interposition. In 1985, after an experimental study, DeMeester et al.[50] proposed a new physiologic approach to the problem of DGER with the duodenal switch procedure. More recently, Madura and Grosfeld[51] advocated the use of simple biliary diversion. Overall, these procedures are used only in a fraction of the patients showing severe DGER.

Total Duodenal Diversion

The technique that is most often used currently was described by Holt and Large[52] (Figure 12.1). The standard operation is performed through an abdominal incision. When the diversion is performed in patients who have not undergone a previous gastrectomy, it includes resection of

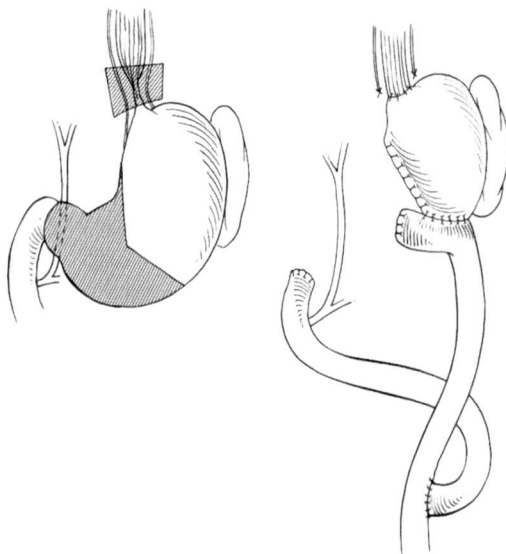

Figure 12.1. On the left is illustrated truncal vagotomy, gastric antrectomy, and when necessary, segmental esophageal resection for a nondilatable stricture. On the right, reconstruction is shown using the 45-cm-long Roux-en-Y gastric drainage procedure to divert biliary and pancreatic secretions away from the stomach. (Reprinted from Payne.[25] Used with permission of Mayo Foundation.)

the mobile part of the duodenum, an antrectomy (gastric division following a vertical line extending from the angle of the lesser curvature), and a bilateral truncal vagotomy. The digestive tract continuity is restored using an end-to-side gastrojejunostomy on a 45- to 60-cm Roux-en-Y jejunal limb. Some authors suggest closure of the diaphragmatic crura with an anti-reflux fundoplication. This may be seen as a therapeutic overkill when acid and bile exposure have been eliminated. Most authors agree on the necessity to perform a bilateral truncal vagotomy, as antrectomy and duodenal diversion is considered as an ulcerogenic operation. This is evidenced by frequently documented postoperative stomal ulcers as complications of TDD.[53]

Total duodenal diversion is considered a safe operation. No mortality is reported when TDD is used for severe esophagitis lesions. Postoperative morbidity ranges from 9 to 27%. The higher complication rate was seen when resection of an esophageal stricture was added. In general, TDD is very effective in controlling the reflux symptoms and healing related esophagitis. Most of the strictures are under control early after the operation or at the most within a year postoperatively, after 1–3 dilation sessions. Only 5% of all patients require resection of their esophageal strictures. Fekete et al.[54] reported partial regression of Barrett's mucosa in 20% of their patients. Most authors, however, report no change of Barrett's metaplasia in the esophagus after TDD.

The results of TDD are frequently expressed in general terms, looking mostly at the overall functional results. After a few years of enthusiastic use of TDD, several reports emphasized the side effects and the postoperative complaints of the operation, namely, postprandial epigastric fullness, dumping, weight loss, or bile vomiting. These symptoms were very similar to the duodenogastric reflux symptom complex that led to surgery. The postoperative assessment criteria used in these patients is mostly subjective, with the terminology of excellent, good, fair, or poor, which roughly encompasses the Visick grading system. This enables a relatively accurate comparison between the reported series. Ellis and Gibb[55] observed significant improvement in 73–100% (mean 90%) of 14 patients in a series of TDD reported between 1955 and 1992. This represents a total of 293 patients treated for DGER. More recently, there have been reports of good to excellent results in 76–97% of patients.[56–58]

When the same operation is used to treat biliopancreatic gastritis, the results are less encouraging. Madura[59] found that only 54% of 527 patients treated in such manner between 1980 and 1993 reported significant improvement. Hinder[60,61] opted for TDD in association with an anti-reflux procedure whenever possible. He reported that 15–50% of patients operated for duodenogastric reflux complain of significant postoperative symptoms early after a TDD. On longer-term follow-up, 15–20% of patients continue to experience the same symptoms. The discrepancy in the results comparing biliopancreatic reflux esophagitis and biliopancreatic gastritis without esophagitis remains unexplained because the basic pathophysiology is considered to be the same.

The length of the Roux-en-Y limb between the gastrojejunal anastomosis and the jejunojejunal anastomosis has been a matter of controversy. Most authors consider that a 45-cm limb is a minimum.[25] A 50- to 60-cm limb is usually preferred to minimize the risk of persistent or recurrent symptoms.

Why 15–20% of patients still have postoperative symptoms despite good to excellent endoscopic results is still a matter of debate and controversy. Total duodenal diversion is in itself a procedure that causes sufficient foregut modification to explain at least part of the postoperative problems of either dumping or poor gastric emptying. The bilateral truncal vagotomy and the partial gastrectomy are the most frequently suggested culprits in the literature. Denervating the stomach and the proximal foregut does create motility changes. Despite these well-documented effects, vagotomy is considered essential when an antrectomy and interruption of gastroduodenal continuity are the result of the operation.

Early in the assessment of this type of reconstruction, Welch et al.[62] documented in the laboratory the increase in gastric secretion of acid resulting from a Roux-en-Y diversion without antrectomy or vagotomy. If an antrectomy is added to the diversion without a vagotomy, postoperative stomal ulcers on the gastrojejunal anastomosis are almost inevitable. Gustavsson et al.[63] and Davidson and Hersh,[64] however, suggest that the gastric stasis seen after gastrectomy and Roux diversion is not significantly influenced by truncal vagotomy. Most of the time, when TDD is indicated, an antrectomy has already been done, usually with a gastrojejunal reconstruction (Billroth II). This operation has been the leading cause of bile reflux damage in the remaining stomach and in the esophagus.

The antrectomy is essential in order to gain good control of the gastric acid secretion in parallel to the control of the bile injury caused by the diversion. An inadequate gastric resection has been shown to be responsible for some of the worst postoperative gastric emptying problems. A limited antrectomy may result in a "dependent sump" causing early postoperative vomiting whereas the opposite, an extensive two-thirds gastrectomy, usually results in severe postoperative digestive discomfort. Vogel and Woodward[65] reported that revisional surgery for gastric atony after TDD resulted in clinical improvement and normalization of gastric emptying. In these patients, the size of the gastric remnant correlated with the amount of improvement.

The effects of truncal vagotomy on gastric motility may result in various patterns of gastric emptying. However, there was no significant difference in solid meal emptying when Billroth II gastrectomy was performed compared with TDD.[66] Furthermore, there may be no correlation between persistent postoperative symptoms and delayed gastric emptying. Gastric emptying problems are usually found to improve with time.

Duodenal Switch

The postoperative problems encountered after TDD prompted DeMeester et al.[50] in 1987 to propose a new operation to palliate these effects. Based on an experimental study, the "suprapapillary Roux en Y duodenojejunostomy," or "duodenal switch," sought to decrease the symptoms allegedly related to antrectomy, vagotomy, and bypass of the duodenal channel. It was destined more specifically to treat patients who had duodenogastric reflux without previous gastric resection. The intact pylorus and the proximal duodenum, divided above the ampulla, are connected end to end to the jejunum. The excluded duodenum is then reinserted in the digestive continuity by creating a jejuno-jejunal anastomosis 55 cm below the first anastomosis.

After the initial report from DeMeester et al. in 1987, Wilson et al.[67] presented their series of 42 patients operated for biliopancreatic gastritis. Two-thirds of the patients had GERD symptoms. Seventeen of the patients had a previous anti-reflux operation and 12 underwent a Nissen fundoplication at the time of their duodenal switch. For two patients with acid hypersecretion a selective vagotomy was added. The mean follow-up was 2.3 years and 33 of the 42 patients (78%) are reported as having good results. More recently, Klinger et al.[68] emphasized a good clinical outcome in 94% of their 32 patients. Dumping or vomiting as a manifestation of poor gastric emptying did not disappear completely after the suprapapillary duodenal diversion. In the 65 patients reported by Csendes et al.,[69] the entire group had a documented Barrett's esophagus. The duodenal diversion in these patients was in addition to an anti-reflux repair and a highly selective vagotomy. Ninety percent of the patients had a good clinical outcome (Visick I and II) with no reoperation during a mean follow-up of 28 months. Erosive esophagitis accompanying Barrett's esophagus disappeared in 90% of the patients in whom it was originally present. Although the operation did not modify the length of the metaplastic esophagus, the number of patients with mild dysplasia decreased from seven preoperatively to four after the operation. There was no postoperative death. Morbidity was identified in approximately 12% of patients.

Normalization of gastrointestinal hormone secretion and of the gastric emptying pattern is the recognized effect of the duodenal switch operation. The efficacy of the operation in eliminating bile reflux has been clearly documented by using Bilitec® measurements.

Biliary Diversion

This is the most recent operation designed to relieve of bile reflux into the stomach. Basically, the 45-cm Roux-en-Y limb used in this operation is diverting only the bile component through an end-to-side choledochojejunostomy. Digestive tract continuity is restored by an end-to-side jejunojejunostomy 45 cm distal from the ligament of Treitz. Cholecystectomy is added routinely and there is no gastric or vagotomy procedure.

The results of this operation are assessed in two distinct reports by Madura and Grosfeld.[51] The first is a series of 27 patients with bile gastritis, 24 of whom had already had various gastric operations such as Billroth I or II gastrectomies, Roux-en-Y procedure, and vagotomy. Twenty-two of the 26 long-term surviving patients achieved good to excellent results (84.6%) with complete relief of the burning pain, nausea, and bilious vomiting.[51]

In a prospective, nonrandomized observation by Madura,[59] the biliary diversion operation was compared with a classic Roux-en-Y duodenal diversion operation. Fourteen percent of the 16 patients in the biliary diversion group and 37.5% of the 21 patients in the duodenal diversion group had esophagitis. In contrast to the previous report, there was no significant previous surgical history except for a Nissen fundoplication in two patients of the TDD group and in three patients of the bile diversion group. Although the follow-up times were unclear and unequal for both groups, better results were

reported after the bile diversion operation (14 of 16 patients asymptomatic) when compared with the results of the TDD operation (2 of 21 patients asymptomatic). However, these good results did not take into account the fact that four patients in the bile diversion group had to be reoperated for gastroesophageal reflux. No postoperative deaths were reported in either series. Whereas the morbidity rate was 37% in the earlier series, only 1 patient of 16 had a postoperative complication after bile diversion. This difference may be influenced by the absence of previous gastric resection.

Technical Aspects

Long-limb Roux-Y Jejunal Reconstruction after Total or Proximal Gastrectomy

A segment of jejunum used for distal esophageal reconstruction is certainly a most useful tool when it combines the benefits of restoring intestinal continuity and prevention of biliary and pancreatic reflux as in a long-limb Roux-Y. Its size is appropriate and peristalsis is retained.[70] Because the length of a jejunum interposition is limited by its vascular supply, and although it can reach the neck, in most cases it will rarely reach above the aortic arch. A long-limb Roux-Y reconstruction with jejunum is the preferred conduit after a total gastrectomy and short distal esophageal resection. It is also if a total esophagectomy and total gastrectomy are required, where the interposed colon is anastomosed to the efferent limb (Figure 12.2). The variations in the blood supply to the proximal jejunum can be a challenge especially when a long segment is needed (Figure 12.3).

Transillumination is used routinely to examine the vascular supply. There should be no interruption in the vascular arcade of the segment to be used. It is best to start dissection at least 20 cm from the ligament of Treitz. At this level, vascular branches are longer and more amenable to be pedicled for a long segment. In addition, a minimal length of 20 cm is recommended for the afferent limb to facilitate the construction of the jejunojejunostomy, in order to prevent distortion of the loop and obstruction at the anastomotic site. Once the vessels of

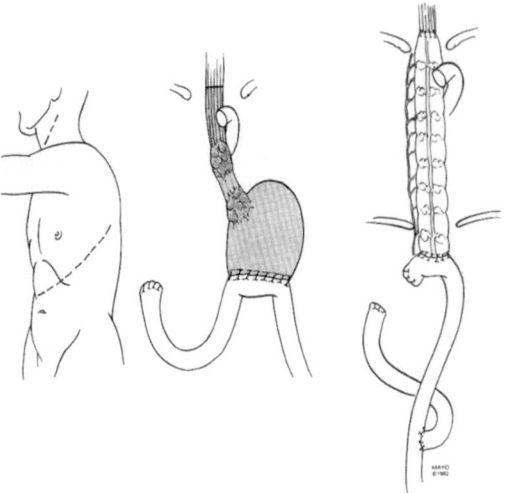

Figure 12.2. In patients requiring total esophagectomy and total gastrectomy, as is required in the patient shown (center), with distal esophageal malignant disease and previous Billroth II procedures, it is preferable to anastomose the interposed colon to a long-limb Roux limb (right) to prevent postoperative oral regurgitation and aspiration of biliary-pancreatic secretions. Such resection and reconstruction can be effected as shown on the left, through a left thoracoabdominal incision and left cervical incision. (Reprinted from Payne.[25] Used with permission of Mayo Foundation.)

the main pedicle have been isolated, temporary occlusion with atraumatic vascular bulldog clamps is used on the branches and arcades to be ligated. The presence of pulsation, peristalsis, and color should be observed and maintained before division and ligation of those vessels (Figure 12.4). The jejunum is then transected using a linear-cutting stapler and the ends are oversewn with interrupted 3-0 silk sutures. The distal cut end of jejunum is brought through a small defect in the transverse mesocolon and anastomosed end-to-side to the distal esophagus in one interrupted layer of inverting 3-0 absorbable monofilament polyglyconate (Maxon®) suture. The anastomosis is constructed as close as possible to the end of the efferent limb to avoid a blind pouch situation. The proximal jejunal segment distal to the ligament of Treitz passes behind and to the left of the efferent limb and an end-to-side jejunojejunostomy is constructed 45 cm distal to the esophageal anastomosis (Figure 12.5). The mesentery is closed to prevent internal herniation.

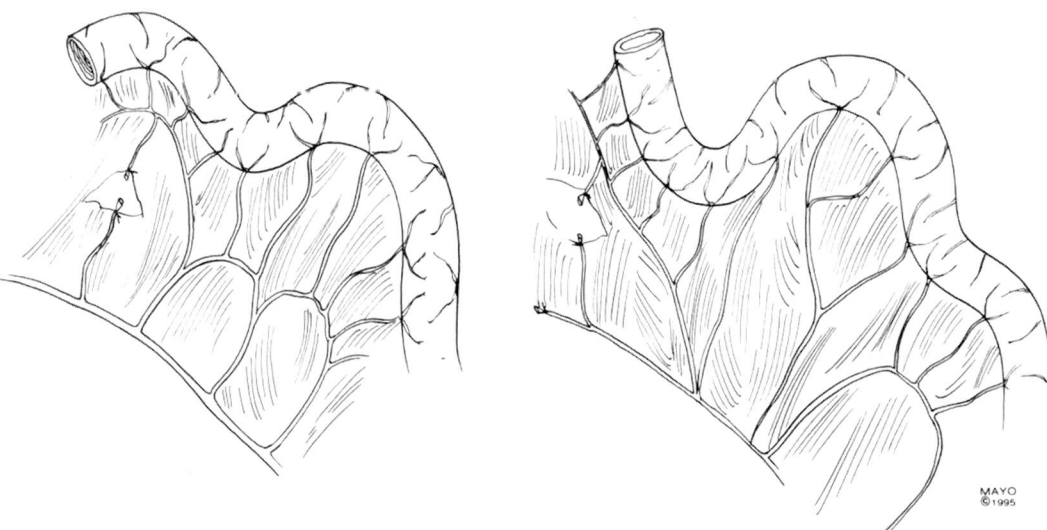

Figure 12.3. Congenital variations in jejunal mesenteric vascular patterns, such as an interruption in the vascular arcade (right), preclude use of portions of the jejunum that would normally be used for esophageal reconstruction (left). (Reprinted from Deschamps.[70] Used with permission of Mayo Foundation.)

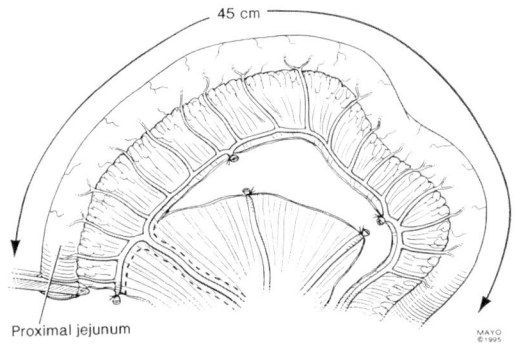

Figure 12.4. After confirmation of viability with trial clamping, division and ligation of the jejunal branches and arcades is accomplished, leaving the main pedicle as the primary blood supply for the efferent loop. Note the uninterrupted arcade and length of the efferent loop, which should be 45 cm. (Reprinted from Deschamps.[70] Used with permission of Mayo Foundation.)

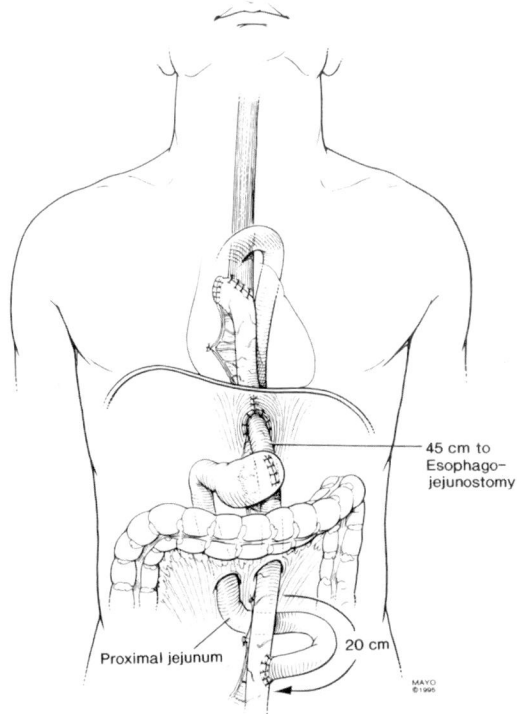

Figure 12.5. Completed long-limb Roux-en-Y reconstruction after total gastrectomy and partial esophagectomy. The efferent loop measures 45 cm in length and passes behind the stomach. The afferent loop measures at least 20 cm and passes behind and to the left of the efferent loop. (Reprinted from Deschamps.[70] Used with permission of Mayo Foundation.)

Conclusion

When the surgeon considers the possibility of a reoperation for a failed anti-reflux procedure, vagotomy and antrectomy with Roux-Y reconstruction is performed mostly as a tertiary procedure when the fundus is inadequate for any type of repair. Despite the potential disadvantage of regurgitation and aspiration of a bland refluxate, it remains a viable alternative to extensive resection.[71]

References

1. DeMeester S, DeMeester T. Esophageal pH studies in esophageal disease. In: Shields TW, LoCicero J III, Ponn RB, eds. General Thoracic Surgery. 5th ed. Philadelphia: Lippincott Williams & Wilkins; 2000:1635–1647.
2. Vaezi M. Duodenogastroesophageal reflux. In: Castell DO, Richter JE, eds. The Esophagus. 4th ed. Philadelphia: Lippincott Williams & Wilkins; 2004:434–450.
3. Ollyo JB, Monnier P, Fontolliet C, et al. The natural history and incidence of reflux oesophagitis. Gullet 1993;3: 3–10.
4. Iascone C, De Meester TR, Little AG, et al. Barrett's esophagus. Functional assessment, proposed pathogenesis and surgical therapy. Arch Surg 1983;118:543–549.
5. Gillen P, Keeling P, Bryne PJ, et al. Barrett's oesophagus: pH profile. Br J Surg 1987;74:774–776.
6. Salo JA, Kivilaakso E. Role of bile salts and trypsin in the pathogenesis of experimental alkaline esophagitis. Surgery 1983;93:525–532.
7. Kivilaakso E, Fromm D, Silen W. Effect of bile salts and related compounds on isolated esophageal mucosa. Surgery 1980;87:280–285.
8. Harmon J, Johnson L, Maydonovitch C. Effects of acid and bile salts on the rabbit esophageal mucosa. Dig Dis Sci 1981;26:65–72.
9. Lillemoe KD, Johnson LF, Harmon JW. Taurodeoxycholate modulates the effect of pepsin and trypsin in experimental esophagitis. Surgery 1985;97:662–667.
10. Salo JA, Kivilaakso E. Role of luminal H+ in the pathogenesis of experimental esophagitis. Surgery 1982;92: 61–68.
11. Safaie-Shirazi S. Effect of pepsin on ionic permeability of canine esophageal mucosa. J Surg Res 1977;27:5–8.
12. Gotley DC, Morgan AP, Ball D, et al. Composition of gastroesophageal refluxate. Gut 1991;32:1093–1099.
13. Stein HJ, Feussner H, Kauer W, et al. "Alkaline" gastroesophageal reflux: assessment by ambulatory esophageal aspiration and pH monitoring. Am J Surg 1994;167: 163–168.
14. Bradley EL III, Isaacs J, Hersh T, et al. Nutritional consequences of total gastrectomy. Ann Surg 1975;182: 415–429.
15. Attwood SEA, Smyrk TC, DeMeester TR, et al. Duodenoesophageal reflux and development of esophageal adenocarcinoma in rats. Surgery 1992;111:503–510.
16. Clark GWB, Smyrk TC, Mirvish SS, et al. Effect of gastroduodenal juice and dietary fat on the development of

Barrett's esophagus and esophageal neoplasia: an experimental rat model. Ann Surg Oncol 1994;1: 252–261.

17. Stein HJ, Barlow AP, DeMeester TR, et al. Complications of gastroesophageal reflux disease. Role of the lower esophageal sphincter, esophageal acid and acid/alkaline exposure, and duodenogastric reflux. Ann Surg 1992; 216:35–43.

18. Vaezi MF, Richter JE. Role of acid and duodenogastroesophageal reflux in gastroesophageal reflux disease. Gastroenterology 1996;111:1192–1199.

19. DeMeester T, Attwood S, Smyrk T, et al. Surgical therapy in Barrett's esophagus. Ann Surg 1990;212:528–542.

20. Topart P, Vandenbroucke F. Biliopancreatic reflux esophagitis. The role of the Roux-en-Y long limb diversion. Chest Surg Clin N Am 2001;11:605–618.

21. Fein M, Ireland AP, Ritter M, et al. Duodenogastric reflux potentiates the injurious effects of gastroesophageal reflux. J Gastrointest Surg 1997;1:27–33.

22. Batzri S, Harmon JW, Schweitzer EJ, et al. Bile acid accumulation in gastric mucosal cell. Proc Soc Exp Biol Med 1991;1997:393–399.

23. Mason RJ, DeMeester TR. Importance of duodenogastric reflux in the surgical outpatient practice. Hepatogastroenterology 1999;46:48–53.

24. Mattioli S, Pilotti S, Felice V, et al. Ambulatory 24-hour pH monitoring of esophagus, fundus, and antrum: a new technique for simultaneous study of gastroesophageal and duodenogastric reflux. Dig Dis Sci 1990;35:929–938.

25. Payne WS. Prevention and treatment of biliary-pancreatic reflux esophagitis. The role of long-limb Roux-Y. Surg Clin North Am 1983;63:851–858.

26. Sears RJ, Champion G, Richter JE. Characteristics of partial gastrectomy (PG) patients with esophageal symptoms of duodenogastric reflux. Am J Gastroenterol 1995;90:211–215.

27. Vaezi MF, Richter JE. Acid and duodenogastroesophageal reflux in postgastrectomy patients: response to therapy. Am J Gastroenterol 1995;90:A80.

28. Champion G, Richter JE, Vaezi MF, et al. Duodenogastroesophageal reflux; relationship to pH and importance in Barrett's esophagus. Gastroenterology 1994;107: 747–754.

29. Stein HJ, Smyrk TC, DeMeester TR, et al. Clinical value of endoscopy and histology in the diagnosis of duodenogastric reflux disease. Surgery 1992;112:796–804.

30. Stein H, DeMeester T. Who benefits from anti-reflux surgery? World J Surg 1992;16:313–319.

31. Mittal RK, Reuben A, Whitney JO, et al. Do bile acids reflux into the esophagus? A study in normal subjects and patients with GERD. Gastroenterology 1987;92: 371–375.

32. Gotley DC, Morgan AP, Cooper MJ. Bile acid concentration in the refluxate of patients with reflux esophagitis. Scand J Gastroenterol 1988;23:587–590.

33. Bechi P, Falciai R, Baldini F, et al. A new fiberoptic sensor for ambulatory entero-gastric reflux detection. In: Katzir A, ed. Fiberoptic Medical and Fluorescent Sensors and Applications. Bellingham, WA: SPIE; 1992;1648: 130–135.

34. Bechi P, Pucciani F, Baldini F, et al. Long term ambulatory enterogastric reflux monitoring. Validation of a new fiberoptic technique. Dig Dis Sci 1993;38:130–135.

35. Kauer WKH, Burdiles P, Ireland AP, et al. Does duodenal juice reflux into the esophagus of patients with complicated GERD? Evaluation of a fiberoptic sensor of bilirubin. Am J Surg 1995;169:98–104.

36. Tolin RD, Malmud LS, Stelzer F, et al. Enterogastric reflux in normal subjects and patients with Billroth II gastroenterostomy. Measurement of enterogastric reflux. Gastroenterology 1979;77:1027–1033.

37. Stein HJ, Hinder RA, DeMeester TR, et al. Clinical use of 24-hour gastric pH monitoring vs. o-diisopropyl iminodiacetic acid (DISIDA) scanning in the diagnosis of pathologic duodenogastric reflux. Arch Surg 1990;125: 966–971.

38. Drane WE, Karvelis K, Johnson DA. Scintigraphic evaluation of duodenogastric reflux. Problems, pitfalls, and technical review. Clin Nucl Med 1987;12:377–384.

39. Kaye MD, Showalter JP. Pyloric incompetence in patients with symptomatic gastroesophageal reflux. J Lab Clin Med 1974;83:198–206.

40. Gillen P, Keeling P, Byrne PJ, et al. Importance of duodenogastric reflux in the pathogenesis of Barrett's oesophagus. Br J Surg 1988;75:540–543.

41. Iftikhar SY, Ledingham S, Steele R, et al. Bile reflux in columnar-lined Barrett's oesophagus. Ann R Coll Surg Engl 1993;74:411–416.

42. DeMeester TR, Costantini M. Function tests. In: Pearson FG, Deslauriers J, Ginsberg RJ, Hiebert CA, McKneally MF, Urschel HC, eds. Esophageal Surgery. New York: Churchill Livingstone; 1995:119–150.

43. Fuchs KH, DeMeester TR, Hinder RA, et al. Computerized identification of pathologic duodenogastric reflux using 24-hour gastric pH monitoring. Ann Surg 1991;213:13–20.

44. Skinner DB. Surgical management after failed anti-reflux operations. World J Surg 1992;16:359–363.

45. Singh S, Bradley LA, Richter JE. Determinants of oesophageal "alkaline" pH environment in controls and patients with gastro-esophageal reflux disease. Gut 1993;34:309–316.

46. DeVault KR, Georgenson S, Castell DO. Salivary stimulation mimics esophageal exposure to refluxed duodenal contents. Am J Gastroenterol 1993;88:1040–1043.

47. Oberg S, Ritter MP, Crooks PF, et al. Gastroesophageal reflux disease and mucosal injury with emphasis on short-segment Barrett's esophagus and duodenogastroesophageal reflux. J Gastrointestinal Surg 1998;2: 547–554.

48. Fein M, Ireland AP, Ritter MP, et al. Duodenogastric reflux potentiates the injurious effects of gastroesophageal reflux. J Gastrointest Surg 1997;1:27–33.

49. Duranceau A, Ferraro P, Jamieson G. Evidenced-based investigation for reflux disease. Chest Surg Clin N Am 2001;11:495–506.

50. DeMeester TR, Fuchs KA, Ball CS, Albertucci M, Smyrk TC, Marcus JN. Experimental and clinical results with proximal and end-to-end duodenojejunostomy for pathologic duodenogastric reflux. Ann Surg 1987;206: 414–426.

51. Madura JA, Grosfeld JL. Biliary diversion. A new method to prevent enterogastric reflux and reverse the Roux stasis syndrome. Arch Surg 1997;132:245–249.

52. Holt CJ, Large AM. Surgical management of reflux esophagitis. Ann Surg 1961;153:555–562.

53. Kennedy T, Green R. Roux diversion for bile reflux following gastric surgery. Br J Surg 1978;65:323–325.

54. Fekete F, Pateron P, Sauvanet A, Kabbej M. La diversion duodenale totale dans le traitement des oesophagites peptiques complexes. Gastroenterol Clin Biol 1997;21: 823–831.

55. Ellis FH Jr, Gibb SP. Vagotomy, antrectomy, and Roux-en-Y diversion for complex reoperative gastroesophageal reflux disease. Ann Surg 1994;220:536–543.

56. Bonavina L, Incarbone R, Segalin A, Chella B, Peracchia A. Duodeno-gastro-esophageal reflux after gastric surgery: surgical therapy and outcome in 42 consecutive patients. Hepatogastroenterology 1999;46:92–96.

57. Washer JF, Gear MWL, Dowling BL, Gillison EW, Royston CMS, Spencer J. Randomized prospective trial of Roux-en-Y duodenal diversion versus fundoplication for severe reflux esophagitis. Br J Surg 1984;71:181–184.

58. Fekete F, Pateron D. What is the place of antrectomy with Roux-en-Y in the treatment of reflux disease? Experience with 83 total duodenal diversions. World J Surg 1992;16:349–353.

59. Madura JA. Primary bile reflux gastritis: which treatment is better, Roux-en-Y or biliary diversion? Am Surg 2000;66:417–424.

60. Hinder RA. Duodenal switch: a new form of pancreaticobiliary diversion. Surg Clin North Am 1992;72: 487–500.

61. Hinder RA, Bremner CG. The uses and consequences of the Roux-en-Y operation. Surg Annu 1987;19:151–174.

62. Welch NT, Yasui A, Kim CB, et al. Effect of duodenal switch procedure on gastric acid production, intragastric pH, gastric emptying, and gastrointestinal hormones. Am J Surg 1992;163:37–45.

63. Gustavsson S, Ilstrup D, Morisson P, Kelly KA. Roux stasis syndrome after gastrectomy. Am J Surg 1988;155: 490–494.

64. Davidson ED, Hersh T. The surgical treatment of bile reflux gastritis. A study of 59 patients. Ann Surg 1980;192:175–178.

65. Vogel SB, Woodward ER. The surgical treatment of chronic gastric atony following Roux-en-Y diversion for alkaline reflux gastritis. Ann Surg 1989;209:756–763.

66. Donovan IA, Drumm J, Harding LK, Alexander-Williams J. Effect of Roux-en-Y reconstruction on the gastric emptying of a solid meal. Br J Surg 1987;74: 491–492.

67. Wilson P, Anselmino M, Hinder RA. The duodenal switch operation for duodenogastric reflux. Prob Gen Surg 1993;10:242–252.

68. Klinger PJ, Perdikis G, Wilson P, Hinder RA. Indications, technical modalities and results of the duodenal switch operation for pathologic duodenogastric reflux. Hepatogastroenterology 1999;46:97–102.

69. Csendes A, Braghetto I, Burdiles P, Diaz J-C, Maluenda F, Korn O. A new physiological approach for the surgical treatment of patients with Barrett's esophagus. Technical considerations and results in 65 patients. Ann Surg 1997;226:123–133.

70. Deschamps C. Use of colon and jejunum as possible esophageal replacements. Chest Surg Clin N Am 1995;5: 555–569.

71. Deschamps C, Trastek VF, Allen MS, Pairolero PC, Johnson JO, Larson DR. Long-term results after reoperation for failed anti-reflux procedures. J Thorac Cardiovasc Surg 1997;113:545–551.

13

Management of the Short Esophagus

Éric Fréchette and André Duranceau

Positioning the esophagogastric junction below the diaphragm without any tension, during a hiatal hernia repair or after an anti-reflux operation, is of the utmost importance in the surgical treatment of these conditions. Although in most patients such a procedure can be undertaken without technical difficulty, a shortened esophagus can occasionally become apparent and can limit the ability of the surgeon to offer a satisfactory repair. The aim of this work is to define the short esophagus and its clinical manifestations in order to allow esophageal surgeons to recognize the entity and address its management with a logical approach.

Evolution of Hiatal Hernia and Anti-Reflux Surgery

The concept of a shortened esophagus is not accepted by everyone, resulting in controversy over the years.[1,2] Although an occasional patient may be seen with an esophagogastric junction clearly irreducible to its proper position under the diaphragm, there are discrepant opinions among surgeons on what constitutes a shortened esophagus and what is the real incidence of the condition in patients with gastroesophageal reflux disease (GERD) and hiatal hernia. There is no exact and reproducible method of measuring the length of the esophagus before and during surgery. The extent to which the esophageal surgeon has to address the

problem is unknown. At present the existence of a short esophagus is based mostly on indirect and circumstantial evidences.

During the last 50 years, the natural evolution of the various anatomic hiatal hernia repairs and, subsequently, of the numerous anti-reflux operations has resulted in identifying failure patterns which were then related to the severity of the disease. How often a failed anatomic repair was the consequence of not recognizing a short esophagus remains unknown. The inadequate long-term functional results observed with a perigastric fundoplication or a slipped fundoplication, or crural disruption with mediastinal herniation of the repair, raise the hypothesis that such failures might be attributed to a shortened esophagus.[3] In 1950, Norman Barrett wrongly described an intrathoracic stomach when observing a columnar-lined esophagus. He suggested the concept of progressive shortening of the esophagus with distraction of the stomach into the chest. Barrett had coined the term "reflux esophagitis" when ulcers of the esophagus were associated with reflux of gastric content.[4,5] Just previously, Allison[6] had associated the concept of hiatal hernia to the erosive esophagitis observed and to the occasional esophageal stricture, attributing both to gastroesophageal reflux. About the same period that Allison was proposing his anatomic repair, Belsey proposed a partial fundoplication of the gastric fundus on the posterolateral wall of the esophagus. In patients treated by this operation without endoscopic esophagitis, a reflux recurrence rate of 9.5% was observed. When esophagitis without stricture was identified before the operation, 10.3% of these patients had recurrent reflux. If a stricture was present, the operation failed in 45% of the operated population.[7] The repair difficulties and imperfect results obtained when an esophagus is shortened or strictured then led Leigh Collis to propose a lengthening gastroplasty in order to provide good, healthy tissue for the repair while removing tension for its positioning under the diaphragm.[8]

Definition

The abdominal esophagus is said to be from 0.5 to 2.5 cm in length, although Pearl[9] states that it may be as long as 7 cm after mobilization. Allison,[6] taking the level of the lowest connective tissue fibers attaching the esophagus to the diaphragm as the inferior limits of the mediastinum, suggested that there is technically no abdominal esophagus. Despite these views, the surgeon usually has access to an appreciable length of esophagus below the diaphragm.[10]

Thus, if at the time of surgery, after adequate mobilization of the esophagus, the esophagogastric junction cannot be positioned without tension at 2.5 cm or more below the hiatus, the esophagus can be interpreted as being shortened. However, such measurements can be affected by subjectivity and can vary from one observer to another. The degree of esophageal mobilization varies with the approach. Esophageal mobilization at laparotomy succeeds in freeing the distal esophagus from its attachments in the 3-cm trajectory through the tunnel of the diaphragm. The left thoracic exposure has always been championed as allowing complete mobilization of the esophagus to the level of the aortic arch. During a laparoscopic approach, as the pneumoperitoneum exerts an upward pressure on the diaphragm, the perceived length of the esophagus is increased. Furthermore, an associated hiatal hernia and the exact position of the esophagogastric junction renders the concept of junction between the esophagus and stomach difficult to clarify. For these reasons, esophageal shortening is documented objectively only when the anatomic esophagogastric junction cannot be positioned under the diaphragm.

However, a relative shortening of the esophagus precluding the reestablishment of its normal length during esophageal repairs can be assumed if the durability of the repair and an unacceptable failure rate are documented over time. When the clinical evidence shows that a standard repair performed at a given stage of the reflux disease, or with a given type of hiatal herniation, cannot offer the expected durability of such repairs, this may be seen as indirect evidence of a "shortened esophagus." As an example, the upward migration of a standard repair into the mediastinum may suggest an undiagnosed short esophagus. Or a large and irreducible hernia, lying in the distal mediastinum, which usually reveals a shortened esophagus on manometric tracings, is considered to be associated with a shortened esophagus. The columnar esophagus with a high stricture on radiological examination and at endoscopy also suggests to the surgeon a shortened esophagus. Despite all these situations in which the esophagus has all the appearances of being shortened, proper mobilization at surgery usually allows restoration of the esophagogastric junction under the diaphragm. Full mobilization and reduction of a repair under the diaphragmatic hiatus, however, cannot be interpreted as an esophagus of normal length. In such situations, esophageal wall pathology and the patient's habitus will spell the difference between long-term success or failure.

Etiology

Gastroesophageal reflux disease is the main reason for esophageal shortening. The pathophysiology of the short esophagus associated with GERD follows the sequence of erosion ulcers and inflammation associated with chronic esophageal reflux. These factors have been studied in animal experiments and in human pathological evaluation.[11,12] The squamous epithelium of the lower esophagus has poor defense mechanisms against repeated episodes of gastric refluxes. Chronic exposure to gastroesophageal reflux episodes, particularly when acid is mixed with bile salts and/or pepsin, causes a chemical esophagitis with back diffusion through the epithelium. Edema of the lamina propria occurs initially. The inflammation can reach the muscularis mucosae at a later stage. Most of reflux strictures are caused by fibrosis and scar contraction when damage is present at that depth of the esophageal wall. These strictures are usually easily dilatable. If prolonged exposure causes further inflammation and additional scar formation, the consequences of cyclic esophagitis reach the level of the muscularis propria and the periesophageal tissues. Progressive circumferential contraction creates a more fibrous stricture and, simultaneously, longitudinal contraction results in a shortening of the esophagus. Transmural fibrous damage is frequently seen in scleroderma patients especially when they present with an associated complication in a columnar-lined esophagus.

Other conditions have been incriminated in the formation of a short esophagus. In such circumstances, fibrosis need not be present for the acquired esophageal shortening to occur. Type 3 and type 4 paraesophageal hernias and the periesophagitis after previous anti-reflux operations or after repairs of esophageal atresia are examples of these circumstances.

Clinical and radiological findings may immediately suggest the possibility of esophageal shortening. The presence of a reflux stricture at endoscopy or of a high stricture radiologically are known to jeopardize the success of any standard anti-reflux operation: Donnelly et al.[13] and Orringer et al.[14] have documented that 45–75% of patients with reflux strictures or severe esophagitis who undergo a Belsey Mark IV repair will develop a recurrent hiatal hernia or reflux disease during follow-up. The long columnar-lined esophagus, especially if a high stricture is present on radiological examination, is exposed to the same failure risk.[15,16]

The repair of massive hiatal hernias and redo operations are also known to result in a high failure rate.[17] Long-standing type 3 and type 4 sliding and paraesophageal hernias, even if they do not reveal associated reflux esophagitis, will present some degree of circular and longitudinal esophageal muscle contracture. In many of those situations, it is not the anatomic reduction of the junction that is critical, it is the resulting tension on the repair once the esophagogastric junction has been reduced below the diaphragm.

The prevalence of a short esophagus varies significantly among observers. Ritter et al.[18] reported the condition in 3–14% of patients requiring an anti-reflux operation. But in patients having redo surgery associated with an esophageal stricture, a paraesophageal hernia, or a Barrett's esophagus, a 79-fold increase in the need for an esophageal lengthening procedure has been observed.[17]

Investigation

Gastroesophageal reflux is a normal physiological process occurring daily without causing symptoms. Gastroesophageal reflux disease is the result of the same process but exaggerated in frequency and time of exposure and ending in mucosal complications. There is a lack of correlation between patient's symptoms and the actual severity of reflux disease. Collis[19] and Skinner[20] both drew attention to the fact that patients with severe esophagitis may present without symptoms. Inversely, severe symptoms are often found to be perceived without any evidence of esophageal mucosal damage. For these reasons, standardized objective measurements should confirm the diagnosis and the severity of the reflux problem to be treated.

Radiology

The barium swallow is a simple, noninvasive test that should be used to determine the presence or absence of any anatomic abnormality associated with GERD. Free radiological reflux can be observed and reported by the radiologist with sometimes subjective efforts at quantification. However, GERD cannot be concluded from such observations, because up to 20% of normal individuals will show reflux of barium in their esophagus.[21] When patients show an associated hiatal hernia, they may have a greater chance of having esophagitis at endoscopy.[22]

Hiatal hernias larger than 5 cm sometimes are associated with a shortened esophagus.[23] Any stricture should be described and related to associated abnormalities. Overall, there is very little agreement about the relevance of a hiatus hernia to gastroesophageal reflux. In a patient who underwent a previous hiatal hernia and/or an anti-reflux operation, the exact position of the repair should be clarified. The esophagogastric junction needs to be identified within the configuration of the previous repair. A fundic wrap migration into the mediastinum can remain asymptomatic when the anti-reflux mechanism remains intact. If a total fundoplication is completely everted around the stomach, or if a fundoplication has been completed around the smaller curvature, such observations can be associated with either obstruction or reflux symptoms.

Endoscopy and Esophageal Biopsies

The unequivocal documentation of visual and histological damage on the esophageal mucosa is the mainstay of decision-making when treating GERD. Endoscopic evaluation is of primary importance if a patient is suspected of having a shortened esophagus, and even more so in patients with a failed repair. Preferably the surgeon who will provide the treatment should perform or observe the endoscopic assessment. The identification of severe esophagitis or stricture usually presents no problem. Barrett's esophagus can only be documented with multiple biopsies and the histological identification of intestinal metaplasia in the columnar-lined esophagus. Multiple biopsies and brush cytologies are always needed to rule out malignancy if the esophagus is strictured. Esophageal dilatations, using bougies or balloon dilators, may be necessary to provide an esophageal lumen that will allow a proper examination while at the same time permitting easier food intake.

There are numerous esophageal mucosal damage classifications. They are evidence of the lack of reproducible interpretations among various endoscopists. The MUSE classification proposed by Armstrong et al.[24] has the advantage of visually describing and quantifying the four types of mucosal damage that can be observed at endoscopy: metaplasia (M), ulcers (U), stricture (S), and erosions (E). This classification represents an effort to improve the objectivity of recording and scoring existing lesions.

This classification does not recognize observations that correspond to equivocal evidence of reflux damage, as mucosal hyperhemia. The initial observation by Allison[25] that a fundamental difference exists between esophagitis in squamous mucosa and a columnar-lined mucosa is retained in this classification. The refluxate rarely produces deep damage in a squamous mucosa. In a columnar-lined mucosa, the refluxate causing esophagitis often is seen with deep penetration through the esophageal wall, occasionally resulting in periesophageal reaction and mediastinal fibrosis.

Esophageal biopsies should demonstrate the proven end result of reflux damage. Unfortunately, the endoscopic findings do not always tally perfectly with the histological assessment. Confirmation of esophagitis suggested by endoscopy is obtained in 32–72% of patients.[26] Whether this poor correlation between visual documentation and histological evidence is attributable to sampling errors, to the patchy nature of esophageal inflammation, or simply to overinterpretation remains open to discussion. At present, unequivocal histological evidence of reflux damage includes: acute inflammatory reaction in the epithelium and subepithelium; erosions and ulcerations of the mucosa; a fibrotic stricture especially when associated with mucosal breaks; and histological documentation of a columnar-lined esophagus with incomplete intestinal metaplasia.

Motility Studies

Motor function evaluation is essential in the assessment of GERD. The absence of a lower esophageal sphincter (LES) tone provides important prognostic information regarding the potential for successful management of the condition.[27] The quality of the peristaltic activity as well as the strength of esophageal contractions are also considered important aspects of function before selecting a treatment option.[3,28] Despite the use of this investigative technique in defining unequivocal alterations of esophageal physiology leading to reflux disease, its use remains limited in defining the short esophagus. The direct measurement of esophageal length has been disappointing because esophageal manometry cannot predict which esophagus will remain short after adequate mobilization.[29] Despite the suggestion that a manometrically measured short esophagus is associated with a higher number of lengthening operations, manometry alone cannot predict the need for a lengthening procedure.[23,30] Furthermore, manometric findings are not reliable in predicting the failure of an anti-reflux operation.[31] A clearly hypotensive LES remains unresponsive to any medication. Anti-reflux operations, however, help to reestablish a pressure barrier at the esophagogastric junction. Little,[32] in his review of failed anti-reflux repairs, emphasizes that a persistent hypotensive LES is usually evidence of the failure of the sphincter mechanism to stop reflux, usually associated with a complete disruption of the original anti-reflux operation.

Monitoring Acid and Bile Reflux

Ambulatory 24-hour pH monitoring has become the most objective documentation of acid exposure in the esophageal lumen. It provides valuable information in patients with pathological reflux disease by recording the frequency and duration of acid reflux episodes. The constant monitoring of acid exposure also suggests the severity of reflux-related mucosal damage, a severity that always has to be documented by endoscopy.

Bile reflux documentation using a fiberoptic probe (Bilitec) may also be measured, because mixed acid and alkaline reflux has been shown to be associated with the esophageal wall damages of the more severe forms of reflux disease. At present, however, this test is available in a limited number of centers and has been used mostly to study the pathophysiology of the columnar-lined esophagus.[33] Despite providing more objectivity to the diagnosis and treatment of reflux disease, 24-hour acid and bile monitoring cannot predict a shortened esophagus or the need for an esophageal lengthening operation.

Medical Management

Patients with GERD who are referred for treatment of a suspected short esophagus have usually been treated for a prolonged period of time with medication. Proton pump inhibitors and H_2 receptor blockers are the recognized medications proven to offer relief of symptoms and healing of the esophagitis. However, in patients in whom an absent LES has been documented, medication alone does not offer definitive control of the abnormal refluxate and cannot reconstitute a normal esophagogastric junction. For these reasons, symptoms usually reappear when the medication is discontinued.[34]

Lifestyle changes are essential. Weight reduction by reducing alimentary intake while increasing caloric expenditure by exercise is often met with poor compliance. Smoking cessation and alcohol intake reduction are important as well. When a stricture is present and symptomatic, dilation can be offered while medical therapy is undertaken. Simple bougienage or pneumatic dilation relieves dysphagia in 20–30% of patients after the first dilation session. Slowly progressive dilation sessions usually provide safe reopening of the esophageal lumen. In order not to impose additional healing damage to the esophageal wall, a limit of 10-French size increase per session is considered appropriate. Esophageal perforation from these manipulations is seen in <0.5% of patients.[35,36]

Surgical Treatment

Failed control of symptoms or progression of the damage to the esophageal wall over time are the usual reasons bringing patients for a surgical consideration. The basic principles considered essential when offering patients an anti-reflux repair for complications of reflux disease are: 1) identify and mobilize a proper length of esophagus below the diaphragmatic hiatus; 2) create a tension-free floppy total fundoplication over a large bougie—division of the short gastric vessels is usually necessary for such a technique; 3) closure of the hiatus behind the esophagus to ensure hiatal muscle function—anchoring the repair on the right crus of the diaphragm may be added to ensure that the repair will remain in an intraabdominal position. Protection of vagal nerve integrity is essential. If the esophagus is thickened and the gastroesophageal junction difficult to reduce in a normal intraabdominal position, the abdominal route should be abandoned for a left thoracotomy approach to obtain a safe and full mobilization of the esophagus to the aortic arch. If, after such efforts, the repair cannot be completed with at least 2.5 cm of esophagus under the diaphragm and without tension, the esophagus is considered shortened. These principles apply independent of the selected approach.

Standard Anti-Reflux Repairs

When a stricture is dilatable and the esophagus mobilized to the aortic arch, a proper partial fundoplication can usually be obtained and reduced under the diaphragm.[13,14,37–39] Such repairs include the posterolateral Belsey Mark IV and the posterior gastropexy of Hill.

They were shown to offer satisfactory reflux control in 25–85% of treated patients with a follow-up of 16 months to 6 years. When a total fundoplication of the Nissen type was used to treat a strictured esophagus, the short-term success rate was reported to vary between 88 and 100%.[40–42] However, long-term assessment of reflux-induced esophageal strictures in patients treated by a Belsey repair documented a failure rate of 45% in controlling reflux damage.[14] Subsequent reports on Barrett's patients cohorts treated for their reflux complications by total fundoplication revealed an inappropriate failure rate of the operation.[15,16] Repair of massive hernias using standard operations lead to the same dismal results as reported by Pearson et al.[43] Low[44] concluded that an unrecognized short esophagus with a repair under tension is responsible for this high failure rate: esophageal strictures, the columnar-lined esophagus, the failed repairs, and massive hiatal hernias should be considered as categories of esophageal problems at risk of failure when using standard surgical repairs.

Lengthening Gastroplasties

In 1957, Collis,[8] dissatisfied with the problems generated by the short esophagus, including the frequent periesophagitis present in these patients, introduced the concept of esophageal lengthening using the proximal lesser gastric curvature to create a neoesophagus. The lengthening gastroplasty was seen as an alternative to esophagectomy and reconstruction, a solution which was used more liberally at that time. The repositioning of the esophagogastric junction with the recreation of the angle of His was initially thought to be sufficient to prevent gastroesophageal reflux.[8] No anti-reflux mechanism was then added to the gastroplasty, leading to poor reflux control. Subsequently, the initial Collis gastroplasty was combined to a Belsey-type of fundoplication by Pearson whereas Orringer and Henderson advocated the use of a total fundoplication to wrap the neoesophagus.[43] The indications for using a lengthening gastroplasty with either a partial or a total anti-reflux fundoplication have been summarized by Pearson: chronic damage of reflux disease, reop-

erations for failed previous hiatal hernia repairs or anti-reflux operations, and massive hernias with an intrathoracic stomach. More controversial indications are its use in patients with gross obesity or with asthma and chronic obstructive pulmonary disease.[45]

Collis-Belsey gastroplasty. This repair involves the complete mobilization of the distal esophagus and proximal stomach. A no. 48 or 50 bougie is passed into the stomach by the anesthetist and held against the lesser curvature. A GIA stapler with 4.8-mm staples is applied to create a 4- to 5-cm gastroplasty. This is usually sufficient to obviate tension on the repair. The 270° fundoplication replicating the original Belsey repair is then completed, completely covering the transection margin of the gastroplasty while offering the anti-reflux protection of a partial fundoplication. Using this transthoracic repair, Pearson and Henderson[46] reported satisfactory results in 93% of patients treated for a short esophagus associated with esophagitis or stricture. The success rate of the operation was 80% if the operation was offered to patients with unsuccessful previous repairs. If the operation was used in patients treated previously by esophageal myotomy for motor disorders, the overall results were poor. This operation shows excellent long-term results when used in patients with a massive hernia.[30] The main cause for failure when a Collis-Belsey gastroplasty is used is persistent gastroesophageal reflux.[47]

Collis-Nissen repair. Henderson[48] and Orringer and Sloan[49] suggested the use of a combination of a lengthening gastroplasty with a total fundoplication. They proposed that this was a better anti-reflux operation for reflux disease with a reflux-damaged shortened esophagus. The gastroplasty tube is created just as described with the Collis-Belsey repair, resulting in a 4- to 5-cm gastroplasty (Figure 13.1). The transected fundus is then brought as a total fundoplication around the gastroplasty tube. The fundic wrap is sutured to itself, creating a 3- to 4-cm-long, 360° total fundoplication (Figure 13.2). Stirling and Orringer[50] reported the results of this operation. Eighty-eight percent of the patients in their group had good control of symptoms and 8% required medication despite the operation. Ten years after the operation, 34% of patients assessed by 24-hour

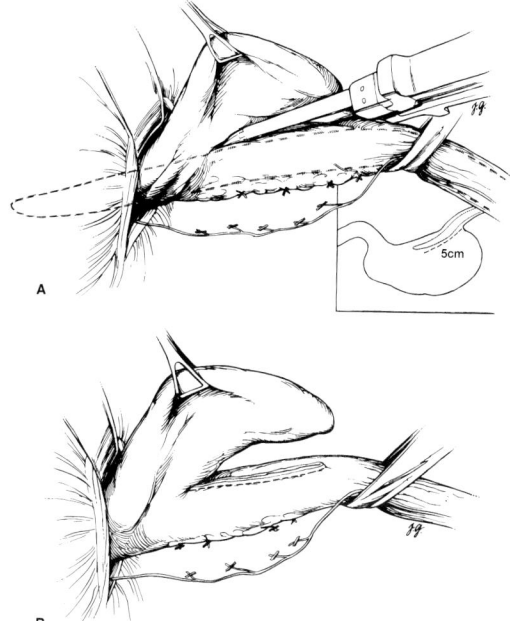

Figure 13.1. The cut Collis-Nissen as described by Orringer requires full mobilization of the gastric fundus and placement of a large bougie along the lesser gastric curvature. A linear cutting stapler is then fired parallel to the bougie to elongate the esophageal tube and enlarge the fundus. (Reprinted from Ferraro P, Duranceau A. Elongation gastroplasty with total fundoplication. Operative Techniques in General Surgery 200;2:24–37, Copyright 2000, with permission from Elsevier.)

pH testing revealed abnormal acid exposure, most of them asymptomatic. When a stricture was present, these authors reported the failure rate for this operation to be 23%.[50]

Uncut Collis-Nissen repair. The uncut gastroplasty was reported by Langer[51] and described by Demos et al.[52] and Bingham.[53] The gastroplasty tube is created from the proximal smaller curvature by the use of a 3-cm linear stapler with 4.8-mm staples, applied along an inlaying no. 48 or 50 bougie held against the small curvature (Figure 13.3). The gastroplasty is created by the apposition of the anterior and posterior wall of the stomach. The gastroplasty tube is not separated from the gastric fundus by transection. The extensively mobilized remaining fundus is then brought around the entire length of the gastroplasty as a total fundoplication and the fundic wrap is sutured immediately anterior to the staple line (Figure 13.4). This repair provides excellent clinical and functional results.

Chen et al.[54] and McDonald et al.[55] reported reflux control in 95% of their patients. The repair remains competent over time, showing an excellent LES gradient but an incomplete relaxation of the sphincter area. A potential weakness of this operation is its obstructive character in patients with poor propulsive capacity. Bingham[53] has also reported the tendency of staples to come out, leaving the mucosal apposition undone and the stomach wrapped around itself. The staple line, in our experience, is well protected by the total fundoplication.

Modified Collis-Nissen repair. When a reoperation becomes necessary after single or multiple previous repairs, the quality of the gastric fundic tissue may not be appropriate for a healthy gastroplasty wrap. In this situation, Jeyasingham's modified cut gastroplasty may be a useful technique as an esophageal-sparing operation. The gastroplasty is fashioned as for the uncut technique, using a 3-cm linear stapler with 4.8-mm staples apposing the anterior and the posterior walls of the proximal stomach

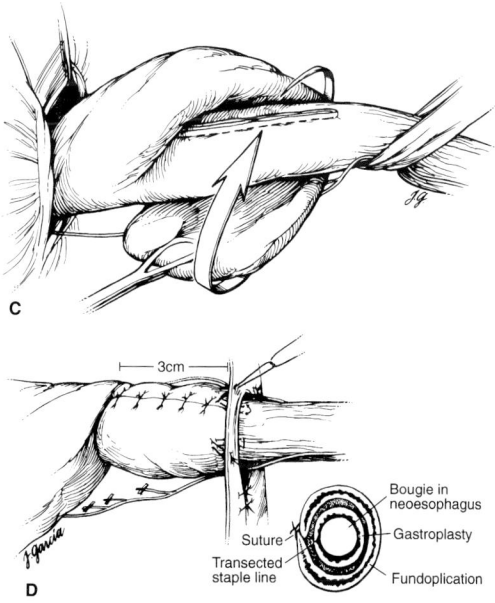

Figure 13.2. After completing the esophageal lengthening portion of the cut Collis-Nissen, a standard total fundoplication is performed with the bougie still in place to appropriately size the wrap. (Reprinted from Ferraro P, Duranceau A. Elongation gastroplasty with total fundoplication. Operative Techniques in General Surgery 200;2:24–37, Copyright 2000, with permission from Elsevier.)

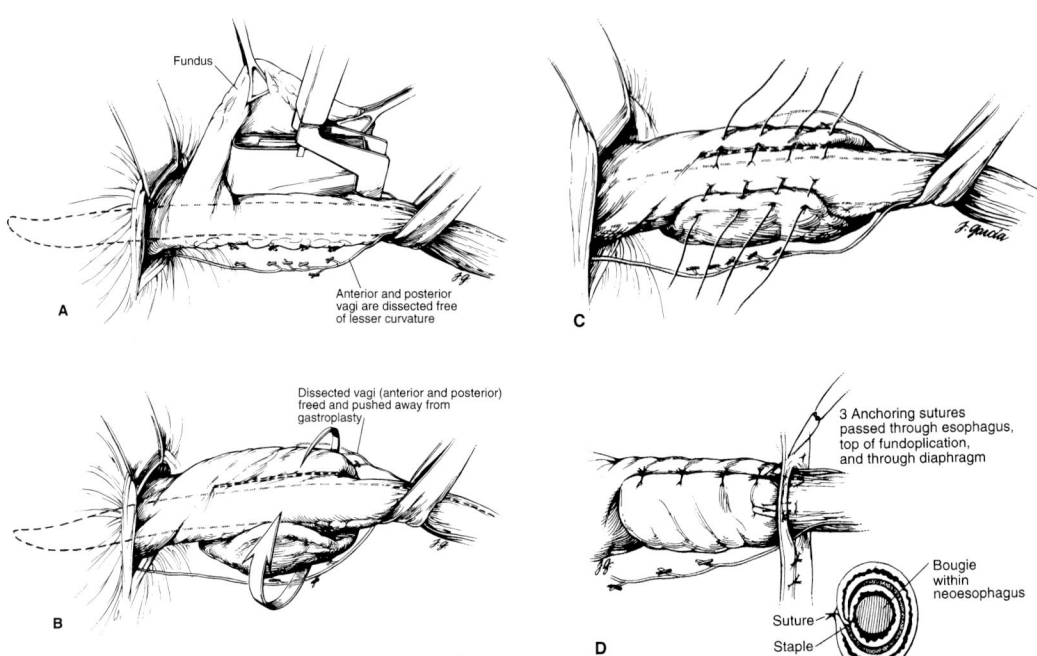

Figure 13.3. An uncut Collis-Nissen is initiated by complete mobilization of the proximal stomach and esophagus. A bougie is positioned along the lesser gastric curvature and a linear stapler (noncutting) is fired parallel to it. This elongates the esophageal tube, around which a fundoplication wrap can be created. (Reprinted from Ferraro P, Duranceau A. Elongation gastroplasty with total fundoplication. Operative Techniques in General Surgery 200;2:24–37, Copyright 2000, with permission from Elsevier.)

Figure 13.4. After the staple line is created for the uncut Collis-Nissen, a fundoplication wrap is created around the extended esophageal tube. (Reprinted from Ferraro P, Duranceau A. Elongation gastroplasty with total fundoplication. Operative Techniques in General Surgery 200;2:24–37, Copyright 2000, with permission from Elsevier.)

parallel to a 48- or 50-French bougie held against the lesser gastric curvature (Figure 13.5). Once the staples are fired, the stomach on the fundus side is opened and the gastrotomy incision is elongated toward the apex of the fundus. The fundus is then closed transversely, as for a pyloroplasty (Figure 13.6). This closure provides a widened fundus with enough anterior and posterior gastric wall to create a 3-cm total fundoplication around the gastroplasty

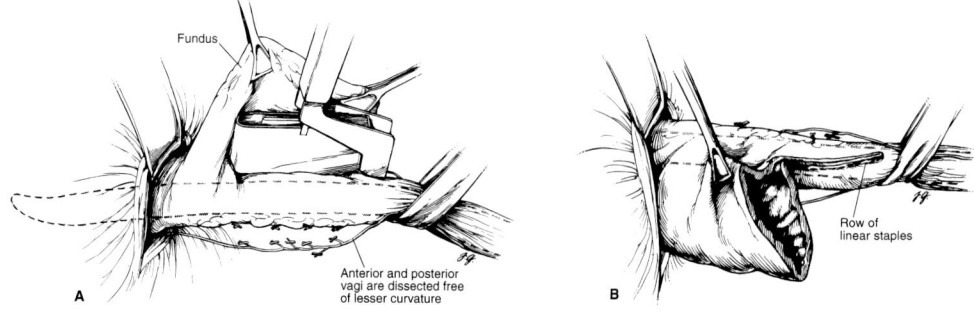

Figure 13.5. A modified Collis-Nissen fundoplasty is initiated after complete mobilization of the fundus and distal esophagus by creating a staple line along the lesser gastric curvature in a manner similar to that used for an uncut Collis gastroplasty. The fundus is opened from the distal end of the staple line toward the tip of the fundus. (Reprinted from Ferraro P, Duranceau A. Elongation gastroplasty with total fundoplication. Operative Techniques in General Surgery 200;2:24–37, Copyright 2000, with permission from Elsevier.)

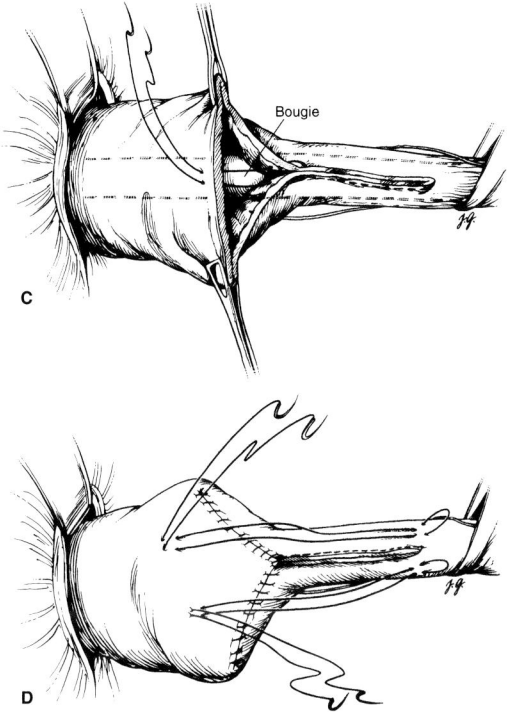

Figure 13.6. After opening the stomach for the modified Collis-Nissen fundoplasty, the fundic incision is closed transversely to widen the fundus. (Reprinted from Ferraro P, Duranceau A. Elongation gastroplasty with total fundoplication. Operative Techniques in General Surgery 200;2:24–37, Copyright 2000, with permission from Elsevier.)

(Figure 13.7). A positive aspect of this repair is the usual better quality of the available tissue provided by the extensive mobilization of the lower gastric body. This "new" stomach wall provides a healthy wrap and a good protection around the gastroplasty tube.[56]

Stricturoplasty and Intrathoracic Fundoplication

Intrathoracic fundoplications were used for the shortened esophagus by Krupp and Rossetti[57] in 1966. They completed a total fundoplication around the lower esophagus and left the repair in the chest. The same type of repair was subsequently used by Woodward as reported by Maher et al.[58] In their review of this technique, they reported good to excellent results in 82% of their patients. An important step that needs to be added to this technique is the essential detail of widening of the diaphragmatic hiatus

to avoid functional obstruction or poor drainage of the supradiaphragmatic stomach.

Thal[59] initially proposed to split the esophageal stricture caused by the reflux and widen the esophagus by pulling the fundus into the chest and applying a fundic patch to cover the opened esophagus. The healing pattern resulted in restricture and this was corrected by adding a skin graft to cover the fundus before the patch closure. But despite protection of the gastric serosa by the graft, free reflux and recurrent esophagitis persisted if an anti-reflux mechanism was not added. A total fundoplication covering the Thal patch was documented to result in satisfactory results in 84% of treated patients.[60]

Both these types of intrathoracic fundoplications, although well known to correct reflux, are not used extensively because of the dangers that have been reported with supradiaphragmatic

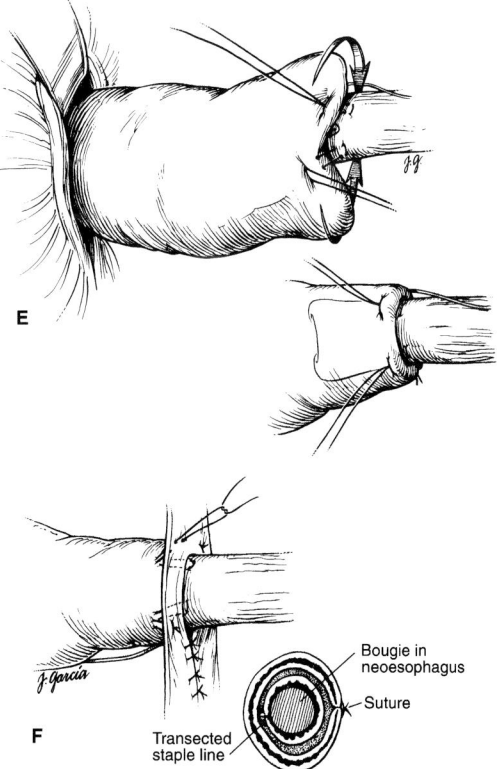

Figure 13.7. Transverse closure of the fundus for the modified Collis-Nissen fundoplasty provides substantial additional fundic tissue, enabling creation of a total or partial wrap around the extended esophageal tube without tension. (Reprinted from Ferraro P, Duranceau A. Elongation gastroplasty with total fundoplication. Operative Techniques in General Surgery 200;2:24–37, Copyright 2000, with permission from Elsevier.)

fundoplications: paragastric hernias, gastric ulcerations, and gastric fistulization with mediastinal structures.

Vagotomy, Antrectomy, and Roux-en-Y Diversion

Multiple failed anti-reflux operations, a short and strictured esophagus, or a failed Collis gastroplasty with either a partial or a total fundoplication may require a more radical approach. Resection of the damaged lower esophagus and reconstruction with the stomach to be left in the distal mediastinum is not an acceptable solution, because restricture by reflux can be expected in nearly 100% of patients so treated. Payne[61] treated this permanent incompetence of the cardia by adding a bilateral truncal vagotomy with an antrectomy for acid suppression and a Roux-en-Y diversion of all pancreatobiliary secretions using a long jejunal limb. Ellis and Gibb[62] and Fekete and Pateron[63] reported their respective experience using this operation. These authors reported a >80% success with this treatment.

Csendes and associates[16] observed an extremely high failure rate when treating Barrett's esophagus patients using conventional anti-reflux repairs. With this observation, they opted for bilateral vagotomy, antrectomy and long-limb Roux-en-Y diversion as primary treatment for these patients. They tried biliary diversion without resection (duodenal switch) but observed a better acid reflux control if an antrectomy was selected. Using this operation, they observed a reduction of low-grade dysplasia in the esophageal columnar-lined mucosa in 50% of treated patients.

Treatment of the Short Esophagus by Minimally Invasive Surgery

Laparoscopic operations to prevent and correct reflux damage to the esophagus have been popularized since the early 1990s. An impressive increase in the number of anti-reflux operations completed per year has been observed with the advent of this new approach. Whereas the indications for anti-reflux surgery have remained unchanged, the mucosal damage severity has been reported to be significantly lower in treated patients.[64]

The shortened esophagus has often been unrecognized with the generalization of anti-reflux operations among a larger number of surgeons able to proceed with the technical aspect of the operation but not always familiar with the pros and cons of various esophageal conditions. Occasionally, this has resulted in disastrous consequences for patients.[65]

The first attempt at creating a lengthening gastroplasty by thoracoscopy was by Demos et al.[66] Swanstrom et al.[67] developed a technique in which the lengthening gastroplasty was created through a right transhiatal thoracoscopy simultaneously to laparoscopic dissection of the proximal stomach. Johnson et al.[68] used the Steichen gastroplasty technique with a transgastric circular stapler to join the anterior and posterior walls of the stomach together around an inlaying bougie held along the smaller curvature (see Chapters 8 and 11). The gastroplasty is then completed with an EndoGIA and the fundoplication created around the gastroplasty. Most authors confirm the feasibility of the technique and satisfactory early results. Few long-term reports are available. Jobe et al.[69] reported on 14 patients treated by a Collis gastroplasty with a fundoplication. With a 14-month follow-up, all patients showed an intact repair. Thirty-six percent of the patients were diagnosed with active esophagitis and 50% of the group was found to have an abnormal 24-hour pH recording. Although feasible, the details of creating a lengthening gastroplasty by laparoscopic and thoracoscopic surgery must be compared with those of the open technique. Only with proper assessment will the functional results and durability of the two approaches become available.

Conclusion

Complicated GERD can lead to a shortened esophagus. The diagnosis can be suspected from the results of preoperative investigation, mostly after documenting the severity of the disease. However, the definitive diagnosis often can be made only at surgery when the surgeon has completely dissected the esophagus and the esophagogastric junction. At present, a high degree of subjectivity is involved in the diagnosis of the short esophagus. Its exact prevalence and incidence among gastroesophageal refluxing patients is still unclear. Most of our knowledge of the condition stems from indirect evidence given by the treatment results of well-defined damage severity in the esophageal wall of patients with severe reflux. Failure to recognize a shortened esophagus will usually result in poor functional results, recurrent hiatal hernias, and progressive reflux damage. Long-term results may well end in resection of the esophagus, exactly what a proper diagnosis and appropriate management should prevent.

References

1. DeMeester SR, DeMeester TR. Editorial comment: the short esophagus—going, going, gone? Surgery 2003;133:364–377.
2. Korn O, Csendes A, Burdiles P, Braghetto I, Sagastume H, Biagini L. Length of the esophagus in patients with gastroesophageal reflux disease and Barrett's esophagus compared to controls. Surgery 2003;133:358–363.
3. Horvath KD, Swanstrom LL, Jobe BA. The short esophagus: pathophysiology, incidence, presentation, and treatment in the era of laparoscopic anti-reflux surgery. Ann Surg 2000;232:630–640.
4. Barrett NR. Chronic peptic ulcer of the oesophagus and oesophagitis. Br J Surg 1950;38:175.
5. Spechler SJ, Goyal RK. The columnar-lined esophagus, intestinal metaplasia, and Norman Barrett. Gastroenterology 1996;110:614–621.
6. Allison PR. Peptic ulcer of the oesophagus. J Thorac Surg 1946;15:308–317.
7. Belsey R. The Belsey Mark IV anti-reflux procedure. In: Zuidema GD, ed. Shackelford's Surgery of the Alimentary Tract. Philadelphia: WB Saunders; 1996:204–213.
8. Collis JL. An operation for hiatus hernia with short oesophagus. Thorax 1957;12:181–188.
9. Pearl RH. Anatomy of the esophagus and posterior mediastinum. In: Nyhus LM, Baker RJ, eds. Mastery of Surgery. Boston: Little Brown; 1984.
10. Skandalakis JE, Gray SW, Skandalakis LJ. Surgical anatomy of the esophagus. In: Jamieson GG, ed. Surgery of the Oesophagus. London: Churchill Livingstone; 1983: 19–35.
11. Gozzetti G, Pilotti V, Spangaro M, et al. Pathophysiology and natural history of acquired short esophagus. Surgery 1987;102:507–514.
12. Lillemoe KD, Johnson LF, Harmon JW. Taurodeoxycholate modulates the effects of pepsin and trypsin in experimental esophagitis. Surgery 1985;97:662–667.
13. Donnelly RJ, Deverall PB, Watson DA. Hiatus hernia with and without stricture: experience with the Belsey Mark IV repair. Ann Thorac Surg 1973;16:301.
14. Orringer MB, Skinner DB, Belsey RH. Long term results of the Mark IV operation for hiatal hernia and analyses of recurrences and their treatment. J Thorac Cardiovasc Surg 1972;53:25.
15. Chen LQ, Ferraro P, Duranceau A. Results of the Collis-Nissen gastroplasty to control reflux disease in patients who have Barrett's esophagus. Chest Surg Clin North Am 2002;12:127–147.
16. Csendes A, Braghetto I, Burdiles P, et al. Long-term results of classic anti-reflux surgery in 152 patients with Barrett's esophagus: clinical, radiologic, endoscopic, manometric, and acid reflux test analysis before and late after operation. Surgery 1998;123:645–657.
17. Urbach DR, Khajanchee YS, Glasgow RE, Hansen PD, Swanstrom LL. Preoperative determinants of an esophageal lengthening procedure in laparoscopic anti-reflux surgery. Surg Endosc 2001;15:1408–1412.
18. Ritter MP, Peters JH, DeMeester TR, et al. Treatment of advanced gastroesophageal reflux disease with Collis gastroplasty and Belsey partial fundoplication. Arch Surg 1998;133:523–529.
19. Collis JL. Peptic stricture of the oesophagus. Acta Chir Belg 1965;S2:41–48.
20. Skinner DB. Symptomatic esophageal reflux. Am J Dig Dis 1966;11:771–779.
21. Ott DJ, Gelfand DW, Chen YM, Wu WC, Munitz HA. Predictive relationship of hiatal hernia to reflux esophagitis. Gastrointest Radiol 1985;10:317–320.
22. Wright RA, Hurwitz AL. Relationship of hiatal hernia to endoscopically proved reflux esophagitis. Dig Dis Sci 1979;24:311–313.
23. Gastal OL, Hagen JA, Peters JH, et al. Short esophagus. Analysis of predictors and clinical implications. Arch Surg 1999;134:633–638.
24. Armstrong D, Blum AL, Savary M. Reflux disease and Barrett's oesophagus. Endoscopy 1992;24:9–17.
25. Allison PR. Reflux oesophagitis its pathology and treatment. Scand J Thorac Cardiovasc Surg 1972;6:318–322.
26. Jamieson GG. Mechanisms of gastro-oesophageal reflux. Aust N Z J Surg 1988;58:193–195.
27. Lieberman DA, Oehlke M, Helfand M. Risk factors for Barrett's esophagus in community-based practice. GORGE consortium. Gastroenterology Outcomes Research Group in Endoscopy. Am J Gastroenterol 1997;92:1293–1297.
28. Pearson FG. Hiatus hernia and gastroesophageal reflux: indications for surgery and selection of operation. Semin Thorac Cardiovasc Surg 1997;9:163–168.
29. Mittal SK, Awad ZT, Tasset M, et al. The preoperative predictability of the short esophagus in patients with stricture or paraesophageal hernia. Surg Endosc 2000;14:464–468.
30. Maziak DE, Todd TR, Pearson FG. Massive hiatus hernia: evaluation and surgical management. J Thorac Cardiovasc Surg 1998;115:53–60.
31. Yau P, Watson DI, Jamieson GG, Myers J, Ascott N. The influence of esophageal length on outcomes after laparoscopic fundoplication. J Am Coll Surg 2000;191: 360–365.
32. Little AG. Failed anti-reflux operations. Pathophysiology and treatment. Chest Surg Clin North Am 1994;4: 697–704.
33. Stipa F, Stein HJ, Feussner H, Kraemer S, Siewert JR. Assessment of non-acid esophageal reflux: comparison between long-term reflux aspiration test and fiberoptic bilirubin monitoring. Dis Esophagus 1997;10:24–28.
34. Lieberman DA. Medical therapy for chronic reflux esophagitis. Arch Intern Med 1987;147:1717.
35. Buchnin PJ, Spiro HM. Therapy of esophageal stricture: a review of 84 patients. J Clin Gastroenterol 1981;3:121.
36. Glick ME. Clinical course of esophageal stricture manage by bougienage. Dig Dis Sci 1982;27:884.

37. Hill LD, Gelfand M, Bauermeister D. Simplified management of reflux esophagitis with stricture. Ann Surg 1970;172:638.

38. Moran JM, Pihl CO, Norton RA, Rheinlander HF. The hiatal hernia-reflux complex. Current approaches to correction and evaluation of results. Am J Surg 1971;121:403–411.

39. Watson A. The role of anti-reflux surgery combined with fiberoptic endoscopic dilation in peptic esophageal strictures. Am J Surg 1984;148:346.

40. Naef AP, Savary M. Conservative operations for peptic esophagitis with stenosis in columnar-lined lower esophagus. Ann Thorac Surg 1972;13:543–551.

41. Safaie-Shirazi S, Zike WL, Mason EE. Esophageal stricture secondary to reflux esophagitis. Arch Surg 1975; 110:629–631.

42. Herrington JL Jr, Mody B. Total duodenal diversion for treatment of reflux esophagitis uncontrolled by repeated anti-reflux procedures. Ann Surg 1976;183: 636–644.

43. Pearson FG, Langer B, Henderson RD. Gastroplasty and Belsey hiatus repair. An operation for the management of peptic stricture with acquired short esophagus. J Thorac Cardiovasc Surg 1971;61:50–63.

44. Low DE. The short esophagus. Recognition and management. J Gastrointest Surg 2001;5:458–461.

45. Pearson FG. Peptic esophagitis, stricture, and short esophagus. In: Pearson FG, Cooper JD, Hiebert CA, Ginsberg RJ, eds. Esophageal Surgery. Philadelphia: Churchill Livingstone; 2002:266–278.

46. Pearson FG, Henderson RD. Long-term follow-up of peptic strictures managed by dilatation, modified Collis gastroplasty, and Belsey hiatus hernia repair. Surgery 1976;80:396–404.

47. Orringer MB, Sloan H. Complications and failings of the combined Collis-Belsey operation. J Thorac Cardiovasc Surg 1977;74:726–735.

48. Henderson RD. Reflux control following gastroplasty. Ann Thorac Surg 1977;24:206–214.

49. Orringer MB, Sloan H. Combined Collis-Nissen reconstruction of esophagogastric junction. Ann Thorac Surg 1978;25:16–21.

50. Stirling MC, Orringer MB. The combined Collis-Nissen operation for esophageal reflux strictures. Ann Thorac Surg 1988;45:148–157.

51. Langer B. Modified gastroplasty: a simple operation for reflux esophagitis with moderate degrees of shortening. Can J Surg 1973;16:84–91.

52. Demos NJ, Smith N, Williams D. A gastroplasty for short esophagus and reflux esophagitis: experimental and clinical studies. Ann Surg 1975;181:178–181.

53. Bingham JA. Hiatus hernia repair combined with the construction of an anti-reflux valve in the stomach. Br J Surg 1977;64:460–465.

54. Chen LQ, Hu CY, Gaboury L, Pera M, Ferraro P, Duranceau AC. Proliferative activity in Barrett's esophagus before and after anti-reflux surgery. Ann Surg 2001;234:172–180.

55. McDonald ML, Trastek VF, Allen MS, Deschamps C, Pairolero PC. Barrett's esophagus: does an anti-reflux procedure reduce the need for endoscopic surveillance? J Thorac Cardiovasc Surg 1996;111:1135–1138.

56. Reilly KM, Jeyasingham K. A modified Pearson gastroplasty. Thorax 1984;39:67–69.

57. Krupp S, Rossetti M. Surgical treatment of hiatal hernias by fundoplication and gastropexy (Nissen repair). Ann Surg 1966;164:927–934.

58. Maher JW, Hocking MP, Woodward ER. Supradiaphragmatic fundoplication. Long-term follow-up and analysis of complications. Am J Surg 1984;147:181–186.

59. Thal AP. A unified approach to surgical problems of the esophagogastric junction. Ann Surg 1968;168:542–550.

60. Maher JW, Hocking MP, Woodward ER. Long-term follow-up of the combined fundic patch fundoplication for treatment of longitudinal peptic strictures of the esophagus. Ann Surg 1981;194:64–69.

61. Payne WS. Surgical treatment of reflux esophagitis and stricture associated with permanent incompetence of the cardia. Mayo Clin Proc 1970;45:553–562.

62. Ellis FH Jr, Gibb SP. Vagotomy, antrectomy, and Roux-en-Y diversion for complex reoperative gastroesophageal reflux disease. Ann Surg 1994;220:536–542.

63. Fekete F, Pateron D. What is the place of antrectomy with Roux-en-Y in the treatment of reflux disease? Experience with 83 total duodenal diversions. World J Surg 1992;16:349–354.

64. Jamieson GG, O'Boyle CJ, Watson DI. Reflux disease without mucosal damage: is there a place for surgery? Chest Surg Clin North Am 2001;11:539–546.

65. Watson DI, Jamieson GG, Devitt PG, Mitchell PC, Game PA. Paraoesophageal hiatus hernia: an important complication of laparoscopic Nissen fundoplication. Br J Surg 1995;82:521–523.

66. Demos NJ, Kulkarni VA, Arago A. Video-assisted transthoracic hiatal hernioplasty using stapled, uncut gastroplasty and fundoplication. Surg Rounds 1994;••: 427–436.

67. Swanstrom LL, Marcus DR, Galloway GQ. Laparoscopic Collis gastroplasty is the treatment of choice for the shortened esophagus. Am J Surg 1996;171:477–481.

68. Johnson AB, Oddsdottir M, Hunter JG. Laparoscopic Collis gastroplasty and Nissen fundoplication. A new technique for the management of esophageal foreshortening. Surg Endosc 1998;12:1055–1060.

69. Jobe BA, Horvath KD, Swanstrom LL. Postoperative function following laparoscopic Collis gastroplasty for shortened esophagus. Arch Surg 1998;133:867–874.

14

Esophagectomy: Indications, Techniques, and Outcomes

Mark K. Ferguson

The need for esophagectomy for managing gastroesophageal reflux disease (GERD) arises in a small minority of patients who experience severe complications of reflux or from anti-reflux surgery. When surgery other than routine fundoplication is necessary for correction of reflux complications, a variety of esophageal-preserving operations is available that minimizes operative risks compared with those associated with esophagectomy. Preservation of esophageal function is an important indication for use of such procedures, because no reconstructive organ can replicate esophageal peristaltic function. In addition, avoidance of esophagectomy helps preserve gastric reservoir and digestive capacities, and eliminates the risk of intrathoracic alimentary tract redundancy that frequently accompanies esophageal reconstructive procedures. Such redundancy can lead to food stasis, early satiety, and weight loss, and contributes to the risk of postprandial aspiration. Because many reconstructive operations include an anastomosis to the cervical esophagus, avoidance of esophagectomy helps preserve swallowing function that can otherwise be altered by injury to regional nerves that coordinate deglutition or by the development of an anastomotic stricture.

Examples of esophageal-preserving operations for reflux-associated problems include patch esophagoplasty operations for treatment of intractable strictures, acid suppression and alkaline diversion for management of primary duodenogastric reflux (see Chapter 12), and esophageal lengthening (gastroplasty) operations for esophageal shortening (see Chapter 13). In some patients, Barrett's esophagus, a complication of reflux, has progressed to high-grade dysplasia or superficial cancer. In such situations, endoscopic mucosal resection or ablative procedures utilizing cautery or laser energy can be used to reduce the risk of invasive cancer while preserving the esophagus. When these procedures are not appropriate for a patient with severe complications of reflux or prior anti-reflux surgery, esophagectomy may be the only therapeutic option remaining.

History

Most early attempts at esophagectomy were performed for esophageal cancer. Bypass operations using skin tubes were developed during the late 19th and early 20th centuries by Mikulicz[1] and Garre[2] for bypass or replacement of the cervical esophagus and by Bircher[3] for bypass of the entire esophagus. Although these surgeons demonstrated that fluids could pass through the skin tubes they had created, successful bypass surgery was not accomplished until 1913 after a transhiatal esophagectomy.[4] Most importantly, quality of life was not maintained with these operations. After >20 years of dismal outcomes of surgically addressing the issue of esophageal obstruction, the first successful transthoracic esophagectomy was performed by Torek in 1913.[5] Even in this patient, no reconstruction was performed; instead, an extracorporeal tube connected a cervical esophagostomy to a gastrostomy to permit the patient to take enteral nutrition.

Another two to three decades were to pass before esophageal resection and reconstruction were performed routinely. Reasons for this included the slow adoption of methods for tracheal intubation for controlled ventilation, lack of understanding of requirements for fluid and electrolyte replacements, and the absence of reliable blood transfusion techniques. The large number of maxillofacial injuries that occurred during World War I stimulated the adoption of endotracheal intubation that had been developed decades earlier.[6] Subsequent anesthetic advances included the introduction of intubation under direct vision, the use of positive pressure breathing apparatus, and the use of curare as a paralytic agent permitting mechanically controlled ventilation.[7-10] Experiences during the Great War also led investigations into transfusion methods and the management of shock, both of which were vital to progress in major operations such as esophagectomy. This growth culminated in the 1930s in the performance of a transthoracic esophagectomy and, for the first time, intrathoracic reconstruction.[11-13]

Even into the 1930s there was considerable debate over what constituted optimal methods of esophageal replacement. In 1934, Ochsner and Owens[14] summarized the extant literature regarding extrathoracic esophageal reconstruction. Skin tubes (dermatoplasty), jejunoplasty, coloplasty, gastroplasty, and hybrid procedures combining two of these techniques all offered mortality rates from 20 to >50%. The procedures were completed in only about half of the patients, and overall good results were reported in only 30–40% of patients. The development of intrathoracic reconstruction techniques using the stomach in the 1930s was enthusiastically adopted, and reports of large series of patients who had undergone successful esophagectomy and reconstruction during the 1940s and 1950s began to appear.[15-19]

Indications

Peptic Stricture

Uncontrolled pathologic gastroesophageal reflux can lead to transmural esophageal inflammation culminating in intractable peptic esophageal stricture and esophageal shortening. This results in ongoing severe reflux symptoms accompanied by dysphagia and weight loss. The incidence of peptic stricture in the era of effective acid suppression medications is estimated to be 1–5% of patients with esophagitis.[20] Initial management of early peptic stricture consists of a careful clinical evaluation including endoscopy with biopsy to rule out cancer, determine whether Barrett's esophagus exists, and obtain a histologic diagnosis. Standard therapy includes intensive acid suppression and dilation, and is successful in about 75% of patients. However, long-term follow-up of such patients is often inadequate, and the true outcomes of medical therapy are not known.[21] Patients with recurrent stricture or ongoing symptoms of reflux in the setting of optimal medical therapy are candidates for anti-reflux surgery. Surgical options include standard partial or total fundoplication, or fundoplication combined with a gastroplasty as an esophageal lengthening procedure. The latter option is often necessary because of esophageal shortening. In rare situations, patch esophagoplasty or antrectomy and Roux-en-Y reconstruction as acid suppression and bile diversion may be indicated.

Indications for esophagectomy in the setting of peptic stricture are fortunately rare. They include nondilatable stricture, perforation during dilation of a stricture, inability to confirm that a stricture is benign, and multiple failed fundoplication operations in the presence of a stricture. The definition of a nondilatable stricture varies, but generally includes strictures for which adequate-sized dilators cannot be passed, failure of resolution of dysphagia after dilation, increasingly frequent dilations to relieve dysphagia, and strictures requiring dilation that have suffered previous perforation. Nondilatable strictures represent the most common indication for esophagectomy in patients with benign strictures.

Gastrointestinal Bleeding

Occasionally severe esophagitis is accompanied by bleeding manifested by guaiac-positive stools, melena, or hematemesis. At times bleeding will be intractable in the setting of optimal medical therapy. In such instances, fundoplication surgery may be recommended to eliminate reflux and permit healing of the raw mucosal surface. On occasions when such interventions fail to control bleeding, it may be necessary to consider esophagectomy for this purpose. Rarely such bleeding is sufficiently massive that desperate surgical measures are required for control. In the presence of uncontrollable bleeding, it is appropriate to consider esophagectomy as a lifesaving maneuver.

Multiple Failed Anti-Reflux Operations

Another indication for esophagectomy for GERD is a history of multiple failed attempts at anti-reflux surgery. Compromise of esophageal blood supply occurs each time the esophagus and stomach are dissected to enable performance of a fundoplication. In addition, accumulated scar tissue as well as anatomic deformities caused by prior operations increase the risk of injury to the vagus nerves and the vagal plexus during dissection. The cumulative effect of these injuries results in loss of peristaltic function (pump function) leading to dysphagia and ineffective esophageal clearance of gastric refluxate. Several reports indicate that satisfactory results after fundoplication surgery occur in only 50–60% of patients who have had two or more prior fundoplications.[22–24] The assessment of esophageal function is more important than merely counting the number of prior operations to determine optimal surgical therapy. Such assessment typically includes endoscopy, manometry, esophageal transit times measured by scintigraphy, gastric emptying time, and, in selected patients, esophageal pH monitoring may also provide useful information. In patients in whom pump function has been lost, strong consideration should be given to performing an esophagectomy.

Complications of Barrett's Esophagus

Reflux is thought to be the primary impetus for the development of Barrett's esophagus. Long-segment Barrett's esophagus is identified in up to 1% of individuals without GERD and in 5–10% of patients with GERD symptoms.[25–27] The incidence seems to increase with advancing age, making it an important concern in the elderly. Barrett's esophagus is an indication for esophagectomy in two classes of individuals. First, in rare circumstances a Barrett's ulcer can develop, which burrows deeply like a gastric ulcer instead of spreading superficially like ulcerations in the squamous esophageal mucosa. Although such ulcers can be controlled with intensive medical therapy, they sometimes extend transmurally and invade other structures, creating a life-threatening situation. In the presence of a deep chronic Barrett's ulcer, esophagectomy should be strongly considered.

The other situation in which Barrett's esophagus is an indication for surgery is when high-grade dysplasia develops. The likelihood of developing high-grade dysplasia is about 1 in every 200 patient years, making the overall risk relatively small.[28] However, when high-grade dysplasia is identified on endoscopic biopsy, there is a 40–50% risk of invasive adenocarcinoma in the esophagus.[29] Moreover, in patients with high-grade dysplasia who are followed in an endoscopic surveillance program, the risk of developing an invasive cancer is about 1 in every 200 patient years.[30,31] Currently the standard therapy for Barrett's esophagus with documented high-grade dysplasia is esophagectomy. However, recent information suggests that the increasing frequency with which Barrett's esophagus is being diagnosed has resulted in a decreasing incidence of high-grade dysplasia.[32] This fact, combined with the development of newer treatment modalities for eradicating high-grade dysplasia, may lessen the need for esophagectomy.

Techniques

Patient Preparation

In many operations performed for failed anti-reflux procedures, the final decision regarding whether to perform another fundoplication or resect the esophagus cannot be made preoperatively, but depends on intraoperative findings. This emphasizes the importance of a thorough preoperative evaluation so that all facts regarding anatomy and physiology are available when a final decision is required during surgery. Both the surgeon and the patient should be comfortable in the knowledge that all appropriate information has been gathered. A thorough discussion with the patient ensures that the patient is aware of possible outcomes of surgery, and that upon awakening the esophagus may have been replaced. In this regard, the colon should routinely be thoroughly prepared so that it is available for use in esophageal reconstruction should the need arise.

Because reoperations are often more arduous than initial operations and require longer recovery periods during which oral alimentation is not possible, the patient's physiologic and nutritional status must be optimized preoperatively. Measures that improve cardiopulmonary function include walking exercise and pulmonary toilet exercises such as coughing and incentive spirometry. Methods of nutritional repletion for patients whose nutritional status is compromised include intravenous alimentation, use of oral supplements, placement of a nasogastric feeding tube, or insertion of an enteral feeding tube.

Approach

The incision(s) used for esophagectomy is tailored to the individual patient's needs first and also to the personal preferences of the surgeon (Table 14.1). In patients in whom possible redo

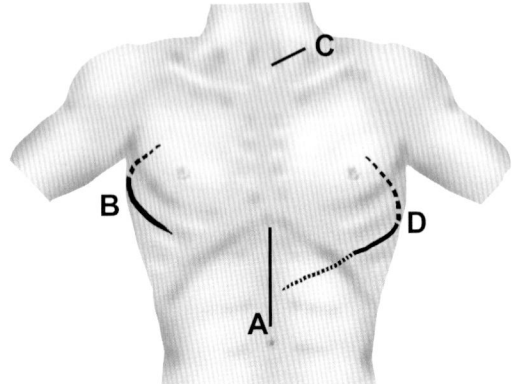

Figure 14.1. Options for surgical approaches to esophagectomy for failed anti-reflux therapy include the transhiatal approach (A + C), an Ivor Lewis resection (A + B), a modified Ivor Lewis esophagectomy (A + B + C), and an exclusive left thoracotomy or left thoracotomy extended across the costal margin into the left upper quadrant of the abdomen (D).

Table 14.1. Options for technical approaches to esophagectomy.

Approach
Left thoracotomy
Laparotomy for transhiatal technique
Left thoracoabdominal incision
Ivor Lewis incisions or modifications thereof
Minimally invasive (especially laparoscopic transhiatal)
Extent of esophageal resection
Distal only
Subtotal (high intrathoracic anastomosis)
Near total (cervical anastomosis)
Options for reconstruction
Gastric pull-up (high intrathoracic or cervical anastomosis)
Short-segment bowel interposition
Long-segment bowel interposition
Composite reconstruction (intrathoracic stomach and bowel or other conduit)

fundoplication is being weighed against possible resection, an approach should be chosen that permits either procedure to be accomplished; either a left thoracotomy or a laparotomy is appropriate in such situations (Figure 14.1). In contrast, a right thoracotomy does not permit adequate visualization of the hiatus and is not appropriate when simultaneous access to the chest and abdomen is required.

When the diagnosis remains enigmatic, especially because of a suspicious stricture, a left transthoracic approach permits optimal visualization of the region of interest and facilitates biopsies. A left thoracotomy permits complete esophageal mobilization and allows an easy approach to the gastroesophageal junction and proximal stomach either through the esophageal diaphragmatic hiatus or through a peripheral incision in the diaphragm. When technically feasible, an esophagectomy and reconstruction may be performed through this incision alone; it provides exposure to enable the surgeon to complete the resection and perform reconstruction with stomach or bowel interposition. If necessary, the left thoracotomy incision may be extended across the costal margin into the left upper quadrant to provide additional exposure to the upper abdomen. However, this incision is associated with a higher frequency of chronic postoperative pain and has an appreciable incidence of chondritis.

A laparotomy incision facilitates dissection of a previously performed fundoplication as long as most of the region of interest remains in the abdomen. If an esophagectomy is found to be necessary, the incision may be used as part of a transhiatal esophagectomy or distal esophagectomy. However, the amount of scarring that is present when end-stage GERD is the indication for surgery sometimes can make adequate and safe dissection of the distal intrathoracic esophagus difficult. Total esophageal replacement is straightforward after completing a transhiatal esophagectomy. Distal esophageal replacement with a short segment of jejunum or colon is technically feasible under some circumstances using the transhiatal approach.

Reoperative surgery for benign esophageal disease, especially recurrent gastroesophageal reflux, is possible in many patients using laparoscopic techniques and has been show to be both safe and effective in the hands of experienced laparoscopic surgeons. Similarly, esophagectomy is now being performed in some centers using a minimally invasive approach exclusively. Current experience with reoperative minimally invasive esophagectomy is quite limited; such experience is likely to grow in the future as surgeons become more adept at this technically challenging approach.

Extent of Resection

Patients operated on for recurrent benign esophageal disease should undergo a so-called "standard" esophagectomy. There is no rationale for an en bloc resection or for an extended or three-field lymph node dissection. The lateral extent of resection is determined by identifying the easiest periesophageal plane to work in that permits esophagectomy. Under most circumstances, this dictates dissection directly on the wall of the esophagus. Entering planes lateral to this exposes the patient to a variety of complications: excess bleeding from damage to surrounding structures such as azygos vein, aorta, and inferior pulmonary vein; pulmonary parenchymal injury with resultant air leak; chylothorax; pericardial injury associated with postoperative arrhythmias or postpericardiotomy syndrome; and recurrent laryngeal nerve injury.

The appropriate proximal extent of resection is controversial. Patients who have failed medical and conservative surgical management of GERD likely have increased sensitivity to refluxate. This may be manifest as an increased susceptibility to tissue injury and/or a heightened sense of pain and discomfort during esophageal exposure to the refluxate. Limiting the resection to a distal esophagectomy with a low intrathoracic esophagogastric anastomosis predisposes patients to continued reflux because it is difficult to create an effective anti-reflux mechanism in this situation. As a result, most experts recommend performing a near total esophagectomy, creating a high intrathoracic or cervical anastomosis, if the stomach is to be used for reconstruction. It must be kept in mind that, after one or more prior fundoplication operations, the viability of the gastric fundus may be compromised. This increases the risk of anastomotic leak or gastric fundic necrosis when the stomach is used for total esophageal replacement.

Alternatively, a distal esophagectomy with short-segment jejunal interposition may be performed. Because the peristaltic activity of the jejunum is preserved in this setting, it helps prevent reflux of gastric contents into the esophagus. The jejunum is also relatively resistant to acid-peptic injury when used for short-segment esophageal reconstruction. A short-segment colon interposition is not quite as good an alternative for esophageal reconstruction. The colon lacks true peristaltic properties, and therefore does not provide as much protection for the esophagus from gastric contents. However, the colon is very resistant to acid-peptic injury, which makes it the favorite organ among some surgeons for short-segment esophageal reconstruction.

There is no controversy regarding the appropriate distal extent of esophagectomy. All of the squamous mucosa must be removed, necessitating division of the esophagus below the anatomic and histologic squamocolumnar junction. It is useful to visually inspect the margin to ensure this has been accomplished; if a question remains, frozen section confirmation that the distal margin is free of squamous mucosa is appropriate. If residual squamous esophageal mucosa is allowed to remain it will constantly be exposed to gastric acid and digestive peptides, resulting in pain, ulceration, stricture formation, or perforation.

Procedure

Decision making regarding the optimal incision to use is complex and is discussed earlier in this section. Once the decision has been made to proceed with esophagectomy, the distal esophagus is mobilized and the esophagus and stomach are freed from the diaphragmatic crura. The order in which this is accomplished depends on the approach being used. The proximal stomach is mobilized but no major blood supply (left gastric artery, right gastric artery) is divided at this point. Any prior fundoplication wrap is undone. This is usually accomplished with careful dissection of adhesions between the esophagus and stomach, dividing the fundoplication sutures as they are encountered. Meticulous dissection usually succeeds in completely unwrapping the stomach, reestablishing the normal size and contour of the gastric fundus. Under some circumstances it is not possible to delineate the two portions of the wrap that make up a total fundoplication. If a plane between the esophagus and the wrap can be established, the wrap is divided with a linear cutting stapler (Figure 14.2).

If the stomach can be returned to its normal anatomy, all options outlined above for the extent of resection and the organ used for reconstruction remain available. If the amount of scarring, ulceration, fistula formation, or other pathologic abnormality is so extensive that the gastric anatomy cannot be reestablished, this usually necessitates partial gastrectomy as part of the esophagectomy, and precludes use of the stomach as an organ to replace the full length of the esophagus. In such a situation, the stomach remnant can be used as a pull-up for partial esophageal replacement or a short (or long) segment bowel interposition may be performed.

Near total esophagectomy. For a near total esophagectomy and reconstruction with a gastric pull-up, the esophagus is mobilized circumferentially from the thoracic inlet to the esophagogastric junction. The vagus nerves are divided inferior to the azygos arch to minimize the risk of injury to the recurrent laryngeal nerves. The stomach is mobilized completely, with division of the left gastric vessels and left gastroepiploic arcade. The blood supply is based on the right gastric artery and the right gastroepiploic vessels. Under circumstances in which prior fundoplication surgery has failed, the short gastric vessels will have been divided previously. This permits development of collateral circulation in the wall of the stomach and may provide for a better overall blood supply than is normally the case when preparing the stomach for use in reconstruction in a previously unoperated patient. Prior division of short

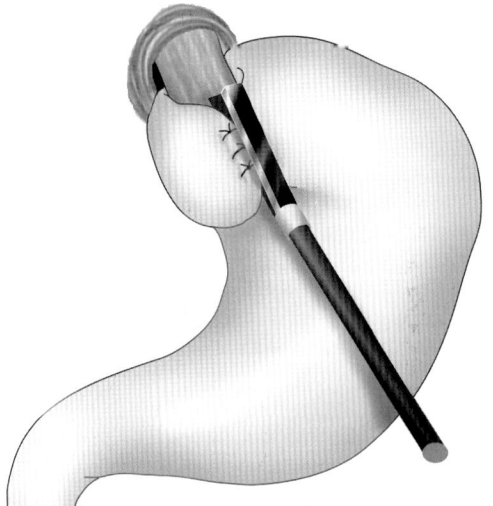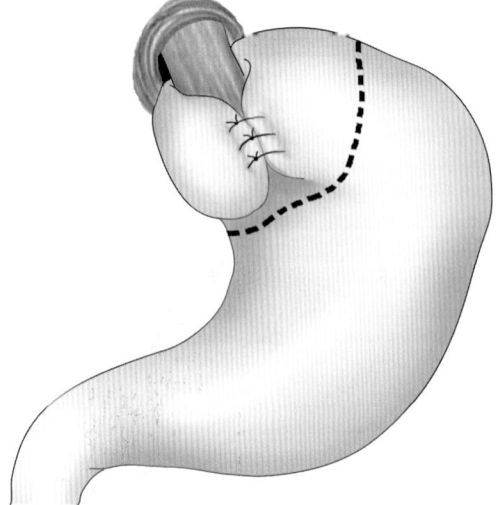

Figure 14.2. Management of a prior fundoplication. Options include dissection of the wrap (not shown), cutting across the wrap (left), and proximal gastrectomy (right).

gastric vessels is often associated with the development of adhesions between the stomach and spleen that require careful dissection and division. The first and second portions of the duodenum are widely mobilized (Kocher maneuver) permitting the pylorus to reach almost to the diaphragmatic hiatus. A gastric drainage procedure (pyloric dilation, pyloroplasty, pyloromyotomy) may be performed.

The esophagus is divided from the stomach with a linear cutting stapler in one of two ways: by simple transection below the squamocolumnar junction, or by creating a gastric tube by resecting the lesser gastric curvature and the esophagogastric junction en bloc. The stomach is brought through the posterior mediastinum, the shortest available route, and is anastomosed to the esophagus either at the apex of the thorax or in the neck through a cervical incision. An anastomosis to the esophagus at the apex of the right hemithorax or in the neck is performed. If the operation is being performed through the left chest and a high intrathoracic anastomosis is considered, the esophagus is brought medial to the arch of the aorta before performing the anastomosis. Unless there is sufficient length of esophagus to then pull both the stomach and esophagus down lateral to the aortic arch to permit suturing the anastomosis, the surgeon should consider a cervical anastomosis instead. Therefore, the surgeon must ensure there is adequate length of the gastric tube before dividing the esophagus proximally.

Partial esophagectomy. The esophagus is mobilized proximally to a region where the muscular thickness and mucosa are normal, usually at or inferior to the level of the inferior pulmonary veins. This assessment may be aided by intraoperative endoscopy. The esophagus is divided from the stomach below the squamocolumnar junction (distal to the esophagogastric junction); it is not advisable to create a gastric tube. As mentioned previously, in patients in whom normal gastric anatomy cannot be restored, it may be necessary to resect the proximal stomach. Additional gastric mobilization is normally not necessary. A gastric emptying procedure may be performed.

If a short-segment jejunal interposition is planned, a segment of proximal jejunum based on the third or fourth branch of the superior mesenteric artery is prepared (Figure 14.3).

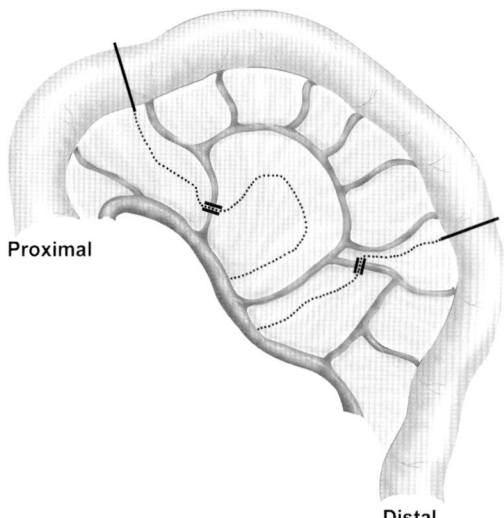

Figure 14.3. The blood supply to the jejunum and construction of a short-segment jejunal graft.

Alternatively, a short segment of colon based on the middle colic artery or on the ascending branch of the left colic artery is prepared (Figure 14.4). The conduit is brought posterior to the stomach and through the esophageal hiatus in an isoperistaltic orientation. An end-to-side proximal anastomosis is usually performed when jejunum is used, whereas an end-to-end anastomosis is performed when the colon is selected. The interposition graft is then drawn into the abdomen to eliminate any redundancy and is anastomosed to the back wall of the body of the stomach. The graft is sutured to the crura with several interrupted stitches to prevent herniation of intraabdominal contents. The stomach is tacked to the diaphragm in a horseshoe shape around the interposition to create a low-pressure anti-reflux barrier. Intestinal continuity is restored.

Postoperative care. A nasoenteral tube is placed to keep the upper gastrointestinal tract decompressed. Some surgeons leave the tube in place until a contrast study, typically performed on postoperative day 5 to 7, shows no evidence for a leak. However, routine postoperative contrast studies are notorious for failing to demonstrate leaks. An alternative management style is to leave the drainage tube in place only if there is clinical suspicion for a leak or delayed gastric

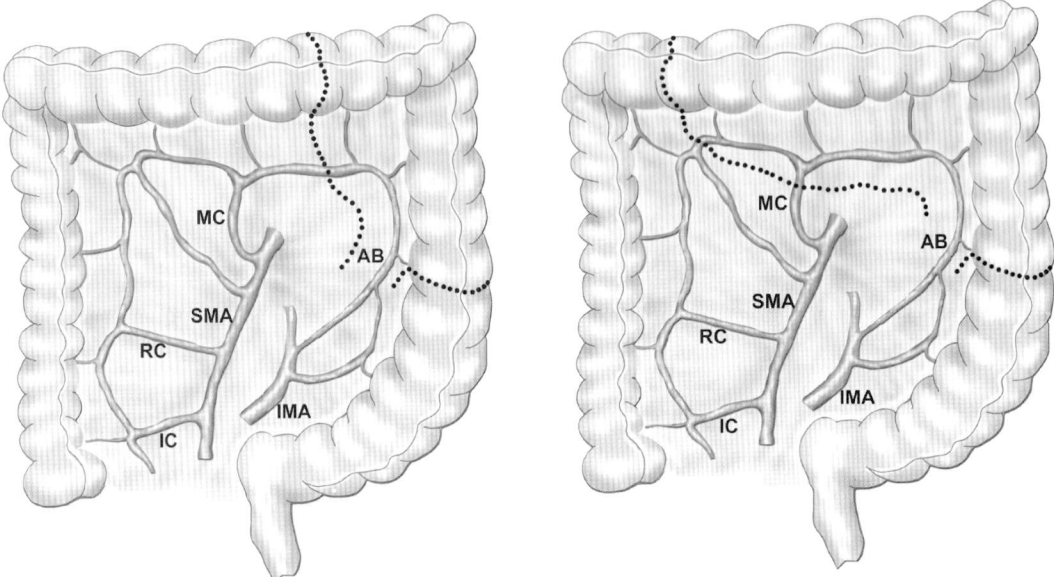

Figure 14.4. The blood supply to the colon includes the ilecolic (IC), right colic (RC), and middle colic (MC) arteries that arise from the superior mesenteric artery (SMA), and the ascending branch (AB) of the left colic artery that arises from the inferior mesenteric artery (IMA). For left colon interposition based on the ascending branch of the left colic artery, a short segment (left) or a long segment (right) may be prepared; the latter requires division of the middle colic artery.

emptying. If the patient is doing well, the drainage tube is removed as soon as bowel activity has resumed, as evidenced by lack of abdominal distension and passage of flatus.

Many surgeons routinely administer intravenous low-dose dopamine (3–5 µg/kg/min) for the first 48–72 hours postoperatively. Patients sometimes experience hemodynamic instability in the early postoperative period because of fluid shifts, myocardial depression, or mediastinal pressure due to the esophageal reconstructive organ. When this happens, the mesenteric vascular bed is the first to be adversely affected by the body's attempt to regulate perfusion. The routine use of dopamine theoretically has the effect of maintaining mesenteric blood flow even if the patient has some depression of myocardial performance or alterations in blood pressure.

Perioperative antibiotics are used routinely, but there is no benefit in administering more than one or two doses postoperatively. Overuse of antibiotics in a prophylactic setting leads to antibiotic resistance. If infection develops, antibiotics are restarted and are tailored to the specific source of infection.

Although there is some controversy regarding the utility of postoperative tube feedings, most surgeons place jejunostomy tubes and use them routinely beginning on the first postoperative day. Tube feedings help maintain nutritional levels and help to prevent bacterial translocation leading to sepsis. Most patients are sent home receiving tube feedings at night whereas eating during the day; the feedings provide a "safety net" so the patients do not have to overeat to maintain adequate nutrition and hydration. This gives them more time to accommodate to the new configuration of their gastrointestinal tract.

The most common complications after esophagectomy are related to pulmonary problems and include pneumonia and respiratory insufficiency. These perturbations result from a number of factors: thoracotomy or upper abdominal incisions causing diaphragmatic dysfunction; fluid shifts postoperatively resulting in pulmonary fluid overload; interruption of pulmonary lymphatics; a space occupying reconstructive organ limiting lung expansion; and recurrent nerve injury preventing patients from generating high airway pressures during cough-

Table 14.2. Operative outcomes after esophagectomy for failed antireflux therapy.

Author	Year	Patients	Leak	Graft Necrosis	Pneumonia	Other	Mortality
Colon/jejunum							
Curet-Scott[33]	1987	32	5	6	5	5	1
DeMeester[34]	1988	24	1	2	—	—	2
Mansour[35]	1997	49	8	2	2	7	3
Thomas[36]	1997	13	2	1	2	4	1
Gandenstetter[37]	1998	17	1	0	1	2	0
Stomach							
Young[38]	2000	29	3	1	2	3	1
Orringer[39]	2001	53	7	0	1	—	2
Totals			12%	5%	6%	6%	5%

ing exercises. Patients are given supplemental oxygen as needed and are asked to do deep breathing and coughing exercises regularly. Use of an incentive spirometer helps the medical staff and the patients assess their performance in deep breathing maneuvers. Optimal pain management is critical in permitting vigorous pursuit of pulmonary toilet exercises.

Delayed gastric emptying, which is manifested by chest pressure, early satiety, and sometimes regurgitation or aspiration, is managed expectantly. Gastric emptying time is substantially reduced with administration of prokinetic agents such as erythromycin, which acts as a motilin receptor agonist. For patients who cannot tolerate or do not respond to erythromycin, metoclopramide may suffice as an alternative.

Outcomes

The results of iterative anti-reflux surgery are well documented in Chapter 11; the success rate for reoperation after a second failed procedure (good or excellent results) is only 50–60%. The outcomes for esophagectomy and reconstruction in well-selected patients surpass that success rate, indicating that esophagectomy should be considered more seriously as the likelihood of success with a redo anti-reflux operation diminishes.

Because they are technically challenging, these operations often engender a higher incidence of postoperative morbidity than do esophagectomies for cancer. The incidence of complications ranges from 25% to almost 60%; typical complications include pneumonia, anastomotic leak, graft necrosis (primarily when bowel interposition is performed), and infection

(Table 14.2).[33–39] The duration of hospitalization usually is measured in weeks, not days, indicating that careful preparation of the patient for a potentially prolonged postoperative course is wise to consider. The mortality rate is as high as 10% but averages about 5%.

At least 50% of patients have residual symptoms long-term after esophagectomy, including dysphagia, early satiety, and regurgitation. Persistent heartburn is very uncommon (Table 14.3).[33,34,36–38] There is no apparent difference between colon interposition and gastric pull-up in terms of long-term symptomatic outcomes. Adverse outcomes are identified more often for physical than for emotional functional components of quality-of-life scales.[38] Interestingly, despite negatively scoring a number of physical components, patients tend to score quality of life overall in a range similar to that reported by people who have not undergone esophagectomy for failed anti-reflux therapy. This outcome helps to underscore the severity of symptoms that patients experienced before definitive treatment by esophagectomy.

Table 14.3. Long-term outcomes after esophagectomy for failed antireflux therapy.

Variable	Incidence (%)
Early satiety	22
Dysphagia	20
Regurgitation	19
Diarrhea	5
Pain	5
Heartburn	2
Aspiration	1
Good/excellent outcome	70

Reports from the late 1980s through 2001 document a success rate of approximately 70% for esophagectomy for failed anti-reflux therapy (Table 14.3).[33,34,36-38] However, interpretation of the long-term results of esophagectomy performed for benign problems is sometimes difficult. Many authors fail to provide true long-term outcomes, reporting only mid-term outcomes, and often many patients are lost to follow-up. Importantly, analyses typically fail to include as a poor outcome patients who suffer operative mortality. As noted earlier, the operative mortality for esophagectomy is not negligible, and far exceeds that documented for more conservative procedures.

Conclusions

Esophagectomy is the final therapeutic option for the management of patients with GERD. It should be reserved for patients with documented "pump failure," severe complications of GERD not amenable to conservative surgical therapy (nondilatable stricture, penetrating ulcers, Barrett's esophagus with high-grade dysplasia), or those with multiple failed attempts at surgical correction of GERD. The final decision regarding the need for esophagectomy often must be made at the time of reoperation. If the problem area is limited to the distal esophagus, partial esophagectomy and jejunal interposition should be considered. Near total esophagectomy is sometimes necessary after multiple failed fundoplication procedures; the frequent need for partial gastrectomy in this setting limits reconstruction options and often necessitates long-segment colon interposition. Long-term outcomes for esophagectomy are not nearly as good as for more conventional surgical approaches to GERD. In appropriately selected patients, however, considerable clinical benefit can be derived. Quality of life in most categories is maintained, and crippling effects of GERD symptoms can be largely eliminated. However, many patients remain somewhat symptomatic, indicating that resection should be reserved for carefully selected patients for whom there are no other viable surgical options. Future efforts at expanding the use of more physiologic alternatives to standard esophagectomy, such as vagal-sparing esophagectomy (see Chapter 15), may further improve the long-term outcomes of esophagectomy for GERD.

References

1. Mikulicz J. Ein Fall von Resection des Carcinomatosen Oesophagus mit Plastischen Ersazt des excirdirten Stuckes. Prager Med Wschr 1886;11:93–94.
2. Garre C. Ueber Oesophagus-Resection und Oesophagoplastik. Langenbeck's Arch Klin Chir 1898;57:719–722.
3. Bircher E. Ein Beitrag zur plastischen Bildung eines neuen Oesophagus. Zbl Chir 1907;34:1479–1482.
4. Denk W. Zur Radikaloperation des Oesophaguskarzinoma. Zbl Chir 1913;40:1965–1968.
5. Torek F. The first successful case of resection of the thoracic portion of the oesophagus for carcinoma. Surg Gynecol Obstet 1913;16:614–617.
6. Rowbotham ES, Magill I. Anaesthetics in the plastic surgery of the face and jaws. Proc R Soc Med 1920–1921; 14:21–27.
7. Magill I. Endotracheal anesthesia. Proc R Soc Med 1928;22:83–88.
8. Gale JW, Waters RM. Closed endobronchial anesthesia in thoracic surgery: a preliminary report. J Thorac Surg 1932;1:432–437.
9. Harroun P, Hathaway HR. The use of curare in anesthesia for thoracic surgery. Preliminary report. Surg Gynecol Obstet 1946;82:229–231.
10. Stephens HB, Harroun P, Beckert FE. The use of curare in anesthesia for thoracic surgery. J Thorac Surg 1947; 16:50–61.
11. Ohsawa T. Surgery of the oesophagus. Arch Jap Chir 1933;10:605–695.
12. Adams WE, Phemister DB. Carcinoma of the lower thoracic esophagus. Report of a successful resection and esophagogastrostomy. J Thorac Surg 1937–1938;7: 621–632.
13. Marshall SF. Carcinoma of the esophagus: successful resection of the lower end of the esophagus with reestablishment of esophageal gastric continuity. Surg Clin North Am 1938;18:643–648.
14. Ochsner A, Owens N. Anterothoracic oesophagectomy for impermeable stricture of the oesophagus. Ann Surg 1934;100:1055–1091.
15. Sweet RH. Surgical management of carcinoma of midthoracic esophagus. Preliminary report. N Engl J Med 1945;233:1–7.
16. Lewis I. The surgical treatment of carcinoma of the oesophagus, with special reference to a new operation for growths of the middle third. Br J Surg 1946–1947;34: 18–31.
17. Garlock JH. Resection of thoracic esophagus for carcinoma located above arch of aorta: cervical esophagogastrostomy. Surgery 1948;24:1–8.
18. Rapant V, Hromada J. Surgical treatment of corrosive stenosis of the thoracic part of the esophagus by a single-stage palliative anastomosis. J Thorac Surg 1950; 20:454–473.
19. le Roux BT. An analysis of 700 cases of carcinoma of the hypopharynx, the oesophagus, and the proximal stomach. Thorax 1961;16:226–255.

20. Loof L, Gotell P, Elfberg B. The incidence of reflux oesophagitis: a study of endoscopy reports from a defined catchment area in Sweden. Scand J Gastroenterol 1993;28:113–118.
21. Ferguson MK. Medical and surgical management of peptic esophageal strictures. Chest Surg Clin North Am 1994;4:673–695.
22. Little AG, Ferguson MK, Skinner DB. Reoperation for failed anti-reflux operations. J Thorac Cardiovasc Surg 1986;91:511–517.
23. Stirling MC, Orringer MB. Surgical treatment after the failed anti-reflux operation. J Thorac Cardiovasc Surg 1986;92:667–672.
24. Pearson FG, Cooper JD, Patterson GA, et al. Gastroplasty and fundoplication for complex reflux problems: long-term results. Ann Surg 1987;206:473–481.
25. Csendes A, Smok G, Burdiles P, et al. Prevalence of Barrett's esophagus by endoscopy and histologic studies: a prospective evaluation of 306 control subjects and 376 patients with symptoms of gastroesophageal reflux. Dis Esophagus 2000;13:5–11.
26. Connor MJ, Weston AP, Mayo MS, Sharma P. The prevalence of Barrett's esophagus and erosive esophagitis in patients undergoing upper endoscopy for dyspepsia in a VA population. Dig Dis Sci 2004;49:920–924.
27. Toruner M, Soykan I, Ensari A, Kuzu I, Yurdaydin C, Ozden A. Barrett's esophagus: prevalence and its relationship with dyspeptic symptoms. J Gastroenterol Hepatol 2004;19:535–540.
28. Conio M, Blanchi S, Lapertosa G, et al. Long-term endoscopic surveillance of patients with Barrett's esophagus. Incidence of dysplasia and adenocarcinoma: a prospective study. Am J Gastroenterol 2003;98:1931–1939.
29. Ferguson MK, Naunheim KS. Resection for Barrett's mucosa with high-grade dysplasia: implications for pro phylactic photodynamic therapy. J Thorac Cardiovasc Surg 1997;114:824–829.
30. O'Connor JB, Falk GW, Richter JE. The incidence of adenocarcinoma and dysplasia in Barrett's esophagus: report on the Cleveland Clinic Barrett's Esophagus Registry. Am J Gastroenterol 1999;94:2037–2042.
31. Spechler SJ, Lee E, Ahnen D, et al. Long-term outcome of medical and surgical therapies for gastroesophageal reflux disease: follow-up of a randomized controlled trial. JAMA 2001;285:2331–2338.
32. Tseng EE, Wu TT, Yeo CJ, Heitmiller RF. Barrett's esophagus with high grade dysplasia: surgical results and long-term outcome—an update. J Gastrointest Surg 2003;7:164–171.
33. Curet-Scott MJ, Ferguson MK, Little AG, Skinner DB. Colon interposition for benign esophageal disease. Surgery 1987;102:568–574.
34. DeMeester TR, Johansson KE, Franze I, et al. Indications, surgical technique, and long-term functional results of colon interposition or bypass. Ann Surg 1988;208: 460–474.
35. Mansour KA, Bryan FC, Carlson GW. Bowel interposition for esophageal replacement: twenty-five-year experience. Ann Thorac Surg 1997;64:752–756.
36. Thomas P, Fuentes P, Giudicelli R, Reboud E. Colon interposition for esophageal replacement: current indications and long-term function. Ann Thorac Surg 1997; 64:757–764.
37. Gadenstatter M, Hagen JA, DeMeester TR, et al. Esophagectomy for unsuccessful anti-reflux operations. J Thorac Cardiovasc Surg 1998;115:296–302.
38. Young MM, Deschamps C, Allen MS, et al. Esophageal reconstruction for benign disease: self-assessment of functional outcome and quality of life. Ann Thorac Surg 2000;70:1799–1802.
39. Orringer MB, Marshall B, Iannettoni MD. Transhiatal esophagectomy for treatment of benign and malignant esophageal disease. World J Surg 2001;25:196–203.

15

Vagal Sparing Esophagectomy

Steven R. DeMeester

End-stage reflux disease is a catch-all phrase used to describe the situation that exists when there is substantial foregut dysfunction in the setting of long-standing reflux disease. It can occur in association with a variety of conditions including scleroderma or other connective tissue disorders, treated achalasia, prior gastric resection or morbid obesity procedures, prior esophagectomy particularly in association with a low intrathoracic esophagogastric anastomosis, repair of congenital tracheoesophageal fistula, or in patients with a history of caustic ingestion. Often patients with end-stage reflux disease have had one or more surgical interventions in an attempt to correct the problem, and many have at least one but more often several of the following abnormalities: severe esophageal body motility dysfunction, stricture, long-segment Barrett's, delayed gastric emptying, large hiatal hernia, or significant esophageal foreshortening.[1]

Management of these patients is complicated and often requires resection rather than attempts at reconstruction, but the treatment in all cases must be individualized. Once the decision has been made that a resection will be necessary to improve the patient's quality of life, the next critical decision is whether to remove the esophagus or the stomach. This decision is based primarily on the severity of injury to the esophagus. In the setting of Barrett's or a severe stricture, generally the best option is esophagec-tomy, whereas if the esophagus has been relatively spared but profound gastric dysfunction is present, then consideration should be given to some type of gastric resection. Many of these patients have had one or more previous surgical procedures on the stomach, esophagus, or both, and the nature of the previous procedure can influence both the choice of resection and the options for reconstruction.

One of the most difficult situations is to recommend resection as the first surgical intervention in a patient. There is a strong temptation to attempt reconstruction in these patients first to see if it gets them by, but often this just sentences the patient to two procedures and two recoveries, and delays their ultimate return to an acceptable quality of life.[2] This is not to imply that resection is always the correct choice, but the decision regarding reconstruction versus resection is complicated, and many factors need to be considered. In some situations, particularly where there has been prior surgery, the final decision regarding resection versus attempted reconstruction can only be made in the operating room after the previous failed procedure has been undone and the amount and condition of residual stomach assessed. Furthermore, initial resection followed by staged reconstruction may be the safest option in some situations, such as in the setting of a redo esophagectomy after a previous limited distal esophagectomy.

Evaluation

The first critical step after meeting a patient with a complex benign foregut problem is a careful evaluation. Upper endoscopy done by the surgeon or at a minimum viewed by the surgeon as it is being done is indispensable for assessing the situation and developing a strategy. Often a motility study is helpful if the status of the esophageal body is in question, and a video esophagram provides invaluable information in these patients about the presence or absence of a stricture, esophageal bolus transport, and the presence and reducibility of a hiatal hernia. Selectively used tests include gastric emptying scans, 24-hour pH monitoring, impedance testing, barium small-bowel follow-through, and abdominal ultrasound or computed tomography scan. A cardiopulmonary evaluation is also advisable in this patient population before embarking on complex foregut surgery.

If esophageal resection is likely to be necessary then the method of reconstruction needs to be determined, and when considering a colon interposition then evaluation with colonoscopy and potentially a visceral arteriogram is recommended. Colonoscopy or an air-contrast barium radiographic study should be performed before use of the colon as an esophageal substitute to rule out polyps, malignancy, or evidence of either inflammatory disease or significant diverticulosis in the area of the colon to be used. Careful consideration should be given before using a colon graft in the presence of any of these abnormalities with the exception of a polyp that has been completely excised. Routine angiography, although not essential, does provide information about anatomic variations that may be present, but most importantly confirms patency of the colonic vessels and the marginal arcade.[3] Most surgeons prefer to use the transverse colon based on the ascending branch of the left colic artery. A stenosis at the origin of the inferior mesenteric artery alters the choice, and either a different graft or use of the ascending colon based on the middle colic vessels would be advisable under such circumstances. Although intraoperative examination of the vascular integrity of the graft can in most circumstances determine the suitability of the graft, it is time-saving to know preoperatively if

there are problems so that a suitable strategy can be prepared.

Operative intervention is undertaken only after a complete assessment of the problem and a frank discussion with the patient about the issues, options, and pros and cons of various therapies have been completed. It is imperative that the surgeon and patient are aligned on the goals of the procedure and the anticipated outcome. Often it is helpful to review all of the patient's symptoms and clarify whether or not that symptom is likely to change or be relieved with the therapy because commonly some symptoms in these complex patients are unrelated to the foregut process. Unrealistic expectations by the patient may lead to dissatisfaction despite what is otherwise a complete success from a surgical standpoint. Furthermore, great caution should be used in regard to promises of pain relief unless there is a clear anatomic or physiologic explanation for the pain which will be corrected by the surgical procedure. Upper abdominal pain seems to be a particularly prominent component of the collection of symptoms often encountered in middle-aged females with a complex foregut problem, and frank discussions before reoperation about the necessity of weaning off narcotics is a critical aspect of the evaluation and care of these patients.

Indications for Vagal-sparing Esophagectomy

A vagal-sparing procedure should be considered in any patient with a benign process that is to undergo esophagectomy. Ideal conditions include achalasia, end-stage reflux disease, and Barrett's with high-grade dysplasia or perhaps intramucosal cancer. Absolute contraindications for a vagal-sparing esophagectomy are the need for a lymphadenectomy because sparing the vagus nerves precludes a lymph node dissection, and prior vagal transection or evidence of gastric dysfunction, particularly a gastric bezoar. Because of the potential for gastric emptying problems, diabetes should be considered a relative contraindication for a vagal-sparing procedure. Other relative contraindications include strictures or a history of caustic injury to the esophagus. In these circumstances, mediastinal inflammation may prohibit safe stripping of the esophagus or may lead to vagal disruption even if the stripping is accomplished safely. We have had one tear in the membranous wall of the trachea in this circumstance, although it was easily repaired via the cervical incision. Nonetheless, in these circumstances, consideration should be given to a formal transthoracic esophagectomy. Prior anti-reflux surgery or other esophageal surgery (repair of perforation, congenital trachea-esophageal fistula, etc.) are also relative contraindications because preservation of the vagus nerves is more difficult in this setting. Lastly, prior gastric surgery such as antrectomy or pyloroplasty may preclude a significant advantage to preserving the vagal nerves, although even in this setting avoidance of postvagotomy diarrhea may be a sufficient reason to spare the vagus nerves if possible.

Surgical Approach

The operation commences in the abdomen, although for redo esophagectomy the best option may be initial transthoracic mobilization of the esophagus and intrathoracic stomach. Until the anatomy is sorted out and a final decision is made regarding resection versus reconstruction, every effort is made to preserve gastric vascularity including the left gastric vessels and the gastroepiploic arcade.

If the fundus is unusable or the gastric vascular supply is inadequate, then the surgical treatment for reflux shifts to either esophagectomy or gastrectomy. In the setting of a recurrent esophageal stricture or long-segment Barrett's with a normal functioning stomach, the best choice is an esophagectomy. In these patients, vagal preservation should be attempted whenever possible. Not only does this reduce the potential for dumping and diarrhea, but it is also the easiest method for removing the esophagus from the mediastinum. With this technique, the esophagus is stripped out without the need for transhiatal dissection.

The hiatus is opened anteriorly with a minimum of dissection and the anterior and posterior vagal trunks encircled with a vessel-loop. The vagus nerves are retracted gently toward the patient's right, and the gastro-esophageal fat pad is dissected beginning on the left of the esophagus and stomach such that it allows the anterior vagus nerve to be brought well over to the right of the esophagus. Failure to do this will lead in most cases to inadvertent injury of the anterior vagus nerve during the subsequent steps of the procedure. Once the anterior vagus is safely over to the right of the esophagus, a highly selective vagotomy is performed starting just above the crow's foot near the antrum. This is necessary if the stomach is to be used as the esophageal replacement, and is beneficial with a colon interposition to reduce gastric acidity and the potential for ulceration in the distal colon graft. The highly selective vagotomy precisely follows the lesser curve of the stomach up to the point where the distal esophagus is reached and the vagus nerves are easily separated from the esophagus. I find that this dissection is facilitated by sequential grasping of the stomach with Babcock clamps along the lesser curve, and by using the Harmonic scalpel for division of the very vascular tissue in this area. Avoidance of a hematoma or bleeding in this area is critical to prevent unintended injury to the distal vagal branches.

At this point, the gastroesophageal junction has been completely exposed and the lesser curve above the crow's foot skeletonized. If the stomach is to be used for esophageal replacement, then the greater curve is mobilized in the same manner as for a standard gastric pull-up. However, if the colon is to be used, then there is no need to mobilize the greater curve completely. Instead, the omentum is detached from the transverse colon and a window created into the lesser sac along the mid-greater curve of the stomach. It is also useful to expose the left crus and divide the most proximal one or two short gastric and posterior pancreatico-gastric vessels to create a passage from the lesser sac to the hiatus for the colon graft. The colon is mobilized in standard manner based on the ascending branch of the left colic artery whenever possible.[4] The necessary length of colon is marked out by measuring the distance from the bottom of the left ear to the xiphoid anteriorly with an umbilical tape and then marking a similar distance on the colon starting from the point where the left colic vessels tether the graft and going proximally. The colon is then divided and placed in the pelvis for later use.

Attention is directed to the left neck and the esophagus is exposed. A Penrose drain encircling the esophagus facilitates traction, and downward blunt dissection is accomplished with a finger to free up the cervical and upper mediastinal esophagus. A gastrotomy is made near the gastroesophageal junction, or alternatively the cardia is divided with a stapler and a small portion of the staple line is opened on the proximal end to provide access to the esophageal lumen. A red-rubber catheter is inserted into the esophagus, or alternatively via a nasogastric tube, one hundred milliliters (ml), of 10% povidone iodine solution is used to irrigate and sanitize the esophagus before stripping it from the mediastinum. A standard vein stripper is passed retrograde up the esophagus and brought out the anterior wall of the cervical esophagus as distally as possible. The esophagus is ligated distal to the exit site of the vein stripper in the neck using a heavy suture, and the cervical esophagus is divided just proximal to where the vein stripper comes out. The divided distal end of the cervical esophagus is suture ligated and tied securely. Several endo-loops help to facilitate a secure ligation. This is a critical step because, if the ligatures slip, the vein stripper will merely pull out, leaving the partially stripped esophagus somewhere in the mediastinum. After changing the vein stripper to the large head, the esophagus is inverted by pulling the vein stripper from below. It is useful to leave a long umbilical tape tied to the cervical end of the divided esophagus to provide access to the tract in the posterior mediastinum after the esophagus has been removed. The esophagus comes out inverted with the mucosa external to the muscular wall, similar to taking off a stocking inside-out. Bleeding usually is minimal and very little force is required to pull the esophagus out. Resistance should raise concern, and excessive resistance should prompt conversion to a transhiatal procedure.

After esophageal stripping, the cardia is divided (if not previously done) distal to the squamocolumnar junction with a stapler and the anterior gastrotomy is closed. The mediastinal tract is sequentially dilated using a 90-mL balloon Foley catheter progressively filled with more saline and pulled through the mediastinum. This dilation procedure prevents mediastinal constriction of the stomach or colon graft. The stomach or colon graft is then pulled up through the posterior mediastinum and a cervical anastomosis is constructed.

When a colon graft is used, the colo-gastric anastomosis will be positioned on the posterior fundus, so it is critical that the colon be brought *behind* the stomach and then guided up through the hiatus into the posterior mediastinum.

When a gastric pull-up is performed, after completing the cervical anastomosis the graft is gently pulled into the abdomen to eliminate redundancy and is sutured to the crura to prevent herniation of abdominal organs into the mediastinum. A nasogastric tube is passed and a feeding jejunostomy tube is placed. When a colon graft has been used, it is pulled gently into the abdomen to eliminate redundancy and divided approximately 10–15 cm distal to the hiatus, taking care not to injure the vascular arcade. A stapled colo-gastric anastomosis is performed to the proximal posterior fundus using a 75-mm GIA stapler, and a nasogastric tube is guided into the stomach. The colon graft is sutured to the crura, and the colo-colostomy is accomplished in standard manner with care taken to avoid traction on the left colic vessels, generally by bringing the right colon up into the left upper quadrant. Finally, the mesenteric defects are closed and a feeding jejunostomy is placed.

Results

At the University of Southern California we have now performed >75 vagal-sparing esophagectomies. In 24 patients the indication was end-stage reflux or Barrett's without cancer. Among these 24 patients, 14 had previous abdominal surgery including 5 with prior fundoplication and 1 with prior vertical-banded gastroplasty for obesity. Nearly half of the patients had an esophageal stricture that had been repeatedly dilated, and 1 patient with Barrett's had undergone photodynamic therapy. Reconstruction was with a colon graft in 22 patients (Figure 15.1) and a gastric pull-up in 2 (Figure 15.2). One colon graft was removed for ischemia. However, because the entire stomach is preserved with this procedure, the patient was later reconstructed with a gastric pull-up without difficulty. One patient with extensive prior abdominal procedures and diabetes had limited dumping symptoms, and one patient had diarrhea that resolved spontaneously. Two patients had delayed gastric emptying symptoms. One

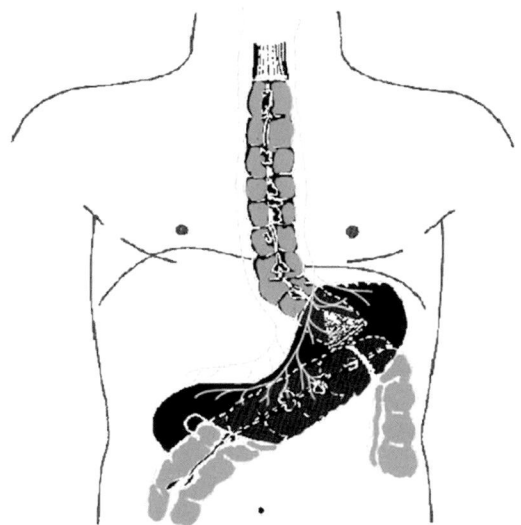

Figure 15.1. A vagal-sparing esophagectomy with colon interposition. Note that the colon graft replaces the esophagus and is anastomosed to the entire, innervated stomach.

We have previously evaluated gastric function and confirmed vagal integrity in a series of 15 randomly selected patients at a median of 20 months after vagal-sparing esophagectomy and colon interposition.[5] The indication for the procedure was benign disease in seven and Barrett's with high-grade dysplasia or intramucosal cancer in eight patients. Outcome was assessed on the basis of symptoms, Congo red gastric staining, basal and sham meal-stimulated gastric acid output, basal and sham meal-stimulated pancreatic polypeptide response, standardized meal consumption, and nuclear medicine gastric emptying half-time. These results were compared with the symptomatic and functional outcome in 10 patients after standard esophagectomy with colon interposition, 10 patients after standard esophagectomy with gastric pull-up, and 23 control subjects. We found that postoperative dumping and diarrhea were significantly decreased in the vagal-sparing group compared with the standard esophagectomy with colon interposition. Furthermore, secretory studies confirmed intact vagal innervation after the vagal-sparing esophagectomy, and in contrast to the other

had had two prior fundoplications but the other had not undergone any prior esophageal surgery. Both had a vagal-sparing esophagectomy with colon interposition, and both ultimately required revision consisting of a proximal gastrectomy with colo-antral anastomosis and pyloroplasty.

Three patients developed an ulcer in the distal colon just proximal to the colo-gastric anastomosis related to acid production by the intact and innervated stomach. For this reason we now include a highly selective vagotomy along the lesser curve of the stomach in these patients. There have been several patients that were taken for a vagal-sparing esophagectomy but during the operation dense scarring around the hiatus precluded vagal preservation and a transhiatal resection was performed. One such patient had had a congenital tracheoesophageal fistula repaired and then subsequently underwent a Nissen for severe reflux as a child, and subsequently presented to the University of Southern California with end-stage reflux. Interestingly, two other patients that had a congenital tracheoesophageal fistula repaired with subsequent end-stage reflux were successfully resected using a vagal-sparing technique, so this procedure is an option in some of these patients.

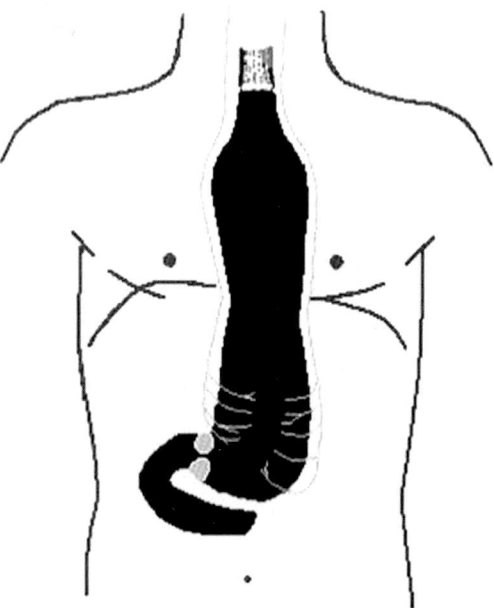

Figure 15.2. Figure 15.2. A vagal-sparing esophagectomy with gastric pull-up. A highly selective vagotomy along the lesser curve preserves antral vagal innervation and no pyloroplasty is performed.

types of esophagectomy gastric emptying studies and meal consumption were similar in normal subjects and patients after vagal-sparing esophagectomy. We concluded that vagal preservation was beneficial and warranted when possible in patients with benign disease or early esophageal cancer.

Summary

End-stage reflux disease can occur as a consequence of a variety of conditions, and typically these patients are quite complex. Many will have had one or more procedures on their esophagus or stomach, and most have a number of symptoms and several esophageal and/or gastric functional abnormalities. The decision to resect the esophagus for benign disease is not easy, but often provides the patient with the surest relief of their symptoms and the greatest likelihood of a good quality of life. An important principle is to minimize the potential for long-term morbidity, and thus preservation of the vagal nerves when feasible is a worthwhile objective. In an early series of these procedures in a complex group of patients, we have had excellent symptomatic and functional results with little dumping or postvagotomy diarrhea. In patients with extensive scarring around the hiatus, the potential for vagus nerve disruption during the

esophageal stripping process is real, and can lead to problems with delayed gastric emptying. Furthermore, patients undergoing reconstruction with a colon interposition after a vagal-sparing esophagectomy should have a highly selective vagotomy to minimize the potential for ulceration in the distal colon secondary to gastric acidity. Alternatively, patients could be kept on acid-suppression medication. Over time the best indications and most important contraindications of a vagal-sparing esophagectomy will become apparent, and the subset of patients with benign or early-stage malignant disease most likely to have the best outcome with this procedure will be defined.

References

1. Gadenstatter M, Hagen JA, DeMeester TR, et al. Esophagectomy for unsuccessful anti-reflux operations. J Thorac Cardiovasc Surg 1998;115:296–301.
2. Watson TJ, DeMeester TR, Kauer WK, et al. Esophageal replacement for end-stage benign esophageal disease. J Thorac Cardiovasc Surg 1998;115:1241–1249.
3. Peters JH, Kronson JW, Katz M, DeMeester TR. Arterial anatomic considerations in colon interposition for esophageal replacement. Arch Surg 1995;130:858–863.
4. DeMeester SR. Colon interposition following esophagectomy. Dis Esophagus 2001;14:169–172.
5. Banki F, Mason RJ, DeMeester SR, et al. Vagal-sparing esophagectomy: a more physiologic alternative. Ann Surg 2002;236:324–336.

16

Future Directions of Therapy for GERD

M. Brian Fennerty and Mark K. Ferguson

This book has been devoted to a critical appraisal of treatment options for gastroesophageal reflux disease (GERD) and failed anti-reflux therapy and has provided a physiologic basis for managing the postoperative syndromes associated with surgical anti-reflux therapy. In this final chapter, we would like to explore what we feel are future prospects for the various management options for patients with newly diagnosed, persistent, or recurrent GERD. Much of what we hypothesize is speculative but these thoughts are meant to encourage the reader to consider what we may be able to offer and how we might approach these patients in the near future.

Physiologic Evaluation of Suspected GERD

The accuracy of intraesophageal pH monitoring will improve as longer monitoring periods become the norm with increased battery capacity of these devices. Furthermore, the patient acceptance of this technique will become substantially better with the tubeless "capsule" systems that are becoming increasingly available. However, the real advance in physiologic testing of the GERD patient will likely come with improvements in and increased availability of esophageal impedance testing.[1] Impedance testing not only detects acid reflux events but also detects nonacidic reflux events as well,

and can evaluate air and liquid esophageal exposure during a reflux event. This technology should ensure that nonacidic reflux causing reflux-type symptoms is accurately diagnosed, and should also help identify the truly functional heartburn patient who will not respond to any of the usual treatment options for GERD (pharmacologic, endoscopic, and surgical anti-reflux therapies).

Medical Therapy for GERD

Pharmacologic therapy of GERD with antisecretory agents originated in the mid-1970s when histamine-2-receptor antagonists first became available.[2,3] However, healing of esophagitis was obtained in only 40–50% of patients and a similar number of patients continued to have symptoms of reflux. Omeprazole was released in 1989 as the first proton pump inhibitor (PPI) for clinical use. Three other first-generation PPIs subsequently became available but all were similar in efficacy, healing esophagitis in approximately 80% of GERD patients with a similar number achieving acceptable symptom relief.[2–4] When a more potent PPI, esomeprazole, was introduced, its use was associated with healing of esophagitis and symptom relief in nearly 90% of patients with GERD.[5] Physicians recently have come to realize that many patients require more frequent dosing (twice daily) or higher doses to achieve and maintain healing and symptomatic remission.[6]

Most importantly, we have learned that these potent antisecretory agents often do not eliminate all symptoms of GERD, especially regurgitation. Thus, medical therapy as it currently stands is not an ideal treatment for GERD in all patients with this disorder and has not proven to be superior to surgery for this condition, having been outperformed by anti-reflux surgery in several studies.[7-10]

What does the future hold for pharmacologic anti-reflux therapy? In the antisecretory arena, longer-acting (e.g., tenatoprazole) and more rapid-acting (i.e., the newly launched immediate release omeprazole and the forthcoming acid pump antagonists) all appear promising.[11,12] Longer-acting agents may prevent breakthrough symptoms with once-a-day dosing and rapid onset agents may allow PPIs to be effective in on-demand situations. It is clear that antisecretory agents are treating the effects of reflux, not the underlying mechanism of reflux.[13] Prokinetic agents that increase gastric emptying (i.e., tegaserod) may be valuable adjuncts to PPI therapy or effective in managing regurgitation or other symptoms that PPIs are relatively ineffective in controlling. Gamma-aminobutyric acid agonists (e.g., baclofen) or other neuromodulators may become useful in treating GERD via their inhibition of transient lower esophageal sphincter relaxations, the primary mechanism for a reflux event. Agents that improve tissue resistance by affecting the "tight-junctions" between cells are being developed and may prove to be very effective in symptom control and healing when reflux cannot be eliminated surgically.

Endoscopic Anti-Reflux Procedures

It is expected that the number of commercially available endoscopic anti-reflux techniques will markedly expand in the next few years. Almost all of these new devices will be injection-type techniques with the remainder being plication devices. Among the injection techniques, most of the new devices likely will utilize already approved human biological substances largely borrowed from the cosmetic surgery arena. Plication technology will continue to evolve into smaller, less cumbersome devices.

We soon will have results of sham-controlled clinical trials evaluating all of the currently Food and Drug Administration cleared or approved endoscopic anti-reflux devices, and this will set the standard for the entire field as it relates to accurately measuring efficacy.[14] There will be continued refinements in the techniques of use for all of these devices, and newer iterations of the devices will optimize the efficacy as well as safety of these procedures.[15-17] It will be interesting to see results of the current endoscopic anti-reflux procedures in patients with more severe reflux anatomy and physiology (those with larger hiatus hernias, more severe esophagitis, presence of Barrett's esophagus) as well as those with atypical GERD symptoms (i.e., cough, hoarseness, asthma).

Newer Indications for Surgical Therapy

Surgical anti-reflux therapy expanded greatly with the introduction of laparoscopic surgical techniques. Initially patients were recommended for laparoscopic fundoplication surgery who fit traditional criteria for open surgery. Patient selection criteria rapidly expanded to include patients whose symptoms were well controlled on pharmacologic therapy but for whom surgery seemed to provide a better lifestyle solution. Recent reports advocate surgical anti-reflux therapy for patients with Barrett's esophagus and no dysplasia as a means for reducing the risk of adenocarcinoma, irrespective of their symptom status. That this practice cannot be sustained on a cost-effectiveness basis is apparent given the fact that millions of people in the United States alone are likely to be candidates for such a procedure. A recent meta-analysis indicates that the risk of developing adenocarcinoma is not reduced by fundoplication surgery.[18]

Newer methods for evaluating patients with GERD and Barrett's esophagus may help physicians better select which patients should be treated more aggressively. In patients diagnosed with Barrett's esophagus, biological characterization of their risk of developing dysplasia or adenocarcinoma may be achieved through use of proteomics, gene analysis, or other advanced techniques. Patients who are stratified into a low-risk group will be initially managed conservatively, whereas those identified as being at high risk for dysplasia or cancer will be treated surgically. The results of surgery in eliminating progression in Barrett's esophagus are best when reflux is reduced to levels experienced by a normal population. Thus it will be necessary to periodically monitor the efficacy of fundoplication surgery through pH or other monitoring. What to recommend for patients with symptomatic relief but who are documented as having abnormal esophageal exposure to acid or other refluxate will be problematic.

Centers of Surgical Excellence

A very large number of fundoplication procedures currently are being performed in Western societies, with an appreciable rate of subsequent surgical failure, and a strong association between failure rates and degrees of surgical experience. In many regions of Europe, surgical therapy is performed primarily in centers of excellence in which a high degree of surgical experience is concentrated. No such centers have been mandated in the United States, and most surgical procedures for GERD are performed in community hospitals by surgeons with moderate levels of experience. Given the high cost of GERD therapy, particularly among patients with failed therapy for GERD, important cost savings will be realized when centers of excellence are established for initial endoscopic and surgical anti-reflux therapy.

Evaluation of the Failed Anti-Reflux Procedure

As has been noted throughout this book, surgical anti-reflux procedures, when performed by an experienced surgeon, are effective in eliminating the symptoms of GERD in the vast majority of patients treated in this manner. Furthermore, because most patients treated surgically derive a durable effect, anti-reflux surgery provides healing and maintenance of remission.

Despite the high success rate achieved with anti-reflux surgery, many patients still will either fail to achieve an initial symptom response or experience a relapse of their GERD symptoms over time. The initial failure rate with anti-reflux surgery is likely much greater in less-experienced surgeons' hands, whereas later anti-reflux surgery "relapses" seem to occur even in patients treated by the most experienced surgeons. The mechanisms or reasons for persistent or recurrent reflux after anti-reflux surgery are not entirely understood. However, given the rapidly expanding use of this surgical procedure, it is clear that we increasingly have to manage patients who have failed anti-reflux surgery. The management options after failure of anti-reflux surgery are either to reinstitute medical anti-reflux therapy, consider performing one of the emerging endoscopic anti-reflux therapies, or perform a repeat anti-reflux surgical procedure.

In the past, the evaluation of a suspected failed anti-reflux surgical procedure likely consisted of a barium swallow and esophageal manometry. These anatomic and physiologic tests have largely been supplanted by or expanded to also include a careful endoscopic assessment and prolonged ambulatory esophageal pH monitoring. We suspect that endoscopy or another means of directly imaging the suspected failed surgical repair will always remain a critical requirement of any postoperative evaluation strategy. However, it is interesting to speculate that nonendoscopic direct imaging of the surgical repair site might become an option in the not-so-distant future.

Recently, a 14 frame per second dual-headed capsule (PillCam; Given Imaging, Yoqneam, Israel) has begun initial testing as a means of evaluating the distal esophageal mucosa for evidence of esophagitis and or Barrett's esophagus. It is plausible that further developments with this noninvasive, office-based test could conceivably offer both an antegrade and retrograde detailed inspection of the surgical site and provide the necessary information the physician needs to assess competency of the original fundoplication.[19]

Another potential means of imaging the wrap may be through the use of high-resolution computed tomography or magnetic resonance scanners using the newer and increasingly available multichannel systems along with software that allows three-dimensional reconstruction and "fly-through" imaging of the gastrointestinal tract. Although most physicians have become aware of this technology as a means of evaluating the colon (computed tomography or magnetic resonance colonography or "virtual" colonoscopy), this technology can also be used to image the small bowel and stomach/esophagus. It is interesting to speculate that three-dimensional reconstruction with "fly-through" capability may allow for the same comprehensive antegrade and retrograde evaluation of an anti-reflux surgical repair that is currently only available endoscopically. Thus we may be able to obtain endoscopic-quality imaging of the suspected disrupted fundoplication noninvasively.

In addition to this fly-through capability for static constructs, increasing computing memory and speed may eventually permit dynamic evaluation of hollow organs in three dimensions at high magnification over time. The primary limitation of this technique will be the radiation dose required to complete the examination, which we estimate will require a period of 10–20 minutes of real time radiography during which patients are put through a variety of swallowing maneuvers. The information obtained would provide imaging at a level of complexity not currently available in any single test and in a noninvasive manner. The three-dimensional evaluation of a dynamic process, with the ability to reconstruct both the esophageal and gastric lumens (fly-through technology) and the fundoplication wrap ("drive-by" technology), would provide the clinician with the capacity to identify details such as inappropriate motion of the stomach within the wrap or which individual suture is creating excessive narrowing of the gastric lumen.

Although both of these above suggestions for imaging an anti-reflux surgical site may at first glance appear highly speculative, the progress made in gastrointestinal imaging with capsule devices and radiology over the last few years is simply staggering. It is entirely conceivable that comprehensive nonendoscopic imaging of the anti-reflux construct can be obtained with these or other advanced imaging technology in development, and we suspect the only real issue is how soon reliable imaging of this nature will become available for clinical use in evaluating a prior anti-reflux surgical repair.

Endoscopic and Pharmacologic Therapy after a Failed Anti-Reflux Surgery

Once it has been objectively determined through appropriate and increasingly accurate diagnostic testing that the symptoms a patient has in the postoperative state are related to continued or recurrent reflux, the next decision one needs to make is how best to manage the patient's GERD. Options include repeat anti-reflux surgery in a center with skill and experience in this type of surgery, endoscopic anti-reflux procedures, or pharmacologic anti-reflux therapy. The treatment choice in this situation, as noted in Chapter 10, is heavily dependent on the patient's preferences regarding further therapy for GERD as well as their unique physiology and anatomy determined by a careful evaluation. Furthermore, the availability of surgical or endoscopic skill in performing these types of repeat procedures may limit or expand the options offered the patient. It is likely that continued improvements and innovation in surgical, endoscopic, and pharmacologic anti-reflux therapy will further expand the clinician's options in managing these patients.

We are not optimistic that we will see controlled trial information on the effectiveness of endoscopic anti-reflux devices in patients with prior failed anti-reflux surgery. Although the anecdotal experience in this clinical arena is likely to expand exponentially, there are few incentives for device manufacturers to test their technology in this patient population that is difficult to study and treat. It is likely that most of what we learn in using endoscopic anti-reflux devices in the failed anti-reflux surgical patient will be based on "experience" rather than science.

Having said this, we do believe that as we further develop data regarding the impact of the endoscopic anti-reflux procedures on lower esophageal sphincter anatomy and physiology, we will more intelligently apply one or more of the devices in the failed postoperative patient. It is also likely that data derived in this setting will allow us to more accurately predict who is a viable candidate for such therapy as well as which procedure is most likely to succeed. In patients with a more intact postoperative anatomy, we suspect that one of the injection techniques will suffice, whereas those with more disrupted anatomy will require more definitive closure of the hiatus, possibly with one of the plication techniques. What we really need to acquire are data regarding the durability, long-term safety, and cost-effectiveness of the devices in the failed postoperative setting. If these devices prove to be durable as an adjunctive therapy for failed anti-reflux surgery, then even a high initial acquisition cost may not be prohibitive in using them in this clinical setting.

What will drive the choice of treatment for the patient with a failed anti-reflux operation will always be dependent on patient-centered goals of therapy, their unique anatomy and physiology, and the availability of expertise in surgical or endoscopic anti-reflux salvage therapy. However, the options within the realm of pharmacologic and endoscopic anti-reflux therapies and evidence for the success of those options in this clinical scenario will likely greatly expand in the coming years. Physicians caring for patients such as these will need to stay abreast of the developments in this field and not only use the most accurate tools available for evaluating the patients with persistent or recurrent GERD after anti-reflux surgery, but also consider all of the various options available to the patient.

References

1. Sifrim D, Holloway R, Silny J, et al. Acid, nonacid, and gas reflux in patients with gastroesophageal reflux disease during ambulatory 24-hour pH-impedance recordings. Gastroenterology 2001;120:1588–1598.
2. Fennerty MB, Castell D, Fendrick AM, et al. The diagnosis and treatment of gastroesophageal reflux disease in a managed care environment: suggested disease management guidelines. Arch Intern Med 1994;156:477–484.
3. Fennerty MB. Medical treatment of gastroesophageal reflux disease in the managed care environment. Semin Gastrointest Dis 1997;8:90–99.
4. Chiba N, De Gara CJ, Wilkinson JM, Hunt RH. Speed of healing and symptom relief in grades II to IV gastroe-sophageal reflux disease: a meta-analysis. Gastroenterology 1997;112:1798–1810.
5. Castell D, Kahrilas P, Richter J, et al. Esomeprazole (40 mg) compared with lansoprazole (30 mg) in the treatment of erosive esophagitis. Am J Gastroenterol 2002;97:575–583.
6. Klinkenberg-Knol EC, Festen HP, Jansen JB, et al. Long-term treatment with omeprazole for refractory reflux oesophagitis: efficacy and safety. Ann Intern Med 1994;121:161–167.
7. Lundell L, Mietten P, Myrvold H, et al. Continued (5 year) follow-up of a randomized clinical study comparing anti-reflux surgery and omeprazole in gastro-oesophageal reflux disease. J Am Coll Surg 2001; 192:172–179.
8. Spechler JS, Lee E, Ahnen D, et al. Long-tern outcome of medical and surgical therapies for gastroesophageal reflux disease: follow-up of a randomized controlled trial. JAMA 2001;285:2331–2338.
9. Walker SJ, Baxter ST, Morris DI, et al. Review article: controversy in therapy of gastro-esophageal reflux disease – long-term proton pump inhibitor or laparoscopic anti-reflux surgery. Aliment Pharmacol Ther 1997;11:249–260.
10. Spechler SJ. The Department of Veteran's Affairs Gastroesophageal Reflux Disease Study Group: comparison of medical and surgical therapy for complicated gastroesophageal reflux disease in veterans. N Engl J Med 1992;326:786–792.
11. Galmiche J, Bruley Des Varannes S, Ducrotte P, et al. Tenatoprazole, a novel proton pump inhibitor with a prolonged plasma half-life: effects on intragastric pH and comparison with esomeprazole in healthy volunteers. Aliment Pharmacol Ther 2004;19:655–662.
12. Vakil N. Review article: new pharmacological agents for the treatment of gastroesophageal reflux disease. Aliment Pharmacol Ther 2004;19:1041–1049.
13. Robinson M. Prokinetic therapy for gastroesophageal reflux disease. Am Fam Physician 1995;52:957–966.
14. Fennerty M. Endoscopic therapy for GERD: what have we learned and what needs to be done? Gastrointest Endosc Clin North Am 2003;13:201–210.
15. Edmundowicz SA. Injection therapy of the lower esophageal sphincter for the treatment of GERD. Gastrointest Endosc 2004;59:545–552.
16. Kahrilas PJ. Radiofrequency therapy of the lower esophageal sphincter for treatment of GERD. Gastrointest Endosc 2003;57:723–731.
17. Fennerty MB. Endoscopic suturing for treatment of GERD. Gastrointest Endosc 2003;57:390–395.
18. Corey KE, Schmitz SM, Shaheen NJ. Does a surgical anti-reflux procedure decrease the incidence of esophageal adenocarcinoma in Barrett's esophagus? A meta-analysis. Am J Gastroenterol 2003;98:2390–2394.
19. Jobe BA, Kahrilas PJ, Vernon AH. Endoscopic appraisal of the gastroesophageal valve after anti-reflux surgery. Am J Gastroenterol 2004;99:233–243.

Index